DOCTOR, CAN I ASK YOU A QUESTION?

DOCTOR, CAN I ASK YOU A QUESTION?

ARTHUR E. BAUE, M.D.

To order additional copies of this book, contact:
Xlibris Corporation
1-888-795-4274
www.Xlibris.com
Orders@Xlibris.com
24868

Contents

Section H—End of Life Decisions

Section I—Nursing Homes, Hospices and Home Health Care

Section J—Our Health Care System

Section K—Ethical Issues in Health Care

Section L—Recommendations About Health

Section M—Disease Prevention and Health Promotion

DEDICATION

I dedicate this book to my family: my wife Rosemary; our children Patricia Nizen, Chris Baue and Bill Baue; their spouses and our seven grandchildren. Over the years, they tolerated not only the briefcase but its owner and the many days and nights away seeing patients, attending meetings, giving lectures and other activities. Their love and support are what make it all worthwhile.

ACKNOWLEDGEMENT

I greatly appreciate the tremendous help of Mrs. Margaret McLaughlin who prepared all the initial drafts of the text and references and the final references and biobliographic materials. Likewise, Mrs. Patricia Krebs who edited the drafts, produced the final text and made many helpful suggestions. This book would never have been completed without these two very capable women and good friends. I appreciate, also the suggestions and support of my wife Rosemary. It was her idea for this book.

DOCTOR, MAY I ASK YOU A QUESTION? HEALTHCARE FROM THE PATIENT'S POINT OF VIEW

"It is more important (for the doctor) to know the patient who has the illness than to know the illness the patient has."

Sir William Osler

"Beware of young doctors and old barbers."

Benjamin Franklin

"The best doctors in the world are Dr. Diet, Dr. Quiet and Dr. Merryman."

Jonathan Swift

"Today it is Dr. Deductible, Dr. Paperwork and Dr. Bureaucracy (Open your wallet. We are from the insurance company and we are here to help.)

Dale Dauten, King Feature, St. Louis Post Dispatch
November 2, 1998

INTRODUCTION

Does the healthcare system seem to you a maze of managed care, HMOs, medical terminology, specialties, and referrals? How do you get the care you need and should have? How do you find a caring, concerned and competent doctor? How do you *know* the doctor is competent? How long must you wait to see a doctor? If a doctor can do something for you, must he or she do it? What is the "technological imperative"?

You and I may yearn for a simpler day in the past, when every family had a doctor who made house calls and was an advisor for health and illness, but now we must sort through today's healthcare maze. By guiding you through it, I hope that you will receive better support and treatment than was possible in those simpler days.

I write from your point of view with a question and answer format, with a focus on patients' questions that is unique. As a patient from time to time, I can share with you what I expect from my doctors. As someone who has spent a lifetime as a physician and medical administrator, I know the system, its strengths, problems and pitfalls. The questions in this book were asked by my patients, my friends and my family members. My wife has received her share of questions as well from relatives. Married to a surgeon for 49 years, she knows what she can and should expect.

A recent advertisement by the United Health Foundation noted, "There are 126 schools in the country that teach you how to be a doctor, but not one for how to be a patient." I once thought of teaching a course on patients' rights. I have written this book to teach you how to be a patient that understands the healthcare system and a patient's rights and privileges. My aim is to help you elicit clear communication from your doctor in language you understand.

A friend told me that when he developed chest pain his doctor referred him to a specialist who ordered some tests, and after getting the results, sent him to another specialist who recommended a certain treatment. My friend asked: "Could you find out what is wrong with me? What did the tests show? Why this treatment?" When I suggested that my friend ask his doctor about the results, the diagnosis, or the reason for therapy, he responded, "My doctor will not explain it to me the way you will." In the same kind of situation you might have said "I don't want to bother my doctor who is so busy," or "No one will talk to me and explain it to me," or, "I don't know what questions to ask". Some doctors may not communicate to your satisfaction, or you may not be sure how or what to ask. You deserve a doctor you can trust. There are many such doctors. I have worked with them and been treated by them.

I believe that patients, and friends and relatives of patients, have the right, not just the privilege, to ask questions of their doctors and to receive explanations that satisfy and are understood. You have the right to understand your disease and therapy, and the right to know your diagnosis and prognosis. If a doctor doesn't explain this satisfactorily, I suggest that you find a doctor who will.

Recently, friends asked for help because their new granddaughter was found to have a small hole in the heart that caused a heart murmur and episodes of rapid heart beats, or tachycardia. The child was seen and evaluated by an excellent pediatric cardiologist. He told them that the hole in the heart was small and would never be a problem; the rapid heart action was normal. Although the grandparents and parents respected the doctor and his opinion, they were not able to just forget their little girl's problem. They asked for my thoughts. I talked to the cardiologist and agreed with his opinion. However, to help the family become more comfortable, I recommended and arranged for a second opinion, which confirmed the first one. They then accepted the recommendation that no treatment was needed.

No attempt is made to review all diseases, problems or treatment; for this please see the Merck Manual for Patients, the Harvard Medical School Family Health Guide or the Healthwise Handbook. Self-help books are also available, along with monthly health letters such as the Harvard Health Letter, the Johns Hopkins White Papers, the University of California Health Letter and a Mayo Clinic Letter.

This book's information about health and healthcare is designed to help you identify your best options for excellent treatment. The book is divided into sections about doctors, hospitals, the healthcare system, ethics, end of life decisions, government programs and aids, health information, health promotion and disease prevention. Roles of faith, spirituality, life style and a positive attitude are also reviewed.

The book discusses the top ten health stories of 2003, as listed in the Harvard Health Letter (December 2003): 1) obesity, 2) SARS contained, 3) angioplasty best for heart attacks, 4) blood pressure guidelines push diuretics, 5) guidelines are not followed by patients, 6) being old is getting younger, 7) another setback for HRT (hormone replacement therapy), 8) low carbs are big, 9) post Tamoxifen drug halves risk of recurrence of breast cancer, and 10) bumpy ride to genomic era.

The book can be used as both a quick reference and for in-depth reading. References are provided in a bibliography at the end of the book for each chapter for additional reading. Organizations and government agencies, with web-site addresses, are identified for further information. For quick reference, there are an index, a glossary with cross indexing to the pages addressing an issue, and suggestion boxes. Information about health and new challenges for patients and health care is found in the media on a daily basis; thus continuous updating will be necessary. The information in this book is as current as the time of printing.

At one time medicine had little to offer other than comfort. You may remember the late nineteenth-century painting by Sir Luke Fildes titled "The Doctor" that shows an older physician sitting dejectedly by the bedside of a sick child. Modern science and technology allow us to treat many diseases, cure a number of problems and relieve the symptoms of many others. With this has come some dehumanization of medicine. Alvan Feinstein, a Professor of Medicine at Yale, points out that "a clinician's traditional obligations to patients are expressed by the aphorism: "guerir quelquefois, soulager souvent, consoler toujours," (to cure occasionally, to relieve often, to comfort always). Advances in science and technology allow us to provide cures more often than ever before, but patients are distressed by our reduced attention to relief and comfort.

I do not intend to doctor-bash. I am proud of being a physician, and I would choose this profession again. Many thoughtful, considerate, capable and empathetic physicians comfort, support, treat and communicate well with their patients. Other physicians, even though superb technicians, may not have such capabilities. When a physician is busy, concerned, upset or distraught about what is happening to a patient, communication may break down.

After a friend of the late Kingman Brewster, then President of Yale University, had coronary artery bypass grafts at the Yale University School of Medicine, Brewster asked me about a cardiac surgeon on the faculty. The patient and his family had complained that the surgeon did not tell them much when he made his rounds. Brewster concluded that perhaps, for that type of highly technical procedure, an excellent technician was better than a communicator. I think, however, that a surgeon can be both a communicator and an excellent technician. Physicians are busy, sometimes overwhelmed; however, explanations, a review of tests, diagnostic possibilities and treatment options do not take a long time to go over with a patient.

I document my sources for everything written and provide the authors' names and sources of quotations, references, and worldwide websites for more information. I describe evidence for therapy and the studies to support the evidence. When claims are made for health benefits but there is no evidence to support these claims, I say so. I state and identify my own opinions and beliefs. A recent book about foods and health stated on its cover "Prevent Cancer with Strawberries" (page 8) and "Perk up your Love Life with Apricots" (page 104). Inside the book, the authors say, "studies prove—it helps you". What are these studies? Where were they published? Have they been repeated? What is the evidence? The authors don't provide *any* evidence in their book. Why don't they? Could it be that they don't have anything other than anecdotes? Health claims are frequently made without supporting evidence.

Some questions and chapters have a large number of references, web-sites and sources of information because they are the hot topics for the public and press that appear in lay and medical literature. Others, with few references, may be important to you, but little has been written about the subjects. To answer questions on those topics, I rely on my experience as a doctor.

Exciting advances in knowledge about human biology and illness have been made recently, as well as amazing technical advances in diagnosis and treatment of human ills such as laparoscopic operations and dilation of blocked coronary arteries, or angioplasty. There is great interest in alternative medicine, homeopathy, herbal medicine and folk medicine. Many of you may use such treatments. I provide information about Chinese traditional medicine that is part of such therapy. Some excellent books on the subject and contents of alternative or complimentary medicine are available. Andrew Weil's book on *Eating Well for Optimum Health* and also *Spontaneous Healing* are two examples. Weil is a medical doctor who reliably documents his recommendations.

With all the medical advances and the 30+ years of greater life expectancy today, as compared with 1900, come problems. How can we pay for all these things? Who should pay for them? Is healthcare a right or a privilege or a necessity? Why do medicines cost so much? Many of your questions about these matters will be answered in the following pages.

Lee, writing in the Harvard Health Letter, points out that, if you read the front page of a newspaper, you may get the impression that this is the golden age of medicine. Actually, American medicine is falling apart; Medicare is going broke, elderly people skip meals to pay for prescriptions, discouraged doctors are retiring early, and HMOs are denying payment for life-saving therapy. Lee indicates that both messages are correct. Healthcare has never been better, yet there are big problems about who will pay for it. Lee goes on to describe four trends: 1) wonderful new medications (but who really needs them and who will pay for them?); 2) molecular medicine and gene therapy that will advance future care; 3) more responsibility by lay people for their health; 4) increased cost to individuals for their health care.

You can do much to prolong a healthy and meaningful life. Doctors, nurses, hospitals and new drugs can also do many things to maintain your health and prevent disease, and to diagnose and treat disease. Genetic research has great promise. I have written an extensive section of questions and answers about staying healthy, disease prevention, health promotion, diet and exercise—what is real, what can be documented, what you can believe.

We better understand now the relationship between our minds and bodies and our immune systems; between attitude and the response to cancer and other diseases; and the effect of faith and prayer on healing, or, as Herbert Benson states, "the power and biology of belief". I provide sources and abbreviations to follow so that you may find out more about these approaches to healing. The word, 'patient', comes from the Latin verb patior—to suffer. I hope my book will help to prevent and relieve your suffering. Please read on.

Arthur E. Baue, M.D.

ABBREVIATIONS USED

AARP—American Association of Retired Persons
ACP—American College of Physicians
ACS—American College of Surgeons
AHA—American Heart Association
AMA—American Medical Association
CDCP—Center for Disease Control and Prevention
CSPI—Center for Science in the Public Interest
CT or CAT scan—Computerized axial tomographic scan
DA—Department of Agriculture
DEA—Drug Enforcement Administration
DHHS—Department of Health and Human Services
EMT—Emergency Medical Technician
EPA—Environmental Protection Agency
EW—Emergency Ward or Facility
FCC—Federal Communications Commission
FDA—Food and Drug Administration
FTC—Federal Trade Commission
GAO—General Accounting Office
GI—gastrointestinal tract
HCFA—Health Care Finance Administration
HHL—Harvard Health Letter
HHS—Health and Human Services
HMO—Health Maintenance Organization
ICU—Intensive Care Unit
IOM—Institute of Medicine
IV—Intravenous
JAMA—Journal of American Medical Association
JCAHO—Joint Commission of Healthcare Organizations
NAS—National Academy of Science
NCI—National Cancer Institute

NCIPC—National Center for Injury Prevention and Control
NEJM—New England Journal of Medicine
NHLBI—National Heart, Lung, Blood Institute
NIH—National Institutes of Health
NRA—National Rifle Association
OR—Operating Room
PCRM—Physicians Committee for Responsible Medicine
PDR—Physicians Desk Reference
SCCM—Society of Critical Care Medicine
USDA—United States Department of Agriculture
WHO—World Health Organization

Section A

**What are my rights and privileges with doctors?
What should I expect from my doctor and
for my health care?**

FINDING A GOOD DOCTOR—KINDS OF SPECIALISTS.

1. **How do I choose or find a good doctor? How do I know the
    doctor is competent? What are the different kinds of
    doctors or specialists?**

For many people, recommendations for a general doctor or specialist
come from family, friends, neighbors or a hospital, or increasingly,
from an insurance carrier or health maintenance organization (HMO). If you
do not have a doctor, I recommend you find one and make contact while you
are well. If you wait until you are sick or injured, you must rely on the emergency
ward of a local hospital. Your care there may be reasonable but you may wait.
They may be busy with more serious emergencies. They may not know you.

Your initial decision is what type of primary care doctor you seek: a family
practice physician, a general internal medicine physician, a general practitioner
for general health problems or a specialist in a combined program of pediatrics
and internal medicine. Primary care physicians are the doctors you see first

for all health problems. Most healthcare plans allow some choice of primary care physicians. If an HMO or an organized health care practice assigns you to a panel of physicians, make an appointment and talk with one or more of them to decide which you prefer. Find someone you are comfortable with, and then seek their help and care. Family physicians with special training in the care of adults, children and families are specialists and may be board certified in family medicine by the American Board of Family Physicians. They are qualified to give excellent care for all health problems, health maintenance, and disease prevention. They can help you in deciding whether you need the care of specialists. You should have a "primary care" doctor to provide care and coordinate your health care needs.

How do I find a doctor if I do not belong to an HMO?

Local hospitals list medical staff members who will accept new patients. You may respond to hospital commercials such as "call a nurse" to get a doctor's name. Obviously, they push members of their own medical staff. However, they will recommend only someone in good standing at that hospital. Should you require hospitalization, such a doctor will recommend that hospital. The county medical society lists doctors who belong to the society and are available. While membership in the medical societies and the American Medical Association indicates that a physician has not been in trouble, it is no assurance that the doctor is good. Liddane quotes Dr. Tom Dent of the University of California as saying, "Choose a doctor based on ability, affability and availability. Finding the right match provides better collaboration for your health." Steps in finding the right doctors: 1) Decide what is important to you and write it down. 2) Choose a board-certified doctor and check with the Medical Society for any disciplinary actions against him or her. 3) Consider a doctor with teaching responsibilities at a hospital (they stay abreast of treatment). 4) Consider a doctor who practices in a highly regarded group. 5) Ask if the doctor is willing to talk to you for 15 minutes to get acquainted. (A recent review found that female physicians tended to spend more time with patients and communicated more effectively.)

Upon meeting the physician, determine whether he or she meets your needs and expectations in personality, communication, bedside manner and approach to care. Is the physician someone you can trust? A good listener? The physician in turn will determine whether you will be accepted as a new patient.

It is important to ask about coverage or availability of your new doctor. Does your potential doctor belong to a group who cover for each other? Who do you call at night and on weekends? Will your doctor be available or will an answering service tell you to go to an emergency facility? Many physician groups alternate night and weekend calls so that someone is always available. Even a doctor in solo practice may alternate calls with other solo practitioners. No doctor can be available all the time.

Other factors to consider in selecting a doctor include:

— Which hospitals does the doctor use?
— To whom does he or she refer for specialty care?
— How far away is the office? Is it convenient to get to?
— Are the office hours convenient?
— Who covers when the doctor is away? Is he or she ever available at night or on weekends?
— How long has the doctor been in practice and at this location? (an indication of stability)
— Is the office staff helpful and friendly?
— Is the waiting room pleasant, clean and comfortable?
— Is the practice well managed?
— How long does it take to get an appointment? (Immediate availability may be a bad sign.)
— How do I relate to the doctor?
— Do I feel rushed?
— Is the doctor in my health plan?

Should you need a specialist, your primary care physician will recommend someone. If you are in a managed care organization or HMO, they will refer you to one of their panel of specialists. You may have to see that specialist if they are to pay for your care.

Primary care physicians look for specialists who do excellent work; no doctor will refer patients to a specialist who is not capable. Confirm this by asking your primary care physician why he or she is referring you to a certain specialist. You may also check on the capabilities of a specialist through the yearly directory of the American Board of Medical Specialties (ABMS), *The Official ABMS Directory of Board Certified Medical Specialists.* This publication is available in public libraries and online with Lexis-Nexis, and contains physician profiles of 37 specialties, from allergy and immunology to urology, 73 subspecialties and over 510,000 physicians. The directory indicates specialists who have completed board certification. You can go to the American Medical Association at *www.ama.assn.org* or the ABMS at *www.abms.org* for their Directory of Physicians in the United States with information on 813,000 physicians—their medical school year of graduation, year first licensed, primary and secondary specialties and board certification. Most libraries will have this directory.

What is board certification?

The American Boards in different specialties certify doctors who fulfill specific educational requirements, receive special training and pass an extensive examination, for example, in ophthalmology, or treatment of the eye, or orthopedics (bone and joint) surgery. The American Boards are voluntary organizations established by doctors that require excellent education for specialists. They are not regulated by government. No law requires this educational experience. A license to practice medicine in a state requires only a year of internship after medical school. An M.D. degree and a license to practice medicine do not insure competence. For that, graduate medical education or specialty training is required.

In general surgery, five years of residency is required with the fifth year spent as a chief resident. During residency the young surgeon completes a prescribed course, performs a number of surgical operations with supervision, and takes care of patients in various circumstances. The resident must pass an examination with both written and oral components to be certified by the American Board of Surgery. The Board believes that this period of education, experience and examination provides surgeons who are capable of safely taking care of you for general surgery, an appendectomy, for example, and also, colon and rectal and oncologic (cancer) surgery. However, other kinds of surgery require even further training. One year more is required for vascular (blood vessels) surgery, two more years for thoracic surgeons (chest-heart-lungs).

There are 24 specialty boards that belong to the American Board of Medical Specialties (ABMS) and issue certificates in 37 areas of specialization and subspecialty certificates in 75 areas. The Board of Internal Medicine, for example, oversees a subspecialty of cardiology.

Standards for medical education and medical schools are very high. They are reviewed frequently and schools are visited and accredited if they pass the review by the Liaison Committee on Medical Education (LCME), composed of representatives of the American Medical Association (AMA) and the Association of American Medical Colleges (AAMC). The AAMC advocates that physicians be altruistic, knowledgeable, skillful and dutiful. Some doctors are M.D.'s—medical doctors. Some are D.O.'s—doctors of osteopathy. In the past, D.O.'s manipulated bones, muscles and joints in the interest of improving health but do this no longer to any degree. Now equivalent in education and capability, M.D.'s and D.O.'s work closely together in many hospitals and clinics. Do not confuse D.O.'s with chiropractors, however, who are not licensed to practice medicine. Their activities will be reviewed under alternative medicine in chapter 42.

Residency programs are regulated by the Accreditation Council for Graduate Medical Education (ACGME) representing all specialties and medical societies.

The ABMS and AMA sponsor residency review committees which establish requirements for the residencies. The ACGME periodically surveys residency programs and accredits them or may withdraw accreditation. The ACGME requires residents to demonstrate competence in patient care, clinical science, practice-based learning and improvement, interpersonal skills and communication, professionalism and systems-based practice.

What is re-certification?

Most specialty boards have developed programs called re-certification. The idea is this: If a specialist demonstrated his capability in 1990, how do we know he or she has kept up 10 years later? These specialists are asked to demonstrate continuing capability by an examination of current knowledge and abilities, another safeguard these specialties provide for you.

How do I know a specialist is qualified?

The Joint Commission on Accreditation of Health Care Organizations allows no one on the staff of an accredited hospital to do special procedures unless board certified in that specialty, with special training in those procedures. Hospitals must be reviewed and accredited yearly by the Joint Commission in order to qualify to receive Medicare payments. Thus, the voluntary hospital system, the voluntary medical system and its organizations such as the American College of Surgeons, other medical specialty colleges and specialty boards, all were developed by doctors to protect you. You can rely on these organizations for advice, for help in finding specialists, and for assurance that the specialists are well trained and particularly board certified. It is unadvisable to go to an uncertified specialist for an operation or other treatment.

When you are referred to a specialist, do not be embarrassed to ask if he or she is board certified. You can ask them where they had their training and how much experience they have had with your particular problem. You can also ask about the operation you are considering—how many and how often are they performed by this specialist, who should be willing to review this with you. Board certified physicians will be pleased to provide evidence of their capabilities.

How do I know that a doctor is competent?

A busy doctor is usually competent. Beyond that rule of thumb, specialty training and board certification insure some level of competence. The county medical society, the state licensing board and specialty societies (e.g., the

American College of Surgeons) hear grievances from patients and families and will discipline doctors for poor care; for big problems they will revoke his license to practice, and, of course, practicing medicine without a license is a felony. Consumer groups have taken the initiative in trying to uncover information about disciplinary actions. See, for example, *www.questionabledoctors.org.* and Public Citizen, which sells books listing doctors with disciplinary records. The Joint Commission on Accreditation of Health Care Organizations lists the accreditation status of hospitals at www.jcaho.org.

A description of the competent physician has now been approved by the ABMS as follows:

The Competent Physician

He should possess the medical knowledge, judgment, professionalism, and clinical and communication skills to provide high-quality patient care. Patient care encompasses the promotion of health, prevention of disease, and diagnosis, treatment, and management of medical conditions with compassion and respect for patients and their families. Maintenance of competence should be demonstrated throughout the physician's career by lifelong learning and ongoing improvement of practice.

General Competence for Doctors

Accreditation Council for Graduate Medical Education (ACGME)

(Medical Schools)

Patient Care
Medical Knowledge
Practice-based Learning and Improvement
Interpersonal and Communication Skills
Professionalism
System-based Practice

Maintenance of Certification

American Board of Medical Specialties (ABMS)

Evidence of professional standing
Evidence of a commitment to lifelong learning and involvement in a periodic self-assessment process
Evidence of cognitive expertise
Evidence of evaluation of performance in practice

What are all the different kinds of doctors or specialists?

GENERAL AND SPECIALTY DOCTORS

Primary Care Doctors

Family Physicians—(General practitioners) They should be Board Certified in Family Medicine

General Internal Medicine/General Internists—Should be Board Certified in Internal Medicine

Pediatric/Internal Medicine Doctors—They have training in both the care of children and adults—should be certified in Internal Medicine or Pediatrics or both

Specialists
Anesthesiology

General, spinal, epidural anesthesia and pain control, pain clinics, intensive care

Internal Medicine

American Board of Medicine (ABM)—Three to four years of residency— General Internal Medicine

Subspecialties of Internal Medicine

There are subspecialty boards for these specialties after certification by the ABM. Each requires further training.

Cardiology (heart)—Invasive Cardiology (blood vessels)

Gastroenterology (GI) tract—liver, esophagus, stomach and intestines

Pulmonology (lungs)

Endocrinology and Metabolism—thyroid, parathyroid, adrenal and other glands

Geriatric Medicine—the elderly (Gerontology)

Hematology—blood and blood clotting

Dermatology—disease of the skin

Infectious Diseases—all acute and chronic infections

Allergy and Immunology—allergic reactions and resistance to disease

Nephrology—diseases of the kidneys
Oncology—malignant diseases (chemotherapy) and bone marrow
     transplantation
Rheumatology—bones and joints
Arthritis—joint disease
Transplantation Medicine—evaluation for and care during and
     after an organ transplant

Intensive Care Medicine

Doctors who work in ICU's could be internists, surgeons, pediatricians, or anesthesiologists. Special training is required.

Emergency Medicine

Doctors who work in a Hospital's Emergency Department and specialize in emergencies. Special training is required.

Otorhinolaryngology (ENT)

Ears, nose, throat and head and neck surgery

Ophthalmology

Eyes—vision, cataracts, retina problems

Pediatrics

Children usually up to age 16. All of the specialties of Internal Medicine are also found in Pediatrics. In addition, there is:

Adolescent Medicine
Developmental Pediatrics
Medical Genetics
Neonatology (newborns)

Obstetrics and Gynecology

Pregnancy, delivery, female problems or diseases of the uterus, vagina, fallopian tubes and ovaries

Nuclear Medicine

Diagnostic studies using radioactive materials. Therapy for certain tumors.

Radiology (X-ray)

Imaging studies, x-rays, scans, CT, PET, MRI, ultrasound, angiography (blood vessel x-rays), invasive radiology (blood vessel stents, dilatation)

Radiation Oncology

Treatment of cancer by x-ray

Pathology

Diagnosis by microscopic study of tissues and by autopsy
Laboratories to study blood and other tissues and blood banking
Forensic pathology—the study of injuries and crimes, autopsies—medical examiners

Surgery

General Surgery—GI tract, thyroid, adrenal, parathyroid glands—five years of Residency
Thoracic Surgery—lungs and esophagus—two additional years after general surgery
Cardiac Surgery—heart and aorta—two additional years after general surgery (some combine thoracic and cardiac)
Vascular Surgery—blood vessels—one year after general surgery
Urologic Surgery—kidneys, bladder and prostate gland
Neurosurgery—brain and spinal cord, nerves
Plastic Surgery—cosmetic and restorative surgery—five to seven years of residency (may be combined with general surgery)
Transplantation—transplanting abdominal organs-liver, pancreas, kidneys or chest organs, heart and lungs
Colon and Rectal Surgery—after general surgery training
Trauma Surgery—injury—after general surgery training
Oncologic Surgery—cancer—after general surgery training
Pediatric Surgery—children—after general surgery training
Surgical Intensive Care—after general surgery training

Orthopedic Surgery

Bones and joints—fractures, joint replacement, tumors of bones

Psychiatry

General Psychiatry—Alzheimer's disease
Geriatric and Children's Psychiatry

Preparing to see a doctor.

**2.   How should I prepare for an office visit to see my doctor?
Why does the doctor want so much information? What about
going to an emergency facility?**

I hope you have established a relationship with a doctor who knows you
and will see you in the office fairly quickly—the same day if you are
acutely ill. For elective, non-urgent, health procedures, an appointment in a
week or two is reasonable. Such procedures include checkups for high blood
pressure, diabetes, gout or other chronic or persistent illnesses. Schedule the
next visit when you leave your doctor's office.

Keep a symptoms diary to review with your doctor, particularly if your health
problem is complex or mysterious. Weil suggests a daily record of when your
pain or other symptoms occur, how long they last and anything associated with
them such as, stress, eating, exercise, activity or other factors. Describe the pain.
Is it burning or throbbing? Does it feel like muscle or bone or joint pain?

Your mind may go blank in a doctor's office, particularly if the doctor doesn't
make you feel at home. Ronny Frishman, writing in the *Harvard Health Letter* says,
"Don't be a wimp in the doctor's office." He recommends, and I agree: Come to
your doctor with questions and ask them, don't be shy; keep the conversation on
track; take notes; if you are uncomfortable with a recommendation, get another
opinion; let the doctor know your limits; educate yourself.

When you visit your doctor, bring all the pills you take so your doctor knows
about them. Know what you expect from the visit

—   a diagnosis—the cause of your problem
—   prognosis—what will happen in the future
—   reassurance
—   information on any new treatment
—   help with practical problems of living
—   help with feelings of fatigue, depression

During the visit, review each list with your doctor, but get to the point. If he seems in a hurry, tell him that you have a number of things to tell him. Ask him to sum them up for you. Answer all questions honestly. Weil suggests tape recording the visit or bringing a family member or friend to take notes.

If you are referred to a medical center, particularly one associated with a medical school, you may be given an appointment in two months. Medical school doctors spend a lot of their time teaching and doing research and see patients only part of the time. They may not be in a hurry for an elective non-urgent problem. Even though your problem is elective and not urgent, however, you may be worried about it. In that case I recommend you ask for a referral to a similar specialist who is in private practice. You will be seen sooner since such a doctor's total activity is seeing and treating patients.

Sometimes medical schools even fail patients with urgent problems, like a woman I know with prior ulcerative colitis who had previously had her colon removed. She developed severe abdominal pain, cramps, gas, and diarrhea and could not eat. She called a medical school department of surgery on August 10 and, cruelly enough, was given an appointment to see a specialist on September 26. In such a situation the patient should write a personal note to the specialist or ask her doctor to call and make an appointment on an urgent basis.

If you have an urgent medical problem such as severe or sudden shortness of breath, an asthma attack, or abdominal or chest pain, your doctor may recommend that you go immediately to an emergency ward where the doctor is on staff. You may need blood studies, urinalysis, x-rays or an electrocardiogram which can only be done in a hospital. Emergency physicians specialize in treating urgent or emergency problems and will help evaluate you. Most emergency facilities have doctors available in the facility 24 hours a day; a smaller or rural hospital may have a nurse on duty and a doctor who is on call. Don't go to an emergency facility for a chronic problem or use it as your family doctor. If you do, you may impede the prompt treatment of true emergencies.

Depending upon your medical urgency or emergency, your primary care doctor may request a consultation from a specialist such as a surgeon, a cardiologist for your heart, or a pulmonologist for your lungs. The specialist, after seeing you, should give a report immediately to your doctor. This is the role of a consultant—to see you in consultation and report to you and your doctor. If you and your doctor agree with what the consultant has recommended, the consultant will proceed with treatment, hospitalization, or diagnostic tests. If your doctor has not been part of the process, ask the consultant if your doctor knows what is happening.

A doctor may have many patients to see and be on a tight schedule, particularly if a number of you get sick and must see the doctor urgently. You may have to wait, and the doctor also may not have a lot of time to spend with you. It is important to deal with the urgent problem and not with other chronic problems.

It is not necessary for the doctor to act in a hurry. I sat down when talking to a patient after the history was taken and the patient examined. I reviewed what I thought was the problem and what I would recommend doing about it and would ask for questions. I tried to give the impression that you were the only person I was thinking about at that time and I had all the time in the world (which I didn't). If I felt that more time was needed, I would ask you to think about my recommendations (more diagnostic studies or an operation or seeing another specialist), review them with your family, and return to see me again. A doctor should be able to guide you to stick to your problem and not launch into other discussions.

The *Harvard Health Letter* suggests 11 things you should talk to your doctor about: what do you want to do but can't do anymore, what you are afraid of, where you've traveled, a family member with a serious disease, over-the-counter pills you take, medications prescribed by other doctors, medicines you're supposed to take but don't, whether you smoke or drink, and whether you are depressed, stressed, incontinent, or sexually dysfunctional.

Why does the doctor want so much information?

When you first see a doctor, you may be given a patient information form which should be filled out accurately along with insurance or payment information. It may ask what medications you take at home. This is very important. Another form may ask if you have ever been diagnosed or treated for heart disease, blood pressure problems, kidney or bladder disorders, lung disease (asthma, TB), liver problems, diabetes, epilepsy, arthritis, stomach problems, ulcers, bleeding problems and other problems. It may ask if you have ever been hospitalized, and if so for what, and if you have had an operation, and, if so, what kind and the date and any problems associated with the operation or the anesthetic. Your social history is important: information about your marital status, your children, grandchildren, and other relatives. Your work history is important, too. Your medical history should cover any injuries before the onset of your symptoms, any allergies, your smoking history, any regular consumption of alcoholic drinks, any recent weight gain or loss, any skin conditions, hearing or vision problems, bowel or bladder problems, walking difficulties, and sleep habits. Your doctor needs to know how often you have seen a doctor or had medical attention.

In signing a form for assignment of insurance benefits and payment for services, you are agreeing that payment will go to your doctor. Sometimes you are asked for consent in advance for treatment in an institute or clinic where you go, or authorization to release information, or for legal processes. Don't sign this until you see the doctor and know what is involved. How can you consent to treatment when you don't know what it will be? My wife was once asked to sign a treatment authorization, release of information and information for legal processes before she saw the doctor. She refused to do so and said that she would sign when she understood what was involved in treatment and what was to be done with the information. Never agree to treatment and release of information in writing, in advance, if you do not know what they will involve.

APPOINTMENTS.

3. How long must I wait to get an appointment or wait in the office to be seen by my doctor? What if it is an urgent problem? When should I call my doctor?

I never wait more than 5-10 minutes to see my doctor. Does that tell you something? Many patients expect to spend time in a doctor's office waiting beyond the scheduled time for the appointment even though often it should not be necessary to do so. Some doctors are not considerate of your time in the manner of scheduling. A patient should be scheduled for 2:00, another for 2:15, and so on but some offices schedule a number of patients for the same time and they are seen according to their arrival time. If scheduling is left to the office staff, they may protect the doctor so he does not wait. They may believe that his time is more important than yours. This is unfair. Tell your doctor. He may not know what his office staff is doing.

Accurate, timely scheduling requires estimates of the time needed to see each patient, which may be difficult for some doctors. Internists and pediatricians may need to see very sick patients in urgent visits and on hospital rounds. Doctors for whom this is a frequent occurrence should allow open time for these emergencies. Surgeons face a different scheduling problem. Usually surgeons perform operations in the morning and see patients in their offices in the afternoon. Some reverse this, even though it is unfair for a patient to wait without eating or drinking from midnight until the afternoon for an operation. If emergencies intervene or the operation takes longer than estimated, the surgeon may arrive late for office hours. Sometimes this can't be helped; frequently, however, it can. When surgeons schedule an operation, they are asked to estimate the time required. Most surgeons underestimate the time it will take them. They believe they are faster than they are.

One of the biggest hazards to a surgeon's schedule is a "to-follow" operation. This means that one operation have been scheduled for 7:30 or 8:00 a.m., as the first case of the day ("case" is jargon for "operation"). After an operation, it takes a half hour to clean the room and get ready for the next case. If the first operation takes two hours, then the second or "to follow" operation may start at 10:00 a.m. If it takes two hours, this leaves time for lunch for the surgeon and for an appointment with you promptly at 1:00 p.m. as scheduled. If, however, the first or previous operation isn't over until 12 noon, your surgeon then finishes his two hour operation at 2:30 and gets to the office to see you at 2:45 (no lunch for him). You have waited an hour and 45 minutes. This can happen and does. What are your options? First, the surgeon's office staff should keep you apprised of what is happening. Secondly, they should ask if you wish to be seen by a colleague if one is available. Thirdly, they could reschedule your visit if this would be best for you. Finally, if you stick it out, the surgeon should apologize for making you wait. If you are a patient scheduled for an operation to follow an earlier operation, you may wait for hours in the preoperative area until your turn comes. If you come into the hospital at 6:00am on the day of operation, it can be quite disconcerting to have to fast and wait for hours.

During my surgical career, I tried to foresee such problems the day before— a long operation, potential delays, etc—and to be sure that another member of my group practice was in the office to see patients promptly. Patients were also given the option of rescheduling the visit. I tried to see each patient within ten minutes of the scheduled time. It was not always possible. Some patients deserved more time and I provided it for them. If late, however, I felt it was only common courtesy to tell the patient I was sorry to keep them waiting. No doctor is so important, so famous, or so in demand that they should keep patients waiting for more than 10 minutes even one time, certainly not many. You can tell your doctor that such delays are unnecessary.

Most doctors see patients only during the day. A few have evening office hours, more should; I wish I had offered that option to my patients. Some of you may not be able to miss a day's work, even to see a doctor. Some people are not paid if they miss work and unfortunately will not see a doctor until their problem becomes acute, life-threatening, or hopeless.

Many doctors work at a number of hospitals and travel from one to the other and then to their office. The doctor's office staff should be honest about where the doctor is and when he may get to the office. My family members have been told that a doctor was leaving for the office at that moment and would be there shortly only to find out later the doctor had not yet left another hospital which was an hour away. Office staff should be straight forward, honest, supportive and helpful for the patient.

If you are referred to a specialist at a large medical center or to a medical school faculty member, you may be told that the first available appointment is in three months. If your problem is not urgent and you are comfortable with that, go with it. If, however, you feel your medical problem is more urgent or you are anxious about it, say so to the specialist's office. If they will not give you an earlier appointment, go elsewhere. There are many specialists to choose from.

Must you be pushy to get an appointment? Remember, your appointment is being made by a secretary who may have no idea about the urgency of your problem. If you have an urgent problem, be pushy—tell the secretary it is urgent. Tell the secretary that a doctor has referred you. Ask your doctor's office to make the appointment for you. For friends and family, I suggest telling the doctor's office that I have recommended that the patient see the doctor soon. If you see such a doctor, be sure to tell him that his office staff made it difficult to get an appointment.

When should I call my doctor?

For a medical or health problem that bothers you but is not producing severe discomfort or incapacity, it would be best to call and make an appointment. Tell the secretary or nurse what your problem is and how urgent you think it is. If the problem is severe but not an emergency, tell them that and ask for an appointment soon.

If your problem is urgent—shortness of breath, persistent chest pain, or a feeling of sickness—call and ask what to do. Many doctors, particularly pediatricians, set aside some time each day to see sick patients. For fever, call if your child's temperature is over 102 degrees or if yours is over 101 degrees, if a fever persists for a day and you do not know the cause or if it persists over 72 hours and you think you know the cause. Health tips are provided by Consumer Reports on Health. For example, they recommend you should see a physician if any fever lasts longer than three days or is accompanied by frequent, burning or bloody urination, pain in the abdomen, shaking chills or profuse diarrhea lasting more than a day. On nights and weekends the doctor on call may recommend you go to the hospital emergency room. If you have any doubt, call. You can ask for the doctor on call to call you back and you can discuss what to do. For more severe problems, go to the emergency facility to play it safe. Remember though, it is not fair to the emergency facility to go for a chronic problem which has bothered you for some time.

What are same-day doctor visits:

Some medical groups and doctors around the country are trying a no-wait service for patients. You are seen the day you call. No-wait service focuses on the patient which is where it should be. Not only does it make patients happier, but it may make them healthier with earlier diagnosis and care. Wheeler of

Minneapolis Health Partners Clinic found that no-wait service decreased the need for hospitalization and for urgent care center visits and saved money. Medical groups find that scheduling can accommodate a no-wait service; more patients come in on Monday than on Friday, for instance, and scheduling can provide for that. Other trials include group visits for elderly patients with chronic illnesses, regularly scheduled phone calls, e-mailing lab test results and medication changes.

CONTROL

4.   What do the terms "autonomy" or "paternalism" mean in health care? What control do I keep?

Many of you may prefer a paternalistic approach to your care. If you have a doctor you trust, who has taken care of you through various illnesses or even crises in your life, you may tell your doctor "Do what you think is best" or "You know what is best, tell me what I should do." There is nothing wrong with this. This is the paternalistic way medicine was practiced for years. Now the concept of autonomy of yourself, of your body and what happens to you has become widely accepted. You may still decide to do what your doctor thinks is best but you can request an explanation for it. The relationship between you and your doctor is still important. If you do not trust your doctor to do what is best for you, then you need another doctor. Before you change, talk with your doctor about what you expect. He still may be able to provide it.

I have had patients say: "Don't tell me I have cancer, doctor." This may seem like a difficult situation for a doctor but it is necessary to understand such concerns of patients. They fear the worst and are having difficulty facing that possibility. If the diagnosis of malignancy has not been established, then the patient can be told that we don't know yet and we must make sure what the nodule or mass or lump or shadow on x-ray is. The doctor can tell you that you have a tumor, and that tumors can be benign or malignant. If the doctor knows the exact diagnosis, he must be truthful but he need not hit the patient with the whole truth. You could be told: "It is a bad sort of tumor that must be treated." There is no reason why a doctor must deliver to you what you may interpret as a death sentence. You should be given hope for the future no matter how bad your problem is. There is always something to hope for. Some words are worse than others. Cancer may be the worst—a malignancy is synonymous but does not sound as bad. I would never tell you something that was not true. Too much positive spin about treatment may create unrealistic expectations.

But I also want to support you and help you get your problem treated as best as possible. Thus, I don't want you to feel discouraged or helpless. A positive attitude strengthens your immune system and allows you to better combat a disease, even a malignancy (Chapter 17). The *Harvard Health Letter* reviews the gray area of honesty in doctor-patient relationships. We must avoid giving only the bad news and must build trust.

If your doctor is discouraging you, tell him that you want to be positive about this illness. You want to deal with it and overcome it. Tell him you would like him to be positive about it also. The term shared decision-making is used to describe a true partnership between you and your doctor. Now this has gone on to informed choice. Patients vary greatly in how they would like to participate in decisions. Some doctors are providing decision aids (audio-tapes and books) to help you make a choice about therapy.

Another aspect of autonomy is that you are in charge of your body and your health (Chapter 61—informed consent. Chapter 62—a patient's bill of rights). Toward the end of life, it is important to be sure of your rights (Chapter 49— calling it quits) and your decisions before you become incapable of deciding (Chapter 50—living wills).

WHO IS IN CHARGE?

5. Who is in charge of my care and responsible for my treatment? Sometimes I seem to get shuffled from one specialist to another.

You, the patient, are in charge of yourself and your care. The person responsible for recommending diagnostic studies and treatment to you should be identified. This is an important issue if you are referred to or admitted to a hospital and particularly to an intensive care unit. It may also be important if you are in a hospital on a teaching service where physicians assigned as your doctors may rotate every month. Your family should establish who is responsible. If on the staff of the hospital, your primary care doctor could direct your care, but, if not, may not be able to visit you.

You must have a primary care doctor. For problems that require a consultation or detailed diagnostic studies, your primary care doctor may refer you to an internist, a surgeon, or someone in other specific specialties. Your primary doctor will call that physician. The person you go to see is a consultant. The consultant examines you, recommends appropriate studies, and arrives at a conclusion and recommendation for therapy which should be sent back to your primary care physician who will then talk with you about the alternatives. Sometimes, however, the consultant will move ahead and talk with you about proceeding with what is recommended. In either case, the consultant must talk with your primary care physician and send a report to that physician.

Your primary care physician should take responsibility for guiding you through the system, making sure you get enough information to understand your problem, and receive appropriate therapy. If you see a consultant or several consultants, or specialists, and are not happy with what they tell you, ask your primary care physician to help you.

In the event of surgery, the surgeon will be in charge of your care until your discharge from the hospital. At that time the surgeon will arrange follow-up appointments to be sure that you are recovering satisfactorily. These follow-up visits may go on for some months until the surgeon is sure that you have returned to normal. At that time you should be referred back to your primary care physician for continuing care.

In the event of a malignancy, the surgeon may ask to see you yearly to be sure that it has not returned. Your internist would do the same, as would your specialist in lung disease (a pulmonologist); in heart disease (a cardiologist); in kidney disease, (a nephrologists); or any other specialist in internal medicine.

Cancer patients may also see radiation oncologists, trained in x-ray therapy for the treatment of malignancy, and medical oncologists, internists who are experts in cancer therapy. Chemotherapy is the responsibility of medical oncologists who also coordinate patients' care between surgery, x-ray therapy and chemotherapy.

If your problem is pain, your primary care doctor may refer you to a pain clinic or a pain center, usually the responsibility of an anesthesiologist with specific training in the relief of pain. These specialists use nerve blocks, epidural blocks, injections alongside the spine, and other techniques. After treatment, they would get you back again to your doctor for general medical care.

Before, during, and after operation, the surgeon is the "captain of the ship," responsible overall for your care. Anesthesiologists work closely with surgeons. While surgeons administer local anesthetics, injections at the sites of operations or, "freezing, anesthesiologists administer other anesthetics: regional nerve blocks, spinal anesthetics, epidural blocks, or general anesthetics, which put patients to sleep. With a general anesthetic it is a safe practice to put a tube through your mouth and down into your throat, into the windpipe or trachea, to support breathing during the operation. After this, your throat may feel irritated and you may be hoarse for a few days. The anesthesiologist is also responsible for monitoring the depth of anesthesia and your vital signs, blood pressure, pulse, level of consciousness, and so on during the operation. The anesthesiologist is also responsible for getting you to the recovery room where nurses will take over your care and allow you to awaken from the anesthetic, recover and go back to your room.

For an anesthetic in some small or rural hospitals, you may have access only to a nurse anesthetist, a registered nurse (RN) qualified to give most forms of anesthetics after a year or more of special training. In larger hospitals nurse anesthetists work under the supervision of MD anesthesiologists, and in most teaching hospitals only MD anesthesiologists give anesthesia. For major emergencies, trauma and large operations, referral to a large hospital is recommended. Even for small hospitals anesthesiologists believe that they, as medical doctors, should supervise all nurse anesthetists. This is an ongoing debate between the American Association of Nurse Anesthetists and the American Society of Anesthesiologists.

If you have had a large major operation you may go from the operating room to an intensive care unit (ICU) for close observation and support for the next few days or however long support may be needed. You also may go to an ICU from the emergency ward if they believe you had a coronary event or if you have other problems that could require intensive care such as an injury, etc.

In ICUs, your primary care physician will no longer be responsible for your care, but could come to see you from time to time if he/she is a member of the hospital staff. In a surgical ICU, your surgeon is responsible for your care. In other ICUs, physicians trained in intensive care medicine (intensivists) are responsible for all patients in that unit. They may communicate with your surgeon, your internist, your primary care physician, but they will supervise your care, communicate with you and your family and help you to recover and get out of the ICU. It may be difficult for you and your family to know who is in charge. Ask the nurses in the ICU who is directly responsible for your care and ask to speak with that individual. If an intensivist is responsible, your surgeon and other physicians should be kept informed and should be involved in major decisions about your care. The intensivist responsible for your care should meet with your family and be available for questions and concerns. This individual and the nurses in the ICU should be familiar with your wishes and have a copy of your Living Will or Advanced Directive (chapter 50). They should also know who is responsible for you if you become incapacitated. If you and your family believe that you are not getting the information you want, call your own doctor. He should be able to help coordinate your care and information.

Many primary care physicians no longer see you or take care of you in a hospital. Manian describes primary care physicians who see patients only in the office as "officists." This doctor may be assisted by a "screenist"—a nurse practitioner or physicians assistant to answer your phone calls and see you during office visits. The doctor who cares for patients only in a hospital is called a "hospitalist." There are intensivists for ICUs, physiatrists for rehabilitation and finally a SNFist—a doctor who will look after you in a skilled nursing facility, or a SNF.

Some primary care physicians complain that, if they refer you to a large medical center in a big city, particularly to a teaching hospital, the physicians there take over your care and the referring or primary care physician never sees you again. This should not occur. Physicians taking care of you in a tertiary care center, or a major medical center, should always communicate with your primary care physician. When their treatments are concluded, they should send you back to that physician for continuing medical care. If you go to a major medical center, I suggest that you maintain contact with your primary care physician, and ask your doctors in the hospital to do the same.

If you are referred to a major medical center and are hospitalized on the medical service, you may be assigned a consulting physician who is responsible for all the patients on that nursing unit for a brief period of time such as one month. These physicians change every month or so. If you are not sure who is in charge of your care, ask your nurse. You and your family should speak with that doctor. If the doctors change, the new doctor should introduce himself. If you come to a hospital and have a surgical problem but do not know a surgeon, you will be assigned a capable surgeon. This person should introduce himself and be in charge of your care until your discharge from the hospital.

When I go to see my doctor, sometimes I am seen and examined by a nurse. Is that right? I may never see my doctor. What is a Nurse Practitioner?

With additional training and degrees, many nurses become nurse practitioners to help physicians in their practice. Nurse practitioners receive national certification in their specialties, which include internal medicine, pediatrics, geriatrics, school nursing and women's health, and they can acquire superb skills in helping with health care. For many routine matters, a nurse practitioner can take perfectly good care of you. They report to the doctor; for particular problems patients will be asked to stay to see the doctor. I recommend that you rely upon these health care professionals so long as they eventually report to a physician. Nurse practitioners and nurses in general can add immensely to the good care you get from your doctor, but if you do not see your doctor at all, then you can complain.

Some people have recommended or allowed nurse practitioners to practice independently and write prescriptions. This could be acceptable for minor ailments but who is to say what is or when it is a minor illness? Also, it could quickly become a major illness.

What are other kinds of nurses?

RNs may have completed one of two nursing educational programs: three-year diploma programs associated with hospitals and four-year degree programs at schools that award a bachelor of science in nursing. The three-year programs are being replaced by junior college programs with clinical work in hospitals.

Graduates of all nursing programs must take an examination to become an RN. In order to teach nursing, some nurses go on to get a master's or PhD degree in nursing.

RNs are capable of caring for you in a hospital and in the home setting. They plan patient care, give injections and intravenous fluids, do specialized and skilled nursing, supervise licensed practical nurses (LPNs) and nurse's aides, and make certain that doctors' orders are followed. They are responsible for patient care in nursing units—wards, operating rooms and ICUs. A recent study of 6 million patient records showed that patients in hospitals with more RNs had shorter lengths of stay, fewer potentially preventable deaths and lower rates of infection and other complications.

The education of LPNs is not as extensive as that of RN's but they help provide excellent care in hospitals. LPNs must be high school graduates, complete a year of training, and pass a licensing exam. They can take histories, draw blood samples, perform monitoring of vital signs, receive verbal orders, assist with bathing and change dressings, and they are invaluable in nursing home facilities. Nurses' aides assist both RNs and LPNs in a number of ways, among them by taking blood pressure and pulse and measuring heart rate.

What are physician extenders or physician assistants?

Physician assistants, PAs, and surgical assistants, SAs, are college graduates who study in qualifying programs for two to three years after college. They are also called physician extenders and can be very helpful in your care, both in a hospital or a doctor's office. They help doctors in taking a history of your health, doing an initial examination, helping in the operating room, emergency room and intensive care units. There is a National Surgical Assistant Association at 740B2 E. Flynn Lane, Phoenix, AZ 85014, email nsaa@inficad.com.

What are paramedics or emergency medical technicians (EMTs)?

Paramedics or emergency medical technicians (EMTs) have special training to take care of emergencies, to begin resuscitation and transport patients from an accident or from your home to an emergency facility or hospital. EMTs staff ambulances and respond to 911 calls and accidents at home, the workplace or roadways. They are highly trained for emergencies. I, as a physician, step aside when they arrive on the scene. I have seen them work in resuscitation and they are invaluable. They have the equipment to resuscitate patients suffering from cardiac arrest, immobilize fractures, begin intravenous fluids, insert airways, or breathing tubes, extricate passengers from wrecked cars and transport them safely. The many hours of mandatory training required and classifications are determined by the individual states. New York recognizes five EMT levels: First

Certified, First Responder, EMT basic, EMT intermediate, EMT critical care
and the highest level of EMT, a paramedic. Both a written and practical
examination is required of EMT candidates, along with continuing education.

SECOND OPINIONS

6.   What are my alternatives for treatment? When should I get
a second or even a third opinion and how do I get them?

There are always alternatives that you should know about and consider.
Ask the specialist what they are. He should tell you about the risks and
benefits of each. Is the recommended treatment potentially dangerous or
harmful? Are there side effects? Does the treatment work? Is it effective? How
effective? Who says it is effective? Who knows? If the treatment is a drug, is it
approved by the FDA? Is it an experimental drug (see Chapter 61—Informed
Consent)? A good doctor will answer these questions before you ask them. If
you have concerns about the diagnosis of your ailment and recommended
treatment, your own primary care doctor or specialist should welcome a request
for another opinion. Indeed, some HMO's and insurance companies require a
second opinion.

Some patients hesitate to seek a second opinion because they feel they will
insult their doctor. Some doctors may feel threatened by such a request. They
should not be. They should be comfortable with themselves and their opinions.
Zuger points out that Sir Thomas Percival wrote in 1803 that consultations are
necessary in "difficult or protracted cases" and "no important operation should
be determined upon without them."

I always welcomed a request for another opinion, and if a patient seemed
uncertain about a recommendation of mine, I would suggest another opinion.
Our recommendations are called "opinions." They are not facts. They are what
we think is best for you but other good doctors may have other opinions. Most
ailments allow for different treatments. There can be honest differences of opinion
about your treatment.

I will use cancer of the lung as an example. If you develop a cough and a
chest x-ray shows a shadow in your lung, it is important to find out what it is. Is
it benign and harmless, or malignant and harmful? The first step may be a
computerized axial tomographic scan (CT or CAT Scan) to better determine
the location and appearance of the shadow. It may look like a cancer to the
radiologist; that is his opinion. The next step may be a biopsy to obtain a tissue
sample of the nodule. A needle may be put through the chest wall into the
nodule or a small incision may be made to obtain the sample. A pathologist
then will examine the nodule cells through a microscope, to see if they are

similar to lung cancer or not. Pathologists can be wrong, mistaking a benign tumor for a malignant one and vice-versa. This happens very infrequently but if there is any doubt the pathologist should get a consultation. In many hospitals a biopsy of a tumor is always reviewed by other pathologists to be sure they agree.

Now we are getting closer to an exact diagnosis. Can we be 100% certain for you? For many cancers we can be close to 100% certain. If we establish the fact that you have lung cancer then the question is: What do we recommend? Now we need more information. Certain kinds of lung cancer are best treated by chemotherapy and/or x-ray therapy, or radiation therapy, because they have already spread. Is the cancer localized or has it spread to lymph nodes in your chest or elsewhere in your body? We will go back and study your CT scan to look for enlarged lymph nodes and check your liver and adrenal glands, above the kidneys. We will ask whether you have any pain anywhere or headaches which would suggest the possibility of spread of the cancer, or metastases. A positron emission tomography (PET) scan may be recommended. This diagnostic test involves an injection of a small amount of radioactive sugar that goes to tumors and metastases and shows up on an x-ray scan. If you have possible metastases to lymph nodes in your chest, another diagnostic study, a mediastinoscopy may be recommended to you. Through a small incision in your neck, lymph nodes in your chest can be biopsied to see if a tumor is present. If so, a big operation to remove the lung tumor is not worthwhile. The best treatment then would be x-ray treatment and perhaps chemotherapy. If, however, the tumor is localized in your lung with no evidence of spread, then the best treatment is an operation to remove the tumor and surrounding lung tissue. Removal of the entire tumor may require removal of just one lobe of a lung, a lobectomy, or, more drastically, removal of both lobes, a pneumonectomy. The extent of the operation depends on your general health. In order to determine the health of your lungs, your doctor will recommend pulmonary function tests (PFTs) and blood samples to measure how well your lungs provide oxygen to your tissues and remove carbon dioxide. If you have emphysema, another lung disease related to smoking, you may not survive an operation to remove a portion of your lung—or you may require oxygen to breathe for the rest of your life. If you require oxygen after an operation it may not be a happy result for you.

If surgery is indicated, I will tell you that it is the best chance of getting rid of the tumor completely and for a long time. I will tell you that your chances of getting through the operation and recovering your health afterwards are at least 96%. I will tell you about the likelihood of pain in your incision, which usually goes away after several weeks, and other possible, but unlikely, complications such as a cardiac arrest, a wound infection, a breakdown of the bronchus, or the tube to the lobe which was removed, and shortness of breath or a prolonged air leak. I will also tell you that, if nothing is done, the tumor will progress and spread and, within six months to a year, may kill you. I will tell you that you could have x-ray therapy which, over six weeks of daily treatments, will shrink the tumor. The treatments may make it disappear, but it is likely to return in future. You may have other questions. How long will I be in the hospital and how long will I be out of work. How much will it cost? Will my insurance cover it? Many surgeons and teaching hospitals will offer you appropriate treatment even though you cannot pay for it. Then it is your choice. If I have any doubts in my own mind about the best treatment, I will review your problem and all of your studies with my colleagues in our hospital at our weekly chest conference. In attendance are other thoracic, or chest, surgeons; pulmonologists, or lung doctors; pathologists; oncologists, or cancer doctors-for chemotherapy; and radiation therapists. After receiving their joint recommendation, if you still have any concerns about the diagnosis and/or the recommended treatment, you should request a second opinion.

How do I get a second opinion?

Your own doctor or specialist can recommend another doctor for you. You may ask friends, family or others for recommendations. You may ask the county medical society. When you find a doctor who will provide a second opinion, be sure that the doctor has all the information about you—reports, x-rays and scans. When we provide a second opinion, we should not take over your care unless the initial and second opinions are drastically different.

In the event of such a difference, you may to wish to get still another opinion to decide between the differences. Even if the first and second opinions agree, if you are still unsure, you may want a third opinion. It is your health and your body, and you should be able to do what is appropriate and comfortable for you.

If things don't make sense to you, keep asking questions. Some hospitals provide information sheets to help you. The Yale-New Haven Hospital in New Haven, CT, has a brochure, "Making the Right Choice," on obtaining a second opinion. They suggest getting a second opinion if you are having major surgery, to see whether surgery is the only option.

7.   How do I change doctors? What should I do if my doctor withdraws from my care?

If you are unhappy and dissatisfied with your doctor's care, or feel that you and your doctor are incompatible, you may want a change. For continuity of care, find another doctor first. Explain to your new doctor your reasons for making the change and explain them to your former doctor as well. Request that copies of your records be sent to the new doctor.

If your former doctor knows the reasons for your change, that may help him/her. Perhaps, however, you are the problem. Try to assess your attitudes, needs and personality. Perhaps your needs cannot be met by a doctor. Could a clergyman, priest, rabbi, another religious professional or counselor help you?

Your doctor could believe that because of a personality conflict you should turn to another doctor. Your doctor may feel unable to satisfy your needs or demands. Perhaps your doctor believes you should be cared for by a different kind of specialist on a regular basis. If you seem to have a serious psychiatric problem, your doctor may recommend a psychiatrist for your care.

If you have not been completely truthful with your doctor, your doctor may no longer be willing to care for you and tell you to seek care from another physician. If you do not seek care elsewhere, then your doctor may refuse to see you again. Your doctor will put this recommendation in writing as part of your record.

Am I a difficult patient?

If you cannot find a doctor you can get along with, you must ask yourself why. Are you demanding beyond what a doctor can do? Are you angry with the world and yourself? Are you a hypochondriac? Could you have a personality disorder? Do you enjoy being sick? J. E. Groves and E. V. Beresin wrote about patients with personality disorders that keep them from recognizing their problems in "Difficult Patients, Difficult Families." Such patients may be angry, envious and unable to control themselves or to tolerate uncertainty; have grandiose ideas; exhibit outrageous or unfair behavior; or show signs of shyness, seductiveness, rigidity or suspiciousness. These traits are made worse by serious illness and by the need for ICU care. Some patients are problems for even the best of doctors but will accept reasonable explanations and recommendations, followed by a statement such as: "This is all we know and/or this is all we can do." If patients continue asking unending and perhaps unrelated questions, it may be time to ask them to return for another visit when they may have learned more about their problems or even to ask them to consider going to another physician.

How do I know if I am a hypochondriac?

Webster's dictionary describes hypochondria as a mental disorder in which one is tormented by anxiety about one's health and by belief in imaginary ailments. The Greeks, in the 4th century BC, used the term for symptoms such as indigestion, flatulence and melancholy. In women, it was called hysteria. Notable hypochondriacs have included Hans Christian Andersen, Marcel Proust, Leo Tolstoy and Woody Allen; others with obsessions about their health have included Beethoven, Voltaire, Caruso, and John Adams, who predicted his death at age

35 only to live on to age 90. There is no harm in being a bit of a hypochondriac but if it controls your life then you need help from a counselor. Cognitive behavior therapy has now helped hypochondriasis in a controlled trial.

What is Munchausen's Syndrome?

In this severe personality disorder, patients create fictitious illnesses to get treatment and repeated operations, sometimes showing signs of serious illness. The disease is named after Baron Karl Friedrich Hieronymus von Münchausen, an eighteenth century soldier and notorious fabricator who wrote incredible tales of adventure.

I have seen Munchausen's Syndrome patients in emergency rooms complaining of nausea, cramps and abdominal distention. If they have had previous abdominal operations, we would suspect partial small intestinal obstruction and consider another operation. This is exactly what they wish. Sometimes the diagnosis of this syndrome is made because the symptoms are unusual and inexplicable. Gordon recently described a patient who altered her computer pathology reports from previous operations in order to try to convince him to do more surgery. Sanders described a patient who faked seizures and put feces in her I.V. to produce a high temperature. The patient denied having done so and disappeared, leaving behind a fake address and phone number. Munchausen's Syndrome is a strange illness.

8.   Should doctors ever admit they don't know?

Does your doctor seem to know everything? Is he confident and never uncertain? Has he never said, "I don't know?" Is that realistic?

No doctor knows everything. Doctors strive to stay well informed but information on the medical front is increasing exponentially. Your doctor may think you will lose confidence if he says "I just don't know." I believe a doctor should be able to say "I don't know, but we will try to find out" or "Only time will tell." Doctors cannot predict your future with certainty but can give accurate warnings of certain potentially fatal problems. I recently conferred with a patient with cirrhosis of the liver which led to bleeding into the stomach from dilated veins in the esophagus (esophageal varices). I indicated to this patient that if he took one more alcoholic drink, it would lead to another and another and he would be dead in three to six months or fewer from bleeding and liver failure. How could I predict this? My knowledge came from the medical literature on many such patients. The patient stopped drinking and now, two years later, is better.

Predictions about cancer are more uncertain. There is much that we do not know about cancer, and every cancer patient is different. Frequently I observed a problem that I had never seen before and so turned to colleagues in other specialties who could help me. Doctors try to be certain about health, diseases and abnormalities, because the scientific model is to demonstrate or prove certainty. We are uncomfortable with uncertainty because it makes treatment difficult or questionable but I am impressed by how little we know rather than how much we know.

A little humility goes a long way. Do you expect your doctor to know everything? The basic causes of many diseases are not known—arteriosclerosis and cancer among others. Goldstein, Director of the Chronic Fatigue Syndrome Institute, describes commonly misdiagnosed ailments; chest pain, fatigue (chronic fatigue syndrome), headache, impotence, sore throat.

Could my doctor be wrong?

Hopefully, that rarely happens. No doctor is always right, however. Some diseases and human ailments defy an accurate diagnosis for years in spite of the best science and tests available. This is particularly true of vague ailments of fatigue or strange aches and pains. Sometimes a disease begins with mild, non-specific symptoms. Only later as the disease progresses can we make an accurate diagnosis. If your doctor cannot determine what is bothering you or is not treating you to your satisfaction, get another opinion.

I saw this ad or news story about a new treatment. How come my doctor doesn't know about it?

Advertising prescription drugs in the lay press should not be allowed. Advertisements, news articles and television news report so many findings about health that no one can keep up with all of them. Such findings may not be proven. They may not be possible. They may be premature. A self-appointed authority or a company may try to sell a product with no proven benefit. A recent advertisement in *USA Today* quoted "the world's most renowned vitamin researcher." I have never heard of him. Did he appoint himself as the "world's most renowned?" If your doctor doesn't know about certain health products, it may be that they are not worthwhile. (Please read Chapter 10, 11, 42, 66).

GERIATRICS—AGING

9.   I'm getting older. Should I see a specialist for old folks?

The answer to your question is—not necessarily. Your own doctor may be capable of taking care of you. Remember, your doctor is getting older also. The specialty of caring for the elderly is called geriatrics or gerontology and the practitioners are geriatricians or gerontologists. There are not very many of them now. Those with special training or interest in the elderly are primarily in medical schools in a geriatric division of internal medicine.

The best definition of geriatrics I have seen is by Mary E. Tinetti, M.D., Chief, Section of Geriatrics, Yale Medical School. In the Yale Letter of Aging, she writes:

> "If an 80-year-old man tells his cardiologist that he has been having chest pain, the cardiologist will attempt to diagnose the cause of the pain, then prescribe the appropriate treatments. Before deciding how to pursue the cause of the chest pain, the geriatrician will consider the man's other health problems, his general health, diet, exercise, risk factors, his past history of illness and his living circumstances. These may have a relationship to his chest pain."

She goes on:

> "Older adults often have multiple chronic diseases and experience difficulty with one or more activities of daily life. Rather than working alone, therefore, as do most other physicians, geriatricians often use an interdisciplinary approach, working with a coordinated team of nurses, social workers, physical therapists, occupational therapists, and others."

A geriatrician could help you deal with multiple prescriptions, memory difficulties, Alzheimer's disease and early dementia, and could provide a home safety evaluation. To find a geriatrician call the Geriatric Society at 1-800-247-4774 or log on to: *www.americangeriatrics.org.*

Is there anything I can do about aging?

Aging is the natural process of growing older and is not a disease. We can promote healthy aging, decrease its impact and prevent some diseases of the elderly but be careful of anti-aging recommendations in some books, journals, and reports. Ask if they have scientific evidence for their claims or if they are placebos.

Here are six legitimate, sensible recommendations for enjoying a longer, happier and healthier life, from Andrew Weil: 1) keep moving; 2) cover your bases—alcohol—low intake; 3) follow a good, varied diet of fruits and vegetables; 4) keep an active mind; 5) connect with others; 6) cultivate optimism to increase health span as well as life span.

Research on aging now has a higher priority. The National Institute on Aging at the NIH recently gave grants to four universities for research into the basic biological problems of aging. The Ellison Medical Foundation supports basic biological and biomedical research on aging. One recent study turned on the properties of cholesterols, as reported in the Journal of the American Medical Association. The study found that individuals with exceptional longevity, and their children, have larger particles of HDL, or high-density lipoprotein, than LDL, or low-density lipoprotein, with concomitant lesser risk of high blood pressure, heart disease and the metabolic syndrome.

An excellent source of information is the Yale Letter on Aging, from Yale Medicine Publications, P.O. Box 7612, New Haven, CT 06519-0612, or http://info.med.yale.edu/ymm. The writers take up the subject of falls in the elderly and the related problem of osteoporosis. They discuss ways to keep older patients healthy while in the hospital, noting situations where patients may choose the security of the hospital rather than the comforts of home, especially if home care could be a drain on the family. At the Yale New Haven Hospital, teams in the Elderlife program help elderly hospital patients stay healthy, partly through ambulation and other activities to keep them moving.

Setting Priorities for Retirement Years (SPRY), a non-profit foundation in Washington, D.C., is creating a guide to websites with health information for the elderly. Their website is *http://www.spry.org*. The American Association of Retired Persons (AARP) provides information for seniors on public housing, housing for the elderly, Medicaid, Medicare, free meals, food stamps, Social Security, supplemental security income and senior community service employment. The AARP health plan allows subscribers to call nurses for information about any health problem.

A recent Harvard Health Letter discusses prevention and treatment of osteoporosis. Adequate consumption of calcium is important. Adults aged 19 to 50 need 1000 mg of calcium daily, the amount found in about three cups of milk or yogurt. Those 51 and older should aim for 1200 mg of calcium a day through a combination of diet and calcium supplements. Some advise Vitamin D supplements as well.

Alzheimer's disease is a concern of people who are getting older, as is age-related memory loss unconnected with Alzheimer's disease. Early diagnosis and treatment of Alzheimer's disease may help, as reviewed by Cullum and Rosenberg. Early Alzheimer's disease is associated with serious difficulty with recent memory, difficulty carrying out daily tasks and impaired social performance. Another disease of the elderly is Parkinson's, now treatable with medications, an operation or stem cell transplants. Gene therapy is being studied in animals for possible treatment of this disease. For more information see the Harvard Health Letter Vol. 23, June 1999 or contact the National Institute of Neurological Disorders Box 5801, Bethesda, MD 20824, 1-800-352-9424, www.ninds.parkinson.org or the National Parkinson Foundation, Inc., 1501 NW 9th Ave., Miami, FL, 33136-1494, 1-800-337-4545, *www.parkinson.org*. Depression is common in older people but may go unrecognized. Help is available. Suicide threats are an emergency.

Guzmararian, et al found that elderly patients "may not have the literacy skills needed to function in the health care environment". They may not make use of necessary medical care and services, which leads to increased emergency ward use, delay in care with harmful results and less preventive care. The elderly also face problems with medication: overuse, addiction, inappropriate use and inadequate use. The high cost of drugs can discourage some elderly patients from getting prescriptions filled or taking medicines regularly. Review all your medications with your doctor and know what the important ones are.

Sleep may be a problem for the elderly. If so, avoid caffeine in the afternoon and evening, avoid nicotine altogether, don't drink alcohol late at night, don't exercise in the evening, avoid naps in the afternoon, keep the bedroom dark, quiet and not too warm. Do not watch TV in bed.

Few obese people reach 80 years and beyond. Most elderly people are slim and trim. Obesity is associated with diabetes, hypertension, inactivity, and inability to exercise. Animal studies show that decreasing food intake, or caloric deprivation, increases lifespan.

How long can people live? What is the Methuselah factor? Are there pills to help you live longer?

Perhaps biblical times were free of disease or pestilence, allowing the Old Testament figure Methuselah to live 969 years, begetting children up until the end, and Adam to live 930 years. As for us, we have just reached an average life expectancy of 73 years for men and 79 for women. There is talk now about great increases in life expectancy due to better self discipline in maintaining health and scientific control of disease. There are many who seek to live longer and we read now about longevity doctors and how to age in reverse by so-called age protectors. Many scientists believe the biological upper limit of life span to be 120 to 125 years, but not all would accept that limit. In the meanwhile, more people are living to be 90 and 100 or more. The U.S. Census Bureau has predicted that, by 2050, there will be over 834,000 centenarians in this country, up from 64658 as of August 1, 2004.

In certain parts of the world, more people live to be over 100, like males on the island of Sardinia; it is not known if this is due to genetics, diet, climate or red wine. How long will you live? Perls and Silver developed a longevity quiz to help you calculate your estimated life expectancy in *Modern Maturity* for November-December 1999, published by the AARP.

"People who make it past 85 are a hearty group," said Suzman. The medical journal Lancet wrote, "The older you get, the healthier you have been." Perls said, "The genetically weak die off." Warshofsky has described the Methuselah factor as a combination of genetics, moderation, exercise and a positive attitude boosted by natural selection. Home-based programs can reduce the progression of functional decline in physically frail elderly people who live at home. Some people, however, do not want to live a great deal longer and express such wishes in a living will. No one has found the secret of aging without getting old.

A large increase in the number of older people creates concern about Medicare support, the Social Security system, a shortage of geriatricians, where the elderly will live and who will care for them. Some suggest the retirement age be increased to 70.

Social ties reduce cognitive decline in older people. Brisk walking also helps. The Harvard Health Letter advises, "Call up some friends and go for a stroll." After the mid to late 80s, the risk of fatal heart disease and stroke decrease. We all know 80-year-olds who seem much younger. There is chronologic age and then there is biologic age, the age we look and feel and act.

No one knows if gene or hormone therapy will contribute to longevity and well being. However, the possibility exists that the fundamental aging process is under genetic control and could be modulated, counteracting destructive processes we have within us. Oxygen is needed to live but is also dangerous; oxygen free radicals slowly kill us. A gene may inhibit the formation of oxygen free radicals. Body cells have a limited life. After about 50 cell divisions, body cells die in a process controlled by the shortening of the ends of DNA chains, or telomeres. An enzyme telomorase will reverse the process, lengthening telomeres.

According to Pope, "Mainstream scientists agree that aging is not a "disease" that can be "cured" by antioxidant pills, hormone shots, enema regimens or other so called anti-aging substances. Fifty-one top scientists who study aging said: "There are no lifestyle changes, surgical procedures, vitamins, anti-oxidants, hormones or techniques of genetic engineering today that influence the processes of aging. I urge you to avoid buying or using products or other interventions which claim they will slow, stop or reverse aging." Genotology, or anti-aging, is a trillion dollar business. Makers of most anti-aging supplements are 21st century "snake oil salesmen". These supplements include: Herbal Outlook. Liverite, Longevity Signal Formula, St. John's Wort, Kava Kava and Colloidal Silver, Damage Control Master Formula and the Anti-Aging Daily Premium Pax. The American Academy of Anti-aging promotes anti-aging medicines and programs. Where is their evidence? Other claims lacking evidence include Sinatra's special anti-aging edition—"Feel 50 Again;" Mother Nature's Age Erasers in *Prevention Magazine*, "Age-Defying Secrets" from the Editors of *Bottom Line* written by "doctors" and Anti-Aging Prescriptions from the Green Pharmacy. For more legitimate information go to *www.quackwatch.com*; *www.cspinct.org*; *www.ftc.gov*; and *www.fda.gov*. Makers of some products have been fined by the FDA for false or misleading claims.

Is memory loss common with aging? Do medicines help?

Memory loss, or cognitive decline, is common with aging but in itself is not Alzheimer's disease. The cause does not seem to be loss of brain cells but may involve damage to an enzyme receptor and loss of water in the brain, or brain shrinkage. Memory naturally begins a gradual decline sometime in the 50s. Begley lists risk factors for cognitive decline as: the apo4 genes for Alzheimer's disease, high blood pressure, diabetes, heart disease, smoking, alcohol abuse, drugs, low educational level, lack of exercise and social interaction, high stress levels and environmental exposure to neurotoxins.

The Harvard Health Letter describes ways to decrease memory loss and perhaps protect against dementia. They include doing mental exercises, meeting friends, doing different things, decreasing stress, sleeping better, exercising and controlling hypertension. Emmett reports on studies by Fratiglioni et al. indicating that a good network of social interactions helps preserve memory. Living alone is not a problem so long as one has social life. Being alone all the time is bad. Social isolation is associated with cognitive decline, perhaps dementia and Alzheimer's disease. Suzman, cited by Emmett, warns about a possible "chicken and egg" problem. Social isolation could be the first sign of cognitive decline and dementia rather than its cause.

The Institute for the Study of Aging (ISOA) *www.ilcusa.org/publicaitons/ISOA.pdf* and the International Longevity Center USA (ICL-USA) *www.aging-institute-org,* issued a joint report called Achieving and Maintaining Cognitive Vitality with Aging. Copies are available from their web sites. They urge the elderly to use it or lose it by lifelong learning, exercise, daily activities, stress reduction, sleep, emotional stability and adequate nutrition. They list risks for cognitive decline— vascular diseases, smoking, alcohol and lack of exercise and social interaction.

The Harvard Letter points out that there is no memory pill. Schardt reviews so-called memory pills in the Nutrition Action Health Letter and says "don't waste your money" on "Focus Factor," "Senior Moment" (docosahexanoic acid from algae), "Cognita, and "Vinpocetine." He finds little evidence to support the claims for "Cerebroplex." "Gingko biloba" has been touted as a memory enhancer but the evidence is it does not improve memory. The NIH is now carrying out a careful trial. Schardt describes it as a "wallet lightener" as he does phosphatidylserine, a component of the membrane of nerve cells marketed as "Brain Gum," "Brain Sustain" and "Think Young." "Mind-Max," which costs $90/month, may have some benefit. Estrogens may help some women. Vitamin E, an antioxidant does not aid memory.

Alzheimer's disease produces brain injury (death of brain cells or neurons) by three insults: inflammation, oxidative injury and deposit of clumps in the brain of the small protein beta-amyloid (B-amyloid). The Harvard Health Letter lists warning signs as memory loss: forgetting all the time, forgetting how to cook a favorite meal or how to use an appliance, forgetting simple words, getting lost on your own street, forgetting where you are and how you got there; using vague expressions; bundling up when it's hot outside or vice-versa, getting hopelessly lost in familiar ideas; putting things in strange places; going from calm to tears to anger for no reason; becoming fearful, confused, suspicious, overly dependent, or extremely passive; watching television for hours; and sleeping far more than usual. Diagnosis may be difficult at first but symptoms progress rapidly, within six months. The four Alzheimer genes account for only one-quarter of Alzheimer's patients. An experienced clinician can make the diagnosis with about 95% accuracy. A positron emission tomography (PET) scan with a special dye may reveal the disease before symptoms develop.

Emphasis in research and clinical studies has been on trying to slow down the development and progression of the disease. A healthy lifestyle may reduce the risk of developing the disease. This means no smoking, regular exercise, healthy body weight, low cholesterol and blood pressure, a low fat diet with lots of fruits and vegetables, fish one to two times a week, an active social life and use of your mind. Some evidence, not well established in clinical trials, indicates that the following *may* help in putting the disease on hold:

- eating lots of folate and vitamins B_6 and B_{12} in spinach and other leafy green vegetables
- exercising
- stimulating your brain
- taking Ibuprofen—a nonsteroidal anti-inflammatory drug (NSAID)
- taking statins—to lower cholesterol
- taking anti-oxidant vitamin C.

Experimental treatments are being studied. Some with mild cognitive impairment may not go on to Alzheimer's disease.

Weil recommends ten steps to a better memory—

1) give your mind a workout
2) take antioxidants (vitamins C), beta-carotene and selenium—there is some positive evidence
3) take supplemental B vitamins (can't hurt)
4) lower your blood pressure, if high
5) check your medications
6) load up on brain food—cold-water fish, flaxseed (omega-3 fatty acids)
7) keep moving
8) don't skimp on sleep
9) decrease stress
10) pay attention

Rosenfield believes that the risk of Alzheimer's disease can be reduced by exercise, a low fat diet, antioxidants, anti-inflammatory drugs, hormones, gingko biloba and Vitamin E. A new drug for Alzheimer's disease has been approved by the FDA with the trade name Exelon, and the generic name rivastigmine tartrate. It is a brain selective cholinesterase inhibitor which has been found to benefit all three symptom areas: activities of daily life, such as eating and dressing, global functioning including behavior and cognition-thinking and speaking. For more information or help contact The Alzheimer's Association at 1-800-272-3900, *www.alz.org* and the Alzheimer's Disease Education and Referral Center (ADEAR) 1-800-438-4380. *www.alzheimers.org.*

Schardt describes brain boosters as physical activity and mental stimulation and brain busters as alcoholism, depression, diabetes, heart disease, heart surgery, hypertension, sleep apnea and stress.

What is osteoporosis?

Osteoporosis is thinning of the substance of bones by a decrease in mineral density and content, leaving them more porous and brittle with structural weakness and more apt to crack or break. It is the acceleration of the normal changes that occur with age. There are no symptoms until a fracture occurs. Most common are compression fractures of the spine which makes a person shorter and bent forward. Next are fractures of the hip and wrist. Osteoporosis is an under-diagnosed disease and so serious a problem that the NIH has developed a panel on its prevention, diagnosis and therapy. It is more common in women (80%), particularly during and after menopause due to a decrease in production of estrogen which helps maintain bone mass. Risk factors include age (bone lost more quickly than the body forms it); body type (small bodies and so less bone); heredity; race (more common among Asians and whites); estrogen loss (menopause or removal of ovaries); low calcium and vitamin D levels; inactivity; smoking; heavy alcohol consumption; certain medicines; GI surgery and some medical conditions (cancer, anorexia, liver disease, hyperparathyroidism). Millions are affected by osteoporosis.

For prevention, if you are not menopausal: get enough calcium and vitamin D, do weight bearing exercises, don't smoke, and see your doctor if you take steroids, antiepilepsy or thyroid drugs, anti-androgens, heparin, cholestyramine, antacids containing aluminum, methotrexate and cyclosporine. These all erode bone.

If you are menopausal, get a bone density test, consider hormone replacement (17B-estradiol has helped) therapy, be sure of adequate calcium and vitamin D intake and increase your exercise.

If you are over 65: increase your calcium intake to 1500 mg a day and 400-800 IU of vitamin D; exercise; consider medications; get a bone density test.

The U.S. Preventive Services Task Force now recommends routine osteoporosis screening by bone density tests for all women over age 65 and then every 5 years. Medicare will cover this if ordered by a doctor. Calcium in common foods is listed in the Nutrition Action Healthletter Jan/Feb 2002, as is the vitamin D in foods but the easiest solution is to take an ordinary multivitamin with 400 IU of vitamin D or, if you are over age 70, 600 IU.

Several treatments now available for osteoporosis include biphosphonates, (Fosamax—alendronate, Actonel—risedronate), calcitonin (Miacalcin—a synthetic calcitonin), raloxifene (Evista—a selective estrogen receptor modulator—SERMS), estrogen replacement therapy (ERT-HRT) and Forteo (teriparatide), a natural bone building hormone. Zoledronic (Zometa) acid, taken once yearly by IV infusion, may be as good as daily oral medications. More studies are needed to see if it prevents fractures. The long term intake of a diet high in vitamin A (retinol) may promote development of osteoporotic hip fractures in women. The best source of vitamin A is food, not supplements.

I know hip fractures are common in older people. Are there ways to prevent these?

Hip fractures are a major problem for the elderly. The causes are falls and osteoporosis. The Harvard Health Letter and the Yale Letter on Aging provide the following suggestions for preventing falls in the home:

1. Keep your home, particularly stairwells, adequately lighted.
2. Install light switches at the top and bottom of the stairs and near every doorway.
3. Put night lights in hallways, bathrooms and bedrooms.
4. Keep non-skid mats in the bathtub, shower and near the laundry, sink, or any areas that may get wet.
5. Install grab bars in the bathtub or shower area.
6. Wear sturdy shoes with non-slip soles in the house.
7. Don't keep floors highly polished, and remove all scatter rugs.
8. Keep electrical and extension cords away from traveled areas.
9. Keep your home free from clutter.
10. Install handrails on all stairways.
11. Keep active—exercise.
12. Go slowly and do not carry things up and down stairs.
13. Have your hearing, balance and gait checked. If you are unsteady, use a cane or walker.

Six additional tips are:

1. Take a walk.
2. Lower your stroke risk by diet and blood pressure control.
3. Watch out for osteoporosis.
4. Keep your vitamin D intake high.
5. Fall-proof your home.
6. Keep your calcium intake high.

A daily exercise program can improve your balance. Stand and lean your back against a wall and slowly walk your feet out while allowing yourself to slide down the wall, then walk back up to standing (to strengthen thigh muscles); brace yourself on a chair and raise yourself on your toes, up and down (for calf muscles); and finally take a walk. Unsteadiness or dizziness is the third most common problem for the elderly, after headache and low back pain. Usually you can correct it. Lightheadedness may occur if you get out of bed too fast; take a moment to sit. Near-fainting can be helped by sitting or lying down. Our body's gyroscope is in our inner ear, the vestibular apparatus, and close to the cochlea for hearing. Thus, problems with balance and hearing go together, with ringing or buzzing called tinnitus. Problems with the vestibular apparatus may cause three conditions: 1) Meniere's disease—a common cause of vertigo, or spinning dizziness; 2) vestibular neuronitis, which produces vertigo that may last for days to months; and 3) BPPV (a mouthful) benign, paroxysmal positional vertigo—brief, intermittent dizziness brought on by a change in head position. These can all be diagnosed and treated by a doctor. Tinnitus is a more difficult problem to treat. In objective tinnitus produced by various diseases, you can hear actual sounds. In subjective tinnitus, the ringing may be due to the condition of the ears and nerves, to infection or to certain drugs.

Several studies show that wearing an impact-absorbing hip protector will greatly decrease the incidence of hip fractures. These should be required in nursing homes and recommended for many others, particularly if they are unsteady. The problem is getting people to use them.

In Chapter 28, I describe the benefits of an estrogen receptor modulator drug, Raloxifene, in increasing bone density and preventing vertebral fractures in postmenopausal women with osteoporosis. Perhaps it will also decrease the incidence of hip fractures.

Evidence is accumulating now that the statin drugs, developed to decrease cholesterol, also have a protective effect against fractures. The statin drugs may build bone in postmenopausal women. This is true for simvastatin, perhaps for lovastatin and flurastatin, but not necessarily for pravastatin. So far, the evidence is based on observational studies. Randomized prospective trials are needed to prove this.

How long should I drive a car?

Driving an automobile is a symbol of independence and a link with the rest of the world but may be hazardous for the elderly. Starting at age 70, the number of accidents per vehicle-mile-traveled climbs and climbs fast and is very much higher at age 80. Some states require a road test after age 75. The challenge is balancing the need for highway safety and the need for automobility. For the elderly dementia poses one danger as does the sleepiness of Parkinson's disease patients. The Harvard Health Letter lists safe driving tips—

- Maintain a 3-second "cushion" between you and the car in front of you to reduce risk of a rear-end collision. At traffic lights or stop signs, stay far enough behind so you can see the rear tires of the car ahead of you.
- Before driving at night, give your eyes a few minutes to adjust to the dark. Many older people do not drive at night because they can't see as well then. Ask a friend to pick you up.
- Use another route if the minimum speed on the highway feels too fast.
- Clean headlights, taillights, and turn signals. Dirty headlights can be 70% less bright than clean ones.
- Don't stare straight ahead for long periods when driving. Looking to the side every now and then reduces fatigue.
- Be careful of left turns. Improper left turns is one of the most common traffic violations committed by drivers age 55 and over.
- Get a hearing aid. We drive more with our ears than many people realize. Hearing sirens, horns, and other cars is important for safe driving.
- Ask a doctor for help if you're caring for someone who you think shouldn't be driving. A gentle word from a physician can be worth a thousand warnings from a son, daughter or spouse.
- Get a driving assessment. Hospitals and clinics have confidential programs that measure reaction time and other attributes necessary for safe driving. In the Boston area, such testing costs about $150.
- Know when to quit. A car may give you independence and mobility, but if you can't drive safely, it could end your independence and mobility prematurely.

Richard, writing in the Yale Letter on Aging, describes research on how to predict driving risk in the elderly. Here are some signs of increased risk:

Incorrect signaling	Increased agitation or irritation when driving
Trouble navigating turns.	Parking inappropriately
Moving into a wrong lane	Getting lost in familiar places.
Confusion at exits	Near misses
Driving at inappropriate speeds	Ticketed moving violations or warnings.
Delayed responses to unexpected situations	Car accident.
Not anticipating dangerous situations	Confusing the brake and gas pedals
Scrapes or dents on car, garage or mailbox	

TESTS AND TREATMENT

10. Are diagnosis and cure overemphasized by some doctors?

Medical students, residents and practicing physicians are trained to try to make an exact diagnosis of what is bothering you. They listen to what you tell them, they ask questions about your health and they examine you. This allows them to think about the possibilities. Do you have an acute problem such as appendicitis or a chronic problem such as a form of arthritis. Although your doctor may suspect a particular illness, confirmation almost always require some form of laboratory test. For appendicitis, a white blood cell count would be done, a urinalysis to be sure you do not have a urinary tract infection and, for a woman, a pelvic examination to determine whether the pain might be due to a problem with an ovary, a fallopian tube or the uterus. If your health problem is not acute, then other tests or studies might be necessary: x-rays, blood studies, special examinations of your body, and other tests (Chapter 11). The purpose is to make a diagnosis if possible but, even more important, to help you and your doctor learn about any serious medical problems such as a malignant tumor in your brain, your chest, or your abdomen, or heart disease, or one of many other problems. As you may know, a negative test is good news because it means you don't have that disease. Remember also that on occasion a test may be incorrectly positive or negative, a false positive or negative test. It should be repeated.

What if all of tests are negative or normal? Perhaps there is no organic cause for your symptoms. You could have symptoms due to stress or anxiety (functional problems) which should be treated. You also may be developing a disease which is not yet evident. For example, if you have abnormal function of your gall bladder, your initial symptoms of pain below your rib cage on the right side may be non-specific. Studies initially may not show stones in your gall bladder. Stones may only appear later. The question then is how many tests to do if a disease is not yet evident.

Why didn't my doctor find this?

If your doctor sees you shortly after you develop a pain, an ache, or a symptom he may not find the cause of the problem initially. If you continue to have symptoms and the disease develops further, then the cause may be obvious. If your doctor refers you to a specialist later, the specialist may then be able to make the diagnosis. You may wonder why your doctor did not find the cause of the problem. The reason may be that your doctor saw you early in the disease, whereas the specialist saw you when the trouble was more obvious. I was such a specialist for many years, and I was always careful to recognize that when I saw you, your disease had advanced and the tests then were positive. Primary-care doctors may not have the advantage of watching your disease develop further. It is easy to make a diagnosis when the disease becomes obvious.

Diagnosis of some ailments is very difficult even in later stages of the disease. Symptoms may be nonspecific aches and pains that come and go, here and there. This is particularly true with problems related to your joints, or connective tissue diseases like arthritis, or problems related to your nervous system, like multiple sclerosis, lupus erythematosis, auto-immune diseases (Crohn's disease, rhematoid arthritis), early Alzheimer's disease and many others. Gradually, more and more specific tests have been developed for such diseases. Some doctors try to put labels on everything, labels that may later turn out to be wrong. Psychiatrists, for example, may label someone a manic-depressive because they have mood swings. In fact, some months or even years may go by before an exact label is found. This is frustrating for you because you have symptoms which are real and bother you. There may be no good treatment for your symptoms, which is also frustrating.

What about cure?

For some problems you can be cured permanently. Removal of an inflamed appendix or of a gall bladder with stones will bring those problems to an end. With other problems it may not be so.

Dr. Ellen Fox has written about the predominance of the curative model among doctors. She describes this as an emphasis on diagnosis and then cure without as much consideration of your feelings and symptoms other than for leading to a diagnosis. Fox indicates: "in the curative model if your disease cannot be identified or stopped or slowed you could be labeled as untreatable" or "beyond help" or, even worse, incurable.

The other model of care is called the palliative model in which the emphasis is on treatment—relief of symptoms. The World Health Organization (WHO) describes palliative care "as active total care of you as a person if your disease cannot be diagnosed accurately, or if you are not responsive to curative treatment." Fox states: "the emphasis of palliative care is on comprehensive care of the whole patient, including psychological, social, cultural, ethical and spiritual concerns."

A blending of the two models is best for you. If you have a broken arm, you would like it fixed, cured. You don't need an in-depth relationship with the orthopedic surgeon who does the job. If, however, you develop a chronic disease of your joints, like rheumatoid arthritis, you need a caring primary physician and/or rheumatologist who understands you and knows the latest information and treatment for the disease. Rheumatoid arthritis cannot be cured but can be treated to relieve symptoms. If you require admission to a hospital, the emphasis there will be on cure, to help you return home in a healthy state. In your doctor's office, palliation, or relief of symptoms, should predominate.

Many ailments will subside or go away by themselves if you do not develop complications. There may be no cure, but relief of symptoms may be enough for the common cold, the flu, gastroenteritis, muscle and joint strain or sprain, headache and other problems. Only if these symptoms persist is further diagnostic study recommended. How long to wait? There is no exact answer. If you have a persistent cough, a specific kind of a pain, headache or other abnormalities for a week, see your doctor.

Why do doctors order all those tests? Don't they overdo it?

Perhaps, on occasion, they do overdo it. However, many tests may be necessary to:

1) be sure you do not have a dangerous or life-threatening condition (cancer, for example);
2) find the cause of your problem and treat appropriately;
3) be sure that a fracture or other injury is not missed;
4) suggest premalignant changes or an early cancer such as a Papanicolaou (Pap) smear of the cervix, a mammogram to rule out breast cancer, a prostate specific antigen (PSA) blood test to rule out prostate cancer and periodic chest x-rays for smokers or former smokers.

It is often a balance between too many tests and not enough or not the correct test(s). Remember that you can ask your doctor why he is recommending certain tests and on what basis. Routine testing, as part of a periodic health checkup, may not be worthwhile.

Early detection of disease.

An annual examination.

11. Does early detection of disease really make a difference?

For many diseases, early detection provides a better opportunity for treatment and even cure. Many diseases, if treated early, will not produce complications. For example, symptoms of narrowing of a carotid artery in the neck where the blood goes to the brain should be treated promptly, before the patient develops a stroke and paralysis. Such symptoms are brief or transient sudden loss of vision in one eye, an episode of dizziness that comes and goes or transient weakness on one side of the body, called transient ischemic attacks (TIAs). Severe pain in the lower legs during exercise should be treated before there is a threat of gangrene.

A severe headache may suggest a brain tumor or enlargement of a blood vessel, or aneurysm, which requires treatment. Diabetes should be discovered and treated before complications develop. Hypertension may lead to a stroke, unless found and treated. Treatment of these and many other problems can be quite successful. In cancer, an early diagnosis before the tumor has spread to lymph nodes or other organs allows better treatment and a better long-term result. Early diagnosis of Alzheimer's disease allows treatment to slow progression of the disease. The answer is yes: Early detection of disease makes a great deal of difference for you and your health.

Why should I have treatment for a disease if it does not bother me?

Many diseases and health problems may not produce symptoms until disaster strikes. For example, high blood pressure, or hypertension, may not give you trouble until you have a stroke. Diabetes may go undetected until you have a complication such as a circulatory problem in your legs, eyes or kidneys. Pancreatic cancer is all too often a silent killer, showing symptoms of pain, nausea and jaundice only when it is too late. In a number of diseases early treatment will prevent later complications even though you have no symptoms present.

HOW OFTEN SHOULD I SEE MY DOCTOR? What is involved in an annual health checkup? Is it important?

According to old adage, you should see your doctor once a year even if you feel well. The annual physical examination or checkup has become part of our culture, and rightly so. It is important for your doctor to get your history at least once a year, your description of how you feel and of any changes in your health and of anything that bothers you. Your doctor should do a systems review, a thorough review of all systems of your body with questions asked about details of each. (Table I) It is the best chance for early detection of disease. You must tell your doctor about all aspects of your health. Allergies could lead to a fatal reaction if no one knows about them; if you have severe allergies, I recommend that you wear an armband, bracelet or necklace containing that information. You must tell your doctor about diseases that run in your family; a family history of malignant hyperthermia, or extremely high temperature, with anesthesia could be fatal for you if your doctor does not know about it.

The physical examination will help your doctor detect problems like hypertension, heart murmurs, abnormal heart beats, large lymph nodes, a nodule or mass in the breast, an enlargement of an organ in the abdomen or absence of pulses in the legs (atherosclerosis). It is important for your doctor to inspect the skin for possible pre-cancerous tumors or melanomas, to feel for lymph nodes in the neck, arm pits and groins, to check pulses in the feet and neck and to feel the abdomen for the size of the liver, spleen and abdominal aorta, the major blood vessel that goes from your heart to your legs.

What should be done in a good physical exam?

While you are talking, a good doctor will observe you to determine whether you look sick, act sick, are gaunt or look tired; to note the color of your skin and the whites of your eyes, to make sure that they are truly white; and to see if you are well-kept or sloppily dressed, if your hair is combed and even if you wear makeup. On return visits good doctors learn to observe the changes in your appearance that may indicate a change in your health.

After reviewing your problems and observing you, your doctor will ask you to disrobe. Men disrobe to their underwear if their doctor is male. Women should disrobe privately and put on an examination gown. You may ask for a nurse's help. The doctor will come back into the room and begin. A female nurse should always be present when a male doctor is examining a woman. No visitors or family members should be in the room. Pharmaceutical or other business representatives may wish to be present. Do not allow this.

Your blood pressure may have been measured earlier by a nurse or aide. Your doctor will take it again. The examination starts at the top: your head felt for lumps and bumps; your ear canals viewed with an otoscope; the inside of your eyes, the retinas and lenses, seen with an ophthalmoscope. Your tongue and mouth are viewed. Your neck is felt, or palpated, to check for enlarged lymph nodes or glands. A stethoscope over the arteries in your neck is used to check for bruits, or whooshing noises, that may indicate narrowing of a carotid artery, which could lead to a stroke. The movement of your chest with breathing is observed. Your breath sounds are heard on the back of the chest. The axilla (under your arms) is felt for lymph nodes. You lie on your back and your heart sounds are listened to for problems of heart valves, heart rhythm and rate. A woman's breasts are examined to see if a mass can be felt. A man's breasts are also observed. Then a woman's chest is covered and the abdomen examined. The contour is observed. The area under the rib cage is felt for enlargement of the liver, on the right side; of the spleen, on the left side; and of the abdominal aorta in the middle. Also felt are other parts of the abdomen for tenderness or masses, the groins for lymph nodes and pulses and the feet for pulses, to see if the circulation is good. A man then stands so that his groins may be felt for bulges, or hernias, and bends over the table for a rectal exam, done with a gloved finger to feel for enlargement or nodules in the prostate gland and for rectal tumors.

For a woman a pelvic and rectal examination may not be done if she has a regular checkup with her gynecologist. If not, then the examination will be done with the patient lying supine and her legs up in what are called stirrups. The cervix is seen and a Papanicolaou (Pap) smear obtained. All patients are now given cards and equipment to obtain samples of stool for occult blood, small quantities of blood invisible to the naked eye. The presence of blood suggests the possibility of colon cancer and further study is needed.

The skin of the entire body is inspected for moles or nevi, basal cell or squamous carcinomas, and possible melanomas or malignant tumors. Moles, brown spots that are regular in shape, are generally harmless. Basal cell carcinomas, raised irregular nodules, are locally growing malignant tumors that usually do not spread, or metastasize, to other locations. Melanomas, irregular black and gray spots or brown spots with black areas, are very dangerous tumors that spread to lymph nodes and other organs. If you have freckles, red or blonde hair, sunburn easily and have had blistering sunburns, or if you have a family history of skin cancer, you are at increased risk for this disease.

A good physical examination will enable a doctor to address the following questions:

General appearance:	Tense or relaxed, sad, depressed, wasted, uncomfortable, in pain, appearing chronically ill, well developed (wd), well nourished (wn), in no acute distress (nad)? Evidence of weight loss? Any physical abnormalities noted in general appearance?
Vital signs:	Blood pressure, heart rate, pulse Are heart beats regular or not?
Breathing:	how often, difficult?
Head:	Feel for lumps or bumps

Ears:	Snap fingers to check hearing. Any drainage? An otoscope is used to look for wax, perforations or inflammation in the ear canals and ear drums.
Eyes:	Conjunctiva, color: not red (inflammation) or yellow (jaundice)
Pupils:	Size, regularity. Do they react, get smaller with light? Three Rs for pupils—round, regular, reactive Cataracts?
	Using an ophthalmoscope, the doctor looks inside the eyes and determines the appearance of the retina and retinal blood vessels for any signs of diabetes such as yellowish deposits, bleeding areas and dilated blood vessels. Measuring pressure in the eye to check for glaucoma is usually done by an ophthalomologist. Increased pressure is a warning.
Nose:	Drainage or not
Mouth:	Teeth, throat, jaw motion
Face and Neck:	Feel for masses, enlarged salivary glands below the mandible, lymph nodes in the neck, problems in the thyroid gland; listen with a stethoscope over the carotid arteries in the neck for a blowing sound or a bruit indicating arteriosclerosis and narrowing of the vessels which could lead to a stroke
Chest:	Observe configuration, size and shape: An expanded chest suggests emphysema Listen with a stethoscope to the lungs Check heart size by testing for dullness over the chest by thumping, or percussion. Listen to heart sounds for murmurs, rhythm, abnormal sounds
Breasts:	A woman has a breast exam lying down on her back with an arm relaxed over her forehead, relaxing the muscles under the breast. The breast tissue is palpated, nipples observed, and the arm pit (axilla) palpated for lymph nodes or masses.

Abdomen: Configuration is noted, whether distended or flat; palpation at the rib cages for liver and spleen size. The main abdominal blood vessel or aorta is felt for size. Enlargement indicates an aneurysm. The rest of the abdomen is felt for tenderness or masses, a stethoscope used to listen for bowel sounds

Extremities: Appearance, color, and range of motion are noted. Joints observed. Pulses felt in radial artery at the wrist, femoral arteries in the groin and arteries in the feet.

Rectal examination: In men, palpate to determine the size of the prostate gland and presence of nodules, rectal tumors. Note stool color. A sample may be put on paper to test for a slight amount of occult blood.

Pelvic examination: Observe the vagina and cervix, palpate the uterus and region of the tubes and ovaries. This may not be carried out by a primary care physician if a woman sees a gynecologist for periodic pelvic examinations and Pap smears.

What are reasonable screening tests for tumors and for other health problems?

The various screening tests available to detect disease are listed in Table II. Other screening would be considered only for specific purposes or problems and not done on a regular basis. Recommendations by the U.S. Preventive Services Task Force, the American College of Physicians, the American Cancer Society, and other groups, include the following:

Everyone over the age of 35 to 40 should have blood pressure checked at every doctor's office visit and at least once a year. Hypertension is a common abnormality, particularly in males, and can be treated adequately before it results in problems such as stroke or, contributes to arteriosclerosis, heart problems, and other matters. Total cholesterol, high density lipoprotein (HDL) (good cholesterol), low density lipoprotein (LDL) (bad cholesterol) should be measured at age 35 for men and 45 for women and repeated every five years. The National Heart Lung and Blood Institute recommends earlier routine testing: every five years for adults over 20 years of age.

Early treatment of diabetes is important to prevent complications, particularly of the vascular system, the kidneys, and the eyes. A simple dip test for sugar in the urine can indicate the possibility of diabetes.

Immunization should be kept up: a tetanus/diphtheria shot every 10 years, pneumococcal immunization at age 65, and a flu shot each fall, particularly for those over 65.

An annual chest x-ray is important for anyone who smokes or has smoked. Anyone over the age of 40 to 50 would benefit from a chest x-ray every two years.

Women should examine their breasts for lumps monthly, and, after age 40, should have a breast exam by a physician every year and a mammogram every one to two years. Given a family history of breast cancer, more frequent evaluation will help. After age 50, postmenopausal women should have a Pap smear every one to three years to check for malignant cells from the cervix, the mouth of the uterus. Cervical cancer can be detected early by this worthwhile screening test. After age 65, all women who have tested negative may not need it anymore. (Chapter 28—Women's Health)

After age 40, men should have a prostate digital exam every year. It is an open question as to how often men should have a blood test for Prostate Specific Antigen (PSA), a substance indicating the presence of a cancer of the prostate. This substance will appear before a physical examination can indicate the presence of the cancer within the gland. It also allows detection before the cancer spreads outside of the prostate gland into surrounding tissues or to bone. At the present time a positive or higher level of PSA should lead to a biopsy of the prostate by an urologist. If no tumor is found, the test should be repeated in the future. Tests that are more specific for cancer are available now, however. It is estimated that about 65% of men with an elevated PSA do not have cancer.

Observation of your skin, front and back, and mouth and throat for skin tumors and those of the mouth should be done by you frequently and by your doctor yearly. The National Foundation for Cancer Research as a Public Service provides recommendations for cancer detection in Table III. Information can be obtained from them by calling 1-800-321-CURE or by writing to the NFCR, 4600 East West Highway, Suite 525, Bethesda, MD 20814.

Many doctors limit annual or periodic examinations for people aged 65 and older since they are less likely to develop many problems faced by younger people, such as breast and cervical cancer. An older person who has never had skin cancers will very likely not get them. In older people, it is often enough to check appearance, weight, heart rate and blood pressure as well as to take a personal history, with questions like: How are you? Do you have any new symptoms? Is anything bothering you?

Screening for colorectal cancer should include a yearly stool test for blood. Colonoscopy is recommended as a routine screening for everyone over age 45, and then every 10 years if negative; Medicare will pay for this but many insurance programs will not pay for colonoscopy on such a routine basis. Colonoscopic detection of colorectal cancer is uncommon in persons under 45 years of age.

It is important to have a colonoscopy if any change occurs in your bowel movements, if any black (dried) or red (fresh) blood appears in the stool, for instance. People with a family history of colon cancer or a history of colon polyps should have colonoscopy on a regular basis.

All the screening tests present some pros and cons. The general downside to cancer screening is detection of problems that seem malignant but are not, which can lead to unnecessary treatment of a benign condition unless your doctors are very careful. Colonoscopy carries a very small risk of accidental perforation of the colon; and unavailability of the procedure could be another problem. Two other procedures might be done every five years in place of colonoscopy: sigmoidoscopy to detect early cancers in the rectum and lower sigmoid colon, and a barium enema, to detect later cancers. An x-ray scanning called virtual colonoscopy may be about as good as the colonoscopy itself. Evidence is still being evaluated.

Now scans have been recommended and advertised as general screening tests. Total body scans, or full body CTs, can screen for cancer, metastases, organ problems, etc.; electronic beam computed tomography (EBCT) screens for coronary artery disease. Screening without x-ray exposure includes ultrasound magnetic resonance imaging (MRI). The American College of Radiology and the American Cancer Society, however, do not believe there is sufficient evidence to recommend any of these for patients without symptoms.

A huge market now exists for home detection tests for cancer, HIV, diabetes, hypertension and other conditions. Urine tests for small bladder tumors may be available soon. The presence of C-reactive protein (CRP) in the blood may be a sign of heart disease risk; genetic changes in sputum may suggest airway cancer; and protein changes may indicate ovarian cancer. More recently a genetic mutation, the adenomatous polyposis coli (APC) gene, can be detected in the fecal DNA of patients with early colorectal tumors. This exciting test needs further study and development.

Table I

Systems Review

Head:	Do you have any pain, headaches, lumps or bumps?
Eyes:	How is your vision? Has there been any change? Is there anything about your vision or your eyes that is different recently? Any other problems with your eyes?
Ears:	How is your hearing? Have there been any changes? Do you have any pain in your ears? Do you have ringing in your ears and when did it start?

Nose and Throat: Have you had any difficulty with your nose such as your nose being stopped up or a bloody nose from time to time? Do you have sore throats? Is there a change in your voice? Have you noticed any hoarseness?

Neck: Is there any pain in your neck, any limitation of motion, any lumps or bumps that you have noticed?

Chest: Do you have a cough? How frequently? Do you bring up any sputum? Is there ever any blood in it? Do you have chest pain? Where is it? How is your breathing? Have you noticed any shortness of breath? Has there been a change in your breathing? Can you go up a flight of stairs quickly? How far can you walk on the level without getting short of breath?

Heart: Have you had any pain in your chest, particularly pain with exercise that stops when you stop exercising? Any pain in the left side of your lower chest? Pain in the shoulders? A pain in the upper abdomen? Squeezing pain?

Breasts: Have you had any pain or nipple discharge lumps or bumps? Do you examine your breasts yourself?

Gastrointestinal Tract: How is your appetite and swallowing? Do you ever have heartburn? Do you have pain in your abdomen? If so, where is it? high up (may be due to the gallbladder)? in the mid abdomen (may be an ulcer)? Pain on the lower right side may be appendicitis. Pain on the lower left side, low down, may be due to the colon or, in a woman, to the ovaries. How are your bowel movements? Are they regular? Have you been constipated? Do you have diarrhea? Have you ever had black stools or blood in your stools? Describe it. Have you had any pain in your rectum?

Genitourinary Tract Have you had any pain in your flanks, any pain passing your urine?

(Kidneys, Bladder, Prostate Gland): Does urine pass easily? How often must you pass urine? Has there been any burning or blood in your urine? Do you have to get up at night to urinate (nocturia)? Do you have difficulty getting your urinary stream started? Do you notice loss of urine when you cough or laugh (incontinence)?

Male Reproductive System: Have you had any problems with getting an erection or other signs of impotence?

Female Reproductive System: Do you have pain in your abdomen between periods? Are your menstrual periods regular? How much bleeding? Has there been any change? Are you beginning to have irregular menses and at what age? If you are menopausal, have you had any bleeding afterward? Do you have discomfort with sexual intercourse? Do you have bleeding after sexual intercourse?

Extremities, Joints Do you have pain with exercise, any difficulty in motion of any joints or Back: your joints? Do you have pain down your legs or in you back?

Table II

Health Maintenance Studies and Screening Tests

Height and body weight

Blood pressure

Chest x-ray

Mammography—40 and older

Papanicolaou smear (PAP smear)

Prostate exam

Prostate specific antigen levels in the blood (PSA)

Urine test for sugar—blood sugar

Stool for occult blood

Sigmoidoscopy, colonoscopy

Cholesterol and HDL and LDL (high and low density lipoproteins)

Bone density scan—for osteoporosis—women over 65

EKG—periodic—over 40

Thyroid stimulating hormone (TSH)—women over 35—every 5 years for question of hypothyroidsm

Immunizations—influenza, pneumococcus, tetanus—diphtheria booster

Table III

Cancer Detection

		Test or Procedure	
Age	Frequency	Females	Males
18-20	One time	Complete Health Examination	Complete Health Examination
	Monthly	Skin self-exam	Skin self-exam
	Yearly	Pap smear	Testis self-exam
20-40	Every 5 years	Complete Health Examination	Complete Health Examination
	Monthly	Skin self-exam	Skin self-exam
		Breast self-exam	Testis self-exam
	Yearly	Pelvic exam	
		Pap smear	
40-50	Every 3 years	Complete Health Examination	Complete Health Examination
	Monthly	Skin self-exam	Skin self-exam
		Breast self-exam	Testis self-exam
	Yearly	Pelvic exam	
		Pap smear	
		Rectal exam	Rectal exam
		Stool blood test	Stool blood test
	Every 1-2 yrs	Mammogram	
50-65	Every Year	Complete Health Examination	Complete Health Examination
	Monthly	Skin self-exam	Skin self-exam
		Breast self-exam	Testis self-exam
	Yearly	Pelvic exam	
		Pap smear	
		Rectal exam	Rectal exam
		Stool blood test	Stool blood test
		Mammogram	Prostate Specific Antigen Test
	Every 3-5 yrs	Procto-Colonoscopy	Procto-Colonoscopy

MEDI-SPEAK. WORDS I DON'T UNDERSTAND.

MY MEDICAL RECORD.

12. I do not understand many of the words doctors use. Why don't they explain them?

D octors should explain them. A cartoon shows a doctor talking to a patient in his office. The caption is, "Of course you don't understand what I just told you. You're not supposed to understand it." This had been the way that many doctors approached patients in the past but is no longer acceptable. All of you should have explanations in a language you understand.

Thelma and Lois DeBakey, sisters of the heart surgeon, Mike DeBakey have written and spoken extensively about the language that doctors use. They call it Medi-speak or Doctor Speak—a medical foreign language, also called medical jargon. Based on Greek and Latin, it allows doctors to talk and write to each other with precision and exactness. It is not the language that doctors should use with you. You tell your doctor that you have an itch in your rear but he will call it pruritus ani. If your doctor uses medical terms in talking with you, ask him to translate it into ordinary language.

However, you should know terms that describe you and your illnesses. The following tables list and define them.

Your medical record, also called your "History and Physical Examination," contains the following:

1. Chief Complaint: your reason for seeking medical help. This is usually just one sentence, a very brief statement of what is bothering you now, primarily your symptoms, not a diagnosis
2. History of Present Illness: a description of how your present problems came about and how they affect you.
3. Past History: a description of other diseases, illnesses, allergies, operations or injuries you have had that may relate to your present situation.
4. Social History: information about your family, occupation, and other matters important to consideration of your health.
5. Physical Examination/General appearance: Do you look sick? If so, how? The extent of the physical examination will depend on your chief complaint. If the problem is a chronic cough, it is unlikely that your doctor will do a pelvic examination, unless you have not had such an examination for some years.
6. Preliminary Diagnoses: steps to a final diagnosis. The doctor first writes down a working diagnosis or an "impression," the initial impression of

what may be bothering you, and then a "differential diagnosis" to explore other possibilities. Only later will there be a final diagnosis.

7-10. Diagnostic studies will be ordered and results obtained. Doctors' orders for hospital treatment are written in a book for consultation by nurses and aides. Nurses will also keep track of you by notes. Each day your doctor and/or consultants will put information in your chart. You may ask to see them if you wish. Schwartz et al. use the acronym SOAP: S for subjective patients' complaints; O for objective findings on examination or laboratory tests; A for assessment of the illness, diagnosis and prognosis; and P for a plan for further evaluation and/or treatment.

Table 1

Your hospital record is made up of:

1. Chief Complaint—CC·
2. History of Present Illness—HPI
3. Past History—PH
4. Social History—SH
5. Physical Examination—PE
6. Impression (IMP) or working diagnosis. Then a differential diagnosis. Later will come the final diagnosis (Dx)
7. Daily progress notes by physicians
8. Nursing notes
9. Doctors' orders
10. Laboratory results

Table 2

Inflammation or Infection

-itis—is inflammation	-ectomy—if the organ is removed	
Cholecystitis	Cholecystectomy	Gallbladder
Diverticulitis	Colectomy	Colon
Appendicitis	Appendectomy	Appendix
Gastritis	Gastrectomy	Stomach
Esophagitis	Esophagectomy	Esophagus
Pancreatitis	Pancreatectomy	Pancreas
Pyelonephritis	Nephrectomy	Kidney
Cystitis	Cystectomy	Urinary bladder
Encephalitis	Meninges	Covering of the brain
Hepatitis	Hepatectomy	Liver

Cellulitis		Skin
Peritonitis	Lining of abdomen with infection coming from an organ in it	Peritoneum
Colitis	Colectomy	Colon
Pleuritis, or Pleurisy	Lining of the lung and chest wall	Pleura
Pneumonia	Lobectomy or pneumonectomy	Lung
Empyema		Infection in the space between the lung and chest wall
Abscess	A localized infection that can occur anywhere	
Mastitis	Mastectomy	Breast
Thyroiditis	Thyroidectomy	Thyroid gland
	Hysterectomy	Uterus
	Adrenalectomy	Adrenal gland
	Oophorectomy	Ovary
	Hemorrhoidectomy	Hemorrhoids
	Laparotomy	An incision in abdomen
	Thoracotomy	An incision in chest
	Craniotomy	An incision in skull
	Transurethral prostatectomy (TURP)	Prostate removed through urethra
	Laminectomy	An incision to remove a ruptured intervertebral disc Herniorrhaphy Repair of a hernia.

Table 3

Diagnostic Studies

EEG	Electroencephalogram—recording of brain waves.
EKG or ECG	Electrocardiogram—recording the electrical currents and activities of the heart
Mammography	X-ray study of the breast to look for possible cancer
Intravenous pyelogram (IVP)	Dye that appears in the kidneys after injection into a vein in the arm. Tracking the dyes, X-rays show outlines of both kidneys, the ureters, or the tubes which take urine from the kidneys to

	the bladder, and the bladder for stones in the kidneys or other problems.
Barium enema	Injection of the dye barium into the colon through a tube inserted into the rectum. Tracking this white dye, the x-ray shows the outline of the colon and any potential tumors or other problems.
CT scan	A computed tomographic scan, an x-ray or imaging technique, showing details of the inside of the body.
Plain x-rays	For the chest, abdomen, bones and joints and skull.
G.I. series	Ingestion of barium with fluoroscopy to view the esophagus, stomach and duodenum
Small bowel series	X-rays after the G.I. series to show the barium going through the small intestine
Arteriograms	Injection of dye to study blood vessels in the heart, neck, brain, abdomen or extremities
Laminography	Injection of dye around the spinal cord to search for ruptured disks
Magnetic Resonance Imaging (MRI)	An imaging radiologic technique for detailed evaluation of various parts of the inside of the body.
Magnetic Resonance Arteriography (MRA)	An imaging technique for blood vessels
Positron Emission tomography (PET scan)	Injection of a radioactive isotope into the body. Images are taken later showing where the isotope has gone. The isotope would go to a tumor of the lung, for instance, drawn by its high metabolic rate, and would show it as a spot.
Endoscopy	Viewing a body cavity or space with an instrument.
Thoracoscopy	Insertion of a small lighted tube to see the lining of the lung and chest wall.
Peritoneoscopy	Insertion of a lighted tube to see the lining of the abdomen and the organs within it.
Bronchoscopy	Insertion of a tube with a light into the windpipe, or trachea, to show the inside of the trachea and bronchi.
Laryngoscopy	Inspection of the larynx and vocal cords with a mirror and a light, with the mouth open and tongue pulled forward.
Colonoscopy	Insertion of a flexible tube with a light through

	the anus to see the inside of the colon for polyps, tumors and other problems.
Sigmoidoscopy	Insertion of a lighted straight metal tube to see only the lower part of the colon.
Proctoscopy	Insertion of an instrument to show the anus and anal canal.
Cystoscopy	Insertion of a lighted tube to show the lining of the bladder.
Gastroscopy	Insertion of a tube through the mouth and esophagus and into the stomach to show the lining of the stomach. Esophagoscopy uses the same technique to view the inside of the esophagus.
Endoscopic Retrograde Cholangiopancreatography (ERCP)	From a tube through the mouth and stomach and into the duodenum, a smaller tube is put into the common bile duct; injection of dye shows this duct and the pancreatic duct.
Nasogastric tube	A tube through the nose into the stomach
Intubation	Insertion of any tube but usually used to refer to insertion of a tube into the windpipe
Endotracheal tube	Tube inserted into the windpipe to help breathing
Hemodialysis	Artificial Kidney

Table 4

Commonly Used Terms

NPO (nil per os)	Sign placed by the bed of a patient who is not to get anything to eat or drink
Emesis basin	Pan for those who are sick to their stomach.
Emesis	Vomiting.
Ambulate	Take the patient for a walk
Force Fluids	Encourage intake of liquids.
Void	Urinate
IV	Intravenous
OOB	Out of bed
IPPB	Intermittent Positive Pressure Breathing machine to aid breathing
BP	Blood pressure
HR	Heart rate

Medication Schedule for Prescriptions

qid	4 times a day
tid (ter in die)	3 times a day
bid	2 times a day
od or qd	Once a day
qod	Every other day
hs	Before sleep—bedtime
p.c. (post cibum)	After eating food
ut dictum	As directed
ante	Before
prn (pro Renata)	as the occasion arises, occasionally.

Hernias—

Hiatal—stomach pushing up into the chest above the diaphragm
Incisional—a hernia through a previous operative site
Umbilical—at the umbilicus
Femoral—along side the artery and vein to the leg—below the groin
Inguinal—groin

Many medical expressions are abbreviations or acronyms in which the first letters of words or syllables are used as a form of shorthand. Examples include ECG, for electrocardiogram, also called an EKG, or M.S. for multiple sclerosis. Acronyms are common in all aspects of life, particularly with the U.S. Government. The NIH stands for the National Institutes of Health; the FDA for the Food and Drug Administration. Many believe acronyms are overdone but they remain popular in a world in a hurry.

Eponyms name a body part or disease after the person who first described it. Fallot, for example, first described a complex heart defect in the newborn now known as the Tetralogy of Fallot.

Latin or Greek roots are used for many medical expressions and make it easy for physicians, nurses and pharmacists to communicate but may not help patients to understand.

Table 5

Abbreviations	Latin or Greek	English
a.c.	ante cibum	before meals
ad	ad	to; up to
ad lib.	ad libitum	at pleasure

alternis horis	alternis horis	every other hour
aq.	aqua	water
bis	bis	twice
c, c̄	cum	with
caps.	capsula	a capsule
collyr.	collyrium	an eyewash
divid.	divide	divide (thou)
elix.	elixir	an elixir
enem.	enema	an enema
et	et	and
gtt.	gutta(e)	drop(s)
H.	hora	an hour
hor.som., H.S.	hora somni	at bedtime
in d.	in dies	from day to day; daily
inf.	infusum	an infusion
inject.	injecto	an injection
inter	inter	between
lot.	lotio	a lotion
non	non	not
non rep	non repetatur	do not repeat
O.D.	oculus dexter	the right eye
O.L.	oculus laevus	the left eye
omn. hor	omni hora	every hour
omni nocte	omni nocte	every night
pil.	pilula(e)	pill(s)
q.h.	quaque hora	each hour; every hour
q. 2 h.	quaque secunda hora	every 2 hours
q.s.	quantum sufficit;	a sufficient quantity; as much as is sufficient
S.	signa; signetur	write (thou); let it be written; label (thou)
S.A.	secundum artem	according to art
sine	sine	without
ss. ss	semis	a half
suppos.	suppositorium	a suppository
syr.	syrupus	syrup
tabel	tabella (dim of tabula, a table)	a lozenge
talis	talis	such; like this
tinct.	tinctura	a tincture
ung.	unguentum	an ointment

Examples of Acronyms:

ARDS—adult respiratory distress syndrome—lung failure.

FUO—fever of unknown origin.

SBE—subacute bacterial endocarditis—infection inside the heart.

BPH—benign prostatic hypertrophy—an enlarged prostate gland.

TURP—transurethral resection of the prostate—removal of part of the prostate gland

CABG—coronary artery bypass graft.

SOB—shortness of breath.

MI—myocardial infarction—a heart attack.

CA—cancer.

COPD—chronic obstructive pulmonary disease—emphysema.

TIA—a transient ischemic attack—temporary loss of nerve function due to blood vessel disease.

AAA—abdominal aortic aneurysm—enlargement of the main artery in the abdomen.

DNR—do not resuscitate—after a patient stops breathing or her heart stops.

CAD—coronary artery disease.

DNA—deoxynucleic acid.

RNA—ribonucleic acid.

GI—gastrointestinal.

HIV—human immunodeficiency virus—which causes AIDS.

AIDS—acquired immunodeficiency syndrome.

GOVERNMENT AGENCIES:

NIH—National Institutes of Health

NHLBI—National Heart, Lung, Blood Institute

FDA—Food and Drug Administration.

HHS—Health and Human Services

CDC—Communicable Disease Center

HCFA—Health Care Financing Administration (Medicare)

EPA—Environmental Protection Agency

HUD—Housing and Urban Development

OTHERS:

AHA—American Heart Association

AMA—American Medical Association

ACS—American College of Surgeons

DEFINITIONS:

arteriosclerosis—hardening of the arteries—accumulation of cholesterol and
  other materials in the arteries.

emphysema—a disease of the lungs primarily caused by smoking which
  damages the lung causing overinflation with shortness of breath.

stenosis—a narrowing of a blood vessel or the bowel

occlusion—a block in an artery or the bowel

skull—cranium.

vertebra—bones of the neck and back.

maxilla—upper jaw.

mandible—lower jaw.

sternum—bone in the middle front of the chest.

median sternotomy—an incision through the sternum for heart operations.

humerus—the upper arm bone.

clavicle—the shoulder blade.

radius and ulna—the lower arm bones.

carpal bones—the bones of the hand.

phalanges—finger bones.

sacrum, coccyx, pubic bones—the pelvic bones.

femur—the upper leg bone.

acetabulum—femur joint.

patella—knee cap.

tibia and fibula—lower leg bones.

tarsal bone—foot bones.

calcaneus—heel bone.

MY BELIEFS

13. Will doctors always respect my religious, cultural, ethnic beliefs or traditions?

Jehovah Witnesses, Christians who base their religion upon a strict reading
of the Bible, do not accept blood transfusions. If you are a Jehovah Witness
and need a blood transfusion for a major operation, you may decline receiving
blood. No ethical physician will give you blood even though it could be given in
the operating room where no one else would know. This church studies medical
alternatives to blood transfusions, like blood conservation methods for reduction
of postoperative bleeding. With use of such methods, patients may survive open
heart operations without blood transfusions.

Adult Christian Scientists may decide against treatment or an operation even though it may be lifesaving. When an adult does the same for a young child, however, a problem arises. In such circumstances, a court could allow treatment for the child as a ward of the state. I find this acceptable. You may not agree.

Some groups oppose the performance of autopsies or post-mortem examinations. We respect that belief and others as well. Be sure that your physician and nurses know what they are.

As you may know, proof of immunization is required for children to go to school. Exemptions can be obtained for medical, religious or philosophical reasons. Is this a good idea? I believe it is not. The children may be in jeopardy themselves and may infect other kids, as shown in a recent outbreak of measles.

Make your religious preferences or beliefs known when you are admitted to a hospital. Most hospitals have both Catholic and Protestant chaplains available to call on you. Other religious leaders may be available on request. Your family should let your church know that you are in a hospital, otherwise they might not know. Hospitals, in order to protect privacy, no longer provide a list of hospitalized patients to outside agencies. Most hospitals have chapels open for prayer, meditation and religious services.

It is important to consider cultural differences in end-of-life decisions. They require careful communication, knowledge of inequities in care, concern about religion and spirituality, truthfulness, family insistence on decision making and reduced use of hospice care.

Section B

My health. How healthy am I?

RISK FACTORS

14. How do I know how healthy I am?

R eview your own situation: diet, weight, exercise tolerance, and activities. Write it all down, go see your doctor, and get a complete review of your health status.

Many articles rate your risk for heart disease and stroke. If you know your blood pressure, your total cholesterol and high and low density lipoprotein, you can calculate your chances of developing a heart attack or stroke, as exemplified by the Holson study in *Circulation*. 1998 (97;1838), published in a Nutrition Action Health Letter from the Center of Science in the Public Interest. Diabetes, alcohol intake and other factors enter in. Risk factors for death from stroke and heart disease in older adults include relative poverty, lack of physical activity, smoking, and indicators of frailty and disability. Other risk factors are shown in the table.

The damaging effects of stress and mediators activated by stress are well known. See Chapters 76, 84 for detailed reviews of hypertension and blood pressure control, important factors in preventing heart disease and stroke.

Risk factors for development of lung cancer include smoking and exposure to asbestos and to industrial or mining pollutants such as silica. Smoking causes emphysema. Excessive alcohol causes cirrhosis of the liver. Many of these problems and others are reviewed in the following chapters.

Obesity is the most important cause of diabetes. Physical activity decreases the risk as does a diet including whole grain foods. Osteoporosis can be prevented by adequate consumption of calcium and vitamin D. To decrease the risk of colon and rectal cancer, avoid putting on excess weight around the waist, increase exercise and eat more fruits and vegetables. It also helps to get enough calcium and to limit intake of red meat and saturated fat.

Excess weight increases the risk of breast cancer in post-menopausal women. Obesity, alcohol and smoking increase the risk of esophagus cancer whereas a plant-based diet with fiber, vitamin C, folate and beta-carotene lowers risk. On the other hand studies about prostate cancer offer no definite information about the benefits of taking selenium, vitamin E, or lycopene and of consuming less red meat or saturated fat.

What are some of the genetic differences in susceptibility to diseases?

It has been recognized for many years that certain diseases and disorders run in families, among them hemophilia (a blood clotting problem), cystic fibrosis, Parkinson's disease, cardiovascular disease and stroke. Some cancers run in families, including breast cancer associated with BRACI and BRACII genes. (Please see Chapter 28.) Gene expression and abnormal genes or mutations are associated with increased risk of infection and resultant death, which is why some survive a bad infection and others die. There seems to be a gene that protects against heart attacks. We can do nothing about these events but perhaps in the future those with a greater risk can be identified.

The NIH set up the Office of Research on Minority Health after studies showed that the health of minorities in the U.S. was not as good as that of the rest of the population. African-Americans are, generally speaking, in poorer health than others, a problem that began during slavery. It is not known whether the problem is lack of access to medical care, poverty, distrust of the system or lack of culturally compatible physicians.

Table

Risk factors for the development of cardiovascular disease include:

1. Lifestyle—lack of exercise
2. Family history of diseases or deaths
3. Excess weight
4. High blood pressure
5. An unhealthy diet
6. High cholesterol level—and low HDL, high LDL
7. Poor results of a stress test

QUALITY OF LIFE

15. Are doctors really concerned about whether or not I am satisfied with their care?

Yes, they are. Doctors, nurses and hospitals are now sometimes called "health care providers" as if part of a business. In a recent article in the Journal of the American Medical Association, we were referred to "as a service industry which should improve quality, reduce rates, answer questions, assure physical and psychological comfort and offer choices." That is well and good but that takes time and when reimbursement is cut, it is difficult for doctors to provide all of the services requested. Other articles were titled "good customer service as good credit policy" (if you are nice to your patients, they will pay you sooner), or "doctors advised to listen when patients speak on health care" or "satisfied patients will refer patients to you." These articles depict you as a consumer. If you are a consumer, and your doctor is a provider, and this is a service industry, then your doctor could form a union and strike for example, rather than being a professional. But doctors do not want to form unions. (See Chapter 60).

A number of organizations now measure patient satisfaction. The National Committee for Quality Assurance (NCQA), a non-profit group, developed accreditation standards for health plans, relying on its Health plan-Employer Data and Information Set (HEDIS) to measure the quality of care provided. They want to know whether patients are getting immediate services, whether they have a choice of doctors and the skill level of the providers.

The American Medical Association has mounted an initiative to measure physician performance. The Consumer Assessment of Health Plans (CAHPS), with the U.S. Department of Health and Human Services and their agency for health care policy and research, takes patient satisfaction surveys that ask if optimal care is different from what patients seek. The assumption that patients know best may not be totally true or acceptable.

Chung, et al., wrote in a surgical publication about the major factors for patient satisfaction in a plastic surgery clinic. They were waiting time, patient/physician interaction, and speedy and empathic care. Dissatisfaction of families of patients who die in an intensive care unit were related to the type of death, sudden death as compared to death after gradual deterioration; manner of notification of the death, in person or by telephone; and the gender and closeness of the relative to the deceased. Kenagy, et al. wrote that if "other service areas have found ways to improve quality, reduce wages, answer questions, preserve dignity, customize experience, assure physical and psychological comfort and offer choice then all of us in health care have an obligation to study these methods and try to improve." If hotels, airlines, and other service companies treated their customers to the same waiting, inconvenience, unanswered questions and obscure instructions as do many medical centers, they would soon be out of business. Health care organizations need a way to measure patient satisfaction. Greenfield said, "In this environment a specialist who is unavailable or too expensive will simply be replaced."

BETTER HEALTH

16. Are we really healthier now?

Life expectancy was 47 years for a woman born in 1900, compared to more than 75 years—and some say nearly 80—for a woman born in 1988. This gain is due primarily to decreased neonatal and maternal mortality. A male child born in 1990 can also expect to live to age 75. Jane Brody cites national long-term care surveys indicating that every year a smaller percentage of older people are unable to care for themselves. Thus, the elderly population may not be as much of an economic drain as was projected. This is particularly true in health care. Better educated, the elderly are more likely to change lifestyles to improve health.

Public health measures have brought about the improvement in health and increase in life expectancy in the last 100 years. For the increase of 30 years in life expectancy since 1900, 25 are due to advances in public health. JAMA has published CDCP rankings of public health achievements in the U.S. (see the table). The single most important achievement has been vaccination, which completely eradicated smallpox in the world, has almost eliminated poliomyelitis and has controlled measles, mumps, rubella or German measles, tetanus, pertussis or whooping cough, varicella or chicken pox, diphtheria, H influenza type B and hepatitis B. Many other public health measures have improved health and longevity.

In the past, the environment was the primary source of human disease and death, and solving environmental problems has helped control the spread of disease. Helpful measures include water purification, improved sanitation, elimination of mosquitoes and other vectors, adequate nutrition, and vaccination. Infectious diseases have not been totally eliminated, of course, and new diseases are found all the time, among them HIV and AIDS, the various Hanta, Ebola viruses and SARS. Tuberculosis, tetanus, malaria and even typhoid fever are still major problems in some parts of the world. The major risk factors for death and disability worldwide are malnutrition, poor water supply, inadequate sanitation, poor personal and domestic hygiene, unsafe sexual behavior, use of tobacco and alcohol, occupational hazards, hypertension, physical inactivity, illicit drugs and air pollution.

In the western world, human disease now finds its source within the individual, as with the consequences of atherosclerosis, obesity, smoking, alcohol, stress, injury, toxins and carcinogens. Investigators in the past assessed health outcomes by adverse events—deaths, strokes or other serious problems. Now it is better to use gains in life expectancy to measure the effectiveness of health care. Detsky and Redelmeier point out that individuals may be disappointed with what seem to be very small gains in overall life expectancy derived from most modern health care interventions. Present improvements primarily prevent adverse effects of chronic degenerative disease in middle-aged and elderly adults; thus, gains in life expectancy are important for them but more limited in general. For example, in order to increase life expectancy by another 28 years, according to these authors, health care interventions would have the virtual impossible task of reducing mortality from all causes at all ages by 85 percent. It is not unusual for medical therapies to cost $50,000 to $100,000 to achieve a one year gain in life expectancy. Recently it was suggested that quality of life should be used to assess outcomes of health care. The improvement of a patient's perception of their health and function should be the goal of our medical therapy.

Richard Biek, M.D., reports several strange occurrences. When doctors went on strike in Israel in 1955, and recently in California and also in Saskatchewan, death from all causes immediately dropped about 20 percent. In 1975 Israeli doctors went on strike again and deaths immediately dropped 50 percent. Could it be that too much doctoring and health care are not good for you?

What is the recent problem with vaccination?

Recently a scare has arisen about vaccination and its possible link to an increase in cases of autism, a disorder usually appearing in very early childhood characterized by self absorption and social withdrawal. Manning indicated that kids in the U.S. get 21 shots before they start the first grade. Recent headlines read: "Now parents fear shots," and "Are vaccines safe for our kids?" Is autism really on the increase? Manning quoted Rimland, a founder of the Autism Research Institute in San Diego, as saying "It's truly an epidemic." However, some experts, such as Danielson of the Education Department Office of Special Education Programs, said that a few years ago no category existed for reporting autism. The children with autism were always there but not being counted. The apparent increase in autism from 1992-1993 to 1997-1998 may represent not an actual increase but the effect of more reporting of the disorder.

The FDA's Center for Biologics Evaluation and Research (CBER) regulates the quality of vaccines and licenses only those that have been adequately tested. Vaccines are very safe but some side effects occur. Serious reactions, very rare, should be reported to the Vaccine Adverse Event Scoring System (VAERS) at 1-800-822-7967 or *www.fda.gov/cher/vaers/vaers.html* or *www.cdc.gov/nip*. There is also a National Vaccine Injury Compensation Program (1-800-338-2382 or *www.bhpr.hrsa.gov.vicp*).

Autism has developed in some children shortly after vaccination. A few infants have died shortly after vaccinations. Possible associations will now be investigated thoroughly even though vaccinations always involve a chance of coincidental illness, and coincidence may well be at work here. The number of children with autism in California increased rapidly between 1980 and 1994 with no corresponding increase in immunization. If vaccines caused autism, the curves should be similar. Dales et al. found no association between immunization for mumps and measles-rubella and the incidence of autism.

David Satcher, former U.S. Surgeon General, reported recently, in USA Today, that "We will never cease in our efforts to improve the safety of vaccines. To assure optimal health for the American people, safe and effective vaccines must continue to be a national public health priority for each and every American." Satcher and all public health officials are trying to be sure that all American children are vaccinated and also all children elsewhere in the world, and with good reason. Chicken pox vaccine is highly effective, recommended for children 12-18 months old and if used widely could eliminate the disease. The oral poliomyelitis vaccine has virtually eliminated polio in the world but it could come back again if immunization is stopped.

Vaccination has also been used for an outbreak of meningococcal disease, or meningitis, in Quebec Province. Immunization does not increase the risk of juvenile diabetes.

Dr. Glass, a pediatrician, wrote recently that many people do not remember the terrible things that happened before vaccination: babies dying of whooping cough, brain damage from *Hemophilus* meningitis and other scourges. These diseases have not gone away; they are just kept under control by vaccination.

Russia is currently having a diphtheria epidemic due to the lack of shots. As Glass said, "The wolves are still out there." The risk of vaccination, as reviewed by Gellin and Schaffner, is very low and far outweighed by the problems that could occur if a child gets the disease.

A recent study from Vanderbilt University found that roughly 25% of American parents have serious concerns over the safety of vaccination. The American Academy of Pediatrics and Pediatricians in general agree that these are misconceptions with no basis in scientific fact. Anti-vaccination websites are *wrong* in saying that vaccines cause idiopathic disease and erode immunity; that vaccine reactions are under-reported; and that vaccination policy is motivated by the hope of profit. These sites rely heavily on emotional appeal. Vaccination is very safe and very important. It is not totally risk-free, but the benefits far outweigh the risks. The recommended childhood immunization schedule for 2001 is found in the July-August 2001 FDA Consumer.

A global alliance for vaccines and immunization now tries to get affordable vaccines for all. The Gates Foundation gave $1 billion for worldwide vaccines. Ninety percent or more of American children are vaccinated with few complications. Almost all states still mandate vaccination before children go to school. Many states, however, allow personal exemptions from vaccination. There are also religious and philosophical exemptions from immunization laws which are being reviewed to protect children. Feikin et al. found that the risk of measles was 22.2 times greater and pertussis 5.9 times greater in non-vaccinated children. In addition, these non-vaccinated children spread the disease to others. Parents should recognize these risks.

New vaccines are being developed for staphylococcus aureus infection, streptococcus and others. Researchers are trying to genetically engineer apples to produce a vaccine against respiratory syncitial virus (RSV) a common and sometimes deadly virus in children. For children, in particular, a live flu virus administered by spray is being evaluated clinically for safety. A vaccine for Lyme disease was discontinued because of poor demand for it (no profit). The birth dose of Hepatitis B virus vaccine has decreased because of the mercury content of thiomerosal.

Stockpiles of vaccines are running short. Shots for MMR (measles, mumps, and rubella) have been scarce as low profitability has reduced the number of manufacturers. Outbreaks can occur; in 1990, 27,782 kids came down with measles. Some pharmaceutical companies are being encouraged to make vaccines. The Center for Disease Control tries to stockpile some vaccines.

Smallpox vaccination was terminated in 1972. Everyone in the country is now susceptible even those of us who received smallpox vaccination as children many years ago for that vaccination is no longer effective. Because of the possibility that smallpox could be used of terrorism germ warfare with smallpox, should we now seek immunization?

Besides vaccination, the CDCP cites as other great public health achievements improvements in motor vehicle safety, elimination of work-related health problems, control of infectious diseases, declines in death from coronary heart disease and stroke, safer and healthier foods, healthier mothers and babies, access to family planning and contraceptive services, fluoridation of drinking water, and recognition of tobacco as a public health hazard.

What about flu, pneumonia and hepatitis shots?

Flu vaccination remains the best way to prevent and control flu. The CDCP recommend flu and pneumonia vaccination for everyone over 65 years of age, residents of nursing homes and those with underlying health problems. Anyone with congestive heart failure, emphysema and asthma should get a flu shot no matter what age they are. Pneumococcal pneumonia vaccine should also be given every five years to diabetics, alcoholics, and anyone with heart, lung, liver or kidney disease. Flu shots in kids may help protect the elderly.

The AMA recommends flu vaccination for people over 50 years old; residents of long-term care facilities; patients with chronic health problems and immune systems weakened by treatment for HIV and cancer, notably with chemo or radiation therapy; those taking aspirin on a long-term basis; women after the third month of pregnancy; and health care workers. Protection develops about two weeks after the shot and may last a year. The best time to get it is September. If you are older, get to your doctor early, in view of possible delays in supplies and shortages of flu vaccines. Consult your doctor if you have had a reaction to eggs or a previous flu shot or have had Guillain-Barre syndrome.

For more information contact the National Immunization Program Centers for Disease Control and Prevention. (800-232-2522 or *www.cdc.gov/nip/*).

Table

Ten Great Public Health Achievements—U.S. 1900-1999. From 1900 to 1999 the average lifespan in the United States increased by over 30 years, 25 years of which is due to public health.

1. Vaccination—smallpox, polio, measles, rubella, tetanus, diphtheria, H. flu, Hepatitis B.
2. Improvements in motor vehicle safety—safety belts, infant seats, helmets, decreased drinking and driving, engineering efforts.
3. Decreased work related health problems, coal workers' black lung, silicosis, and safer work places.
4. Control of infectious diseases—clean water, better sanitation, antibiotics.
5. Decline in deaths from coronary heart disease and stroke.

6. Safer and healthier foods.
7. Healthier mothers and babies.
8. Access to family planning and contraceptive services.
9. Fluoridation of drinking water.
10. Recognition of health hazards of tobacco use.

FAITH, HOPE AND PRAYER. PLACEBOS.

17. What do faith, hope and a positive attitude have to do with health and healing?

Much is known about the effects of faith, hope and a positive outlook on life in promoting or maintaining health and healing disease. We now have a better understanding of the power of positive thinking, as proposed originally by Norman Vincent Peale. Many physicians, writers and ministers have emphasized mind/body relationships, and the importance of hope and faith in healing.

We have well-documented examples of spontaneous reversal of disease, as well as survival from an injury or disease against all odds. Spontaneous regression of cancer is a biologic phenomenon in which some tumors decrease in size or even disappear. We read about people with cancer who learn that they have three months to live but nine years later write a book about their experience, as did Gregory W. Smith. Is this due to faith, prayer, a positive attitude or some biologic phenomenon which we do not understand? We do not know.

No matter how sick a patient is or how many organs have failed or how many life support systems are required, we can never say with certainty that a patient will die. Ninety-nine gravely ill patients may die, but one may survive. Is this a miracle? You may wish to call it that. I prefer to say that the patient had the resolve, determination, hope, faith and/or physiologic reserve to survive, and that the Almighty acted through natural processes. Just because we do not have scientific evidence for their survival doesn't mean there isn't an explanation. Modern science and molecular biology help us to understand much about life and death, but we are far from knowing everything. We have much to learn, particularly about causes and outcomes of disease.

The following writers explore the phenomenon of spontaneous regression of a disease process.

In Timeless Healing: The Power and Biology of Belief, Herbert Benson, M.D., writes about healing inspired by belief and about "remembered wellness," in which patients get better because they want to. This could be called a placebo effect but it is real and positive. Benson describes three components of "remembered wellness:" belief and expectancy on the part of the patient, belief and expectancy on the part of the caregiver, belief and expectancies from the relationship between the patient and the caregiver. Benson emphasizes his belief that we are wired for God. In his best-selling *The Relaxation Response,* he describes a form of meditation as a way to reduce stress and improve well-being. I also recommend his new book, with Ilene Stuart: *The Wellness Book: A Comprehensive Guide to Maintaining Health and Treating Stress—Related Illness.* Benson, who grew up in an Orthodox Jewish family, states in its final sentences that "my reasoning and personal experience lead me to believe that there is a God. I believe in a scientifically describable biology and evolution and in a world that is, nonetheless, divinely influenced."

My late cousin, the Rev. Garth Ludwig, Ph.D., a Lutheran minister and Professor and Chair of Social Sciences at Concordia University, Irvine, CA, wrote about health, medicine and healing in *The Restoration of Order.* A medical anthropologist and theologian, he notes that Hippocrates used the phrase "Vix trix naturae Medica" as the first to speak about the force that Albert Schweitzer called "The Healer Within." Garth sounds a clear call for Christians to return to the healing ministries of the early church. In his view disease is disorder; healing requires restoration of order in one's life. Disease is the result of separation of the creature from the creator. Garth makes a distinction between disease as an objective phenomenon due to altered biological function of the body and illness which is "a subjective, personal phenomenon in which the individual perceives himself as not feeling well". He describes sickness as a social phenomenon; "a person acts sick". You have seen these distinctions. A person can be cured of an illness by restoring order through faith and belief while still having the disease. Garth calls this "a healthy way to live a disease." Spiritual healing may allow one to live with a disease like rheumatoid arthritis that is not curable at present. He describes the scientific advances of neuropsychiatry and their relationship to our immune system. A positive attitude strengthens our immune system and decreases our susceptibility to disease. Although Garth writes from a Christian viewpoint, other faiths— Judaism, Hinduism, Islam, Buddhism, and Shintoism—all have healing as part of their beliefs and activities. I believe in these approaches. Faith is a powerful healer.

The noted writer on healing Dr. Bernie Siegel, a general surgeon in private practice in New Haven when I was on the faculty at Yale, is a friend and a fine person with a wonderful sense of humor. Observing cancer patients over the years, particularly women with breast cancer, he noticed that those with a positive attitude about life and about the possibility of overcoming their disease were exceptional cancer patients, or as he called them ECAP, doing better and living longer than those who were discouraged or depressed. His approach included "carefrontation," a loving, safe, therapeutic confrontation which facilitates personal change and healing."

Support groups are helpful for patients with cancer. Siegel found a doubling of survival time in women with advanced breast cancer who had a year of group therapy and autohypnosis compared to a control group receiving standard therapy. Three seriously ill women in group therapy were still alive 10 years after the onset of their disease. Information on support groups can be found on the web. (*www.la.wellnesscommunity.org; www.drkoop.com; www.vitaloptions.org; www.acor.org; www.oncolink.upenn.edu/psychosocial; www.intelihealth.com; www.cancercare.org.*

Siegel retired from practice to write and lecture about the importance of hope and a positive attitude about health. I highly recommend his best-selling books, *Love, Medicine and Miracles* and *Peace, Love and Healing.* "Let us choose love and life," he writes at the end of *Love, Medicine and Miracles.*

Neal Weiner, a close friend and Professor of Philosophy at Marlboro College in Vermont, writes about the "Harmony of the Soul-Mental Health and Moral Virtue Reconsidered." He begins with Aristotle and Plato, reviewing traditional ideas and bringing them to the present with Freud, Adler, St. Thomas Aquinas, Sartre, Gregory, MacIntyre, Searle, Veatch and others. Weiner describes good health as right thinking. He considers health a virtue and illness as close to being a vice. This is one of the oldest moral views. It does not mean that illness comes because we must suffer for something that we have done wrong. It means that the classical idea of virtue and the modern idea of mental health are almost astonishingly congruent. For both there is an original harmony of pleasure and function and for both this harmony is disrupted by pain.

Andrew Weil, M.D. has studied and written about the relationship between traditional medicine and alternative or as he calls it complimentary medicine. A "guru" of complimentary medicine, he is also a realist who once said that if hit by a truck he would want to go straight to a modern emergency ward and not to a herb doctor. In his most recent book *Spontaneous Healing,* he writes about our bodies' "natural ability to maintain and heal itself-the motivated patient as a physician." I recommend especially the sections "Optimizing the Healing System" and "Considering the Alternatives." Weil provides many examples of "the faces of healing"—patients he has observed and treated and the role of the mind in healing. He finds that meditation helps the brain (Please see chapter 42). His recommendations for herbal remedies, dietary supplements and diet are the best I have seen, legitimate and reasonable additions to the traditional subject matter of medicine.

Weil writes about the failings of our profession. Here are the complaints he heard most commonly;

"Doctors don't take time to listen to you or answer your questions."

"All they do is give you drugs; I don't want to take more drugs."

"They said that there was nothing more they could do for me."

"They told me it would only get worse."

"They told me I would just have to live with it."

"They said I would be dead in six months".

Reassurance can work wonders. The Mind/body connection is a powerful force. Science has established molecular and cellular evidence of the role that the mind plays in bodily health. The NIH has established 10 centers for mind-body research around the country. Mind/body medicine has been taught at the Harvard Medical School since the time of Oliver Wendell Holmes and Walter Cannon. Mind/body connections can also contribute to the treatment of diseases such as anorexia and bulimia, signs of a troubled body and soul. Mind/body medicine has been found to be cost effective. Religion and spirituality are increasingly applied to medical practice. The health benefits of humor and laughter are also recognized.

What is the wholeness or wholistic medicine?

Wholeness means that physical, emotional and spiritual factors are very important in healing and recovery. Many common folk beliefs or old spouses (wives) tales concern happenings in certain circumstances:

1. Only the good die young.
2. A spouse dies within days or weeks after the death of his or her spouse, a phenomenon especially common among devoted, elderly couples.
3. Someone in fairly good health except for abdominal pain goes into a hospital for surgery, turns out to have abdominal cancer, and dies shortly thereafter.
4. Regression of cancer.
5. Recurrence of malignancy associated with stressful events.
6. Chronic inflammatory diseases brought on by stressful events
7. Pneumonia: the old man's best friend
8. Blood transfusion: a hazard to one's health
9. Obesity: Is pleasantly plump a disease?
10. The influence of background /heredity.

All of these circumstances are related to the immune system. If you let everyone walk over you and do not stand up for your rights, your immune system will be depressed and you may develop an illness and die at a younger age. This has been verified in controlled animal studies. The death of a spouse soon after the death of the other spouse is related to immune suppression. Dying shortly after the discovery of abdominal cancer was once thought to be due to air getting in during an operation. Now we know it is due to the immunosuppression caused by an operation. Stressful events suppress our immune system and allow the possibility of malignancies to begin and grow as do chronic inflammatory diseases initiated by severe stress. Pneumonia is the old man's best friend because elderly individuals frequently suffer from immune suppression.

We recognize now that injury, stress and things that bother us result in suppression of our immune system, which increases our susceptibility to disease. I once performed a coronary artery bypass graft upon a woman who had breast cancer five years earlier. Within a few months of the operation she had metastatic breast cancer throughout her lungs, the result of the immunosuppression of the operation, something that we now understand scientifically. Blood transfusions are also immunosuppressive.

Studies suggest that the spirituality inherent in caring and being cared for can have a healing effect. Family, friends, doctors, nurses and staff along with religious observances, sacraments, prayer, contemplation and meditation all help. The Christian ministry is emphasizing the healing ministry, as does Aldredge-Clanton in "Great Physician, Wisdom Friend, Images of God Influencing the Healing of People with Cancer." Saint Louis Metropolitan Medicine recently ran a series on faith and healing with, "Healthy Mind, Healthy Body" by Moritz. The list continues with "Screening for Spiritual Risk" by Fitchett and "Religion and Health and Is There a Connection"? by Larson and Koenig. Many books have been published recently about mind/body relationships, among them Borysenko's, *Minding the Body, Mending the Mind*; Burke's *Body, Mind and Spirit*; Moore's *Care of the Soul*; Williamson's *Return to Love and Illumination*; Jampolsky's *Love is Letting Go of Fear*; and LeShan's *Cancer as a Turning Point*.

Does a common thread run throughout all of these? I think so and it is a very important for you a patient, to know and understand. Your mind has a very powerful relationship to the health of your body. Hope for the future is critical for us. We must always have hope for the future or depending upon our beliefs, for eternity. We are better off with faith whatever our religious background. Approaching life positively until it comes to an end is healthy and the restoration of order in our lives and right thinking are an important part of good health and a good life.

What does religion have to do with health?

A study by Duke University cited in the Harvard Health Letter showed that those who attended religious services once a week had lower interluekin-6 levels associated with heart disease and immune disorders, lower blood pressure and less likelihood of depression. However, it has been pointed out that people who regularly attend religious services may have healthier life styles. They may not smoke, may drink less alcohol and may exercise more. Prayer seems helpful and intercessory pray for others may have benefit.

What is the placebo effect?

In his recent book *The Power of Hope*, my friend the well-known gastroenterologist Howard Spiro reviews important and positive effects of placebos, inactive substances or sugar pills sometimes used to simulate real medicines in clinical trials. The word "placebo," Spiro points out, means "I shall please" in Latin, and it represents an erroneous translation of "I shall walk before the Lord" in Psalm 1:16:9 as "I shall please the Lord" in the vespers of the office for the dead in the Catholic Church. The vespers were referred to in the twelfth century as placebos, and professional mourners were paid to sing them. Spiro describes a healthy combination of alternative and traditional medicine in the treatment of mind/body and spirit, emphasizing the importance of the doctor-patient relationship and the need for doctors to talk and listen to their patients. He developed the exciting "Humanities in Medicine Program" for students and faculty in the Yale Medical School. His excellent book will help patients and doctors alike.

It has been known for years that if you are given a sugar pill or some other harmless but inactive ingredient you may feel better. If you believe the sugar pill is a worthwhile medicine, it may alleviate your symptoms or even cure a disease. This phenomenon is related to the power of positive thinking. Back when doctors had few remedies, they might give you a placebo, not to trick you but rather to help you believe you would get well.

Placebos are given as part of a randomized prospective trial of a new drug or a new therapeutic agent. Stunkard wrote in 1950 on a method of evaluating a therapeutic agent, a double-blind placebo controlled trial in which neither the researchers nor the subjects know who gets the active agent and who gets the placebo. The placebo is given in exactly the same form as the active ingredient being tested. If you agree to participate in such a trial, you will not know whether you received the placebo or the active substance nor will those in charge of the trial. The information is recorded secretly and the code broken only after the study is completed and those studied have been evaluated for effects and outcome.

In recent drug trials a pharmaceutical company thought they had an exciting and novel compound as an antidepressant which caused almost no sexual dysfunction, a side effect of many other drugs on the market. When the data was analyzed, patients who received a dummy pill did unexpectedly well and almost as well those who received the new drug. Thus, adequacy and effectiveness could not be proven. The placebo effect is of particular interest in psychopharmacology. The placebo effect in patients with depression should be studied as a possible cause of favorable effects.

In a new method to maximize chances of demonstrating efficacy, an "enriched" design or a "run-in trial," all subjects in the initial trial of an antidepressant medicine get a placebo. Only those who do not improve receive the study drug or a placebo at random. Enserink described a third arm in the trial in which subjects receive neither the study drug nor a placebo. Any natural history effect observed in such a trial cannot be distinguished from the Hawthorne effect, or of how an observer affects a study. People who know they are being observed do better. Thus, patients getting active ingredients or placebos may all get better. The enthusiasm and encouragement of the doctor also makes a difference. Injections and operations can also have placebo effects.

FDA regulations set forth five different controls that may be used in a drug trial: placebos, no treatment, active agents, historical controls, and dose comparisons. However, for three decades, the gold standard has been the placebo-controlled double-blind trial.

In spite of flaws and problems with placebo controls, a good alternative is not available. Placebos will continue to be used in the future.

Delap is quoted by Nordenberg as saying, "Expectation is a powerful thing." "The more you believe you're going to benefit from a treatment the more likely it is that you will experience benefit." However, DeLap also said, "We at the FDA don't have an ethical blind spot as some would suggest. Placebos do have a healing power. A patient's right to the best treatment is always paramount."

DENIAL OF DISEASE

18. Are there symptoms I should not ignore?

I remember seeing patients with far-advanced breast cancer who had denied to themselves that anything was wrong. These patients were usually older and lived alone. One woman came to the clinic with breast cancer that had grown through the skin and produced a large infected and foul smelling cancerous ulcer that would have taken months to develop. When did she first notice it? She said that last week she knew something was there. This denial of disease is complex emotionally for such a woman. Doctors must consider those complexities.

Have you had a health problem you tried to ignore? Many people have had that experience. Persistence of symptoms, however, is the most important part of your medical history, or what you tell your doctor about yourself. Certain symptoms are important to recognize immediately because they could represent serious problems.

On the other hand, some of us are chickens; we don't tolerate pain well and seek relief quickly. My wife points out that my own symptoms of what I have ascribed to serious health problems have so far always gone away spontaneously.

As for persistent symptoms, Callahan, in a recent issue of the Reader's Digest, described eight you must not ignore:

1. Leg pain after a long period of travel could indicate blood clots in your legs; such clots could break loose and go to your lungs with a fatal result in the form of a pulmonary embolus or they cause persistent leg swelling.

2. A persistent or lingering cough could indicate a lung tumor, benign or malignant; an infection such as tuberculosis or pneumonia; postnasal drip; asthma; reflux of stomach contents up the esophagus or chronic bronchitis. Some medicines cause coughing.

3. Frequent urination at night—Blood in the urine.
   Men: This is often due to an enlarged prostate gland or an infection in the prostate.
   Men/Women: This could indicate the beginning of diabetes with sugar loss in the urine. It could also indicate an infection or tumor in the bladder. Blood in the urine may indicate a tumor.

4. Difficulty in swallowing could mean at the worst an early cancer of the esophagus. Benign causes could include a stricture, or narrowing, of the lower esophagus from inflammation caused by reflux esophagitis or a hiatal hernia.

5. A change in headache pattern could indicate the beginning of migraine headaches; temporal arteritis, or inflammation of the arteries that come over one side of the head or the other; or an early brain tumor.

6. Severe abdominal pain could be due to a number of serious causes: inflammation of the gallbladder, or acute cholecystitis; inflammation of the colon, or diverticulitis; appendicitis; a perforated ulcer; pancreatitis; or enlargement of the abdominal aorta—an abdominal aortic aneurysm. Such aneurysms can rupture and be quickly fatal.

7. Brief loss of vision in one eye or numbness on one side of the face or body has been called a transient ischemic attack (TIA). Small pieces of blood platelets or clots break off from the carotid arteries in your neck and go to the brain. This requires immediate attention, examination by a physician and perhaps by a vascular surgeon to check for arteriosclerotic narrowing and/or blood clots in the carotid arteries in your neck.

8. Chest pain during exercise may indicate angina pectoris, a problem in blood flow to the muscle of your heart due to arteriosclerotic narrowing. The pain is squeezing in type and goes away when exercise stops. Chest pain that does not go away can mark the beginning of a coronary artery narrowing or occlusion (heart attack) and needs immediate attention. It is best to go to an emergency ward for an electrocardiogram and other

tests to see whether you are having a heart attack that can be treated if caught early.

9. Leg pain in the calf of your leg or the thigh when you exercise which goes away when you stop may indicate narrowing of one or more of the blood vessels to your leg, (called intermittent claudication).

10. Severe persistent pain in the legs or the foot with numbness may indicate block of a major blood vessel and threaten the life of your extremity and should have immediate evaluation by a physician.

11. Vomiting blood could indicate a bleeding ulcer, other abnormalities of the stomach, or esophageal varices—ruptured veins in the esophagus resulting from cirrhosis of the liver, often due to use of alcohol. Vomiting blood is an ominous sign.

12. Black bowel movements or blood in the stool are warnings to see your physician right away. The first concern is cancer of the colon but the cause could also be hemorrhoids or a benign inflammatory condition of the colon.

13. Blurred vision.

14. Shortness of breath, fever and/or a cough with yellow-green discharge.

15. Dizziness and confusion.

16. Unrelieved depression.

Other symptoms which should alert you are: pains in the chest for longer than a few minutes; sexual dysfunction which could be due to diabetes, thyroid problems or tumors; changes in sleep habits; drug reactions; a change in bowel habits; or changes in skin in the form of nodules, pigment spots and frequent bleeding gums.

Some patients are afraid of the truth—afraid that they have a serious problem which will be identified. Thus, they deny symptoms and signs. It is better to seek help earlier.

IF I HAVE PAIN—TREATING SYMPTOMS

19. Shouldn't I be treated if I have pain or symptoms? Why weren't my symptoms treated?

Pain may be sudden and severe, suggesting an acute problem like a heart attack, or gradual and nagging, suggesting a chronic problem like a strain or sprain. Pain has close relationships with our lives and our perceptions of the world in general and our bodies in particular. If something is bothering you, it is bothering you. No one should tell you it is not bothering you. A friend or a spouse may appropriately say, "Try not to let it bother you so much." This is a more sympathetic suggestion but you should not deny the presence of a pain, an ache or anxiety.

It may be extremely hard for your doctor to make a definitive diagnosis, or to find the exact cause, of an initial complaint, which is what we call your symptom. When you feel pain, either physical or emotional, your doctor enters this in the records as a "complaint." Medical histories begin with what we call the "Chief Complaint". Medical students, interns, and residents are taught to record it in your medical record.

Many illnesses begin with a few signs or symptoms that are not recognized initially by the individual. For example, a 60-year-old person notices one day that his bowel movement seems to be darker than usual even though he is not taking supplemental iron by mouth or eating seafood that could darken the stool. Dark stool can signal cancer of the colon, which frequently begins with a small amount of bleeding into the colon. This person, however, does nothing until other symptoms appear: fatigue, weakness, and pale skin and eyes. A simple blood test discloses anemia, most commonly caused in a 60 year-old by carcinoma of the colon. If on the right side of the colon, the ascending colon, the cancer may already have spread to the liver.

A more cautious person who notices dark stool over the next few weeks consults his doctor who tests a stool sample for a trace of blood. Positive results should lead to a study of the lining of the colon by a colonoscopy and/ or by an x-ray study in which barium is put into the rectum. If the colon is normal then other potential causes of slow bleeding from the gastrointestinal tract are sought.

Blood in the stool in a middle aged person is ominous. An ache or a pain somewhere in the body may or may not be harmless. Consider a person who one day experiences sharp pain in the left upper abdomen close to the lower ribs. The doctor first seeks a local and simple explanation. Has the person received a blow there or done strenuous exercise or lifting that could have pulled a muscle or had a paroxysm of coughing? Is the pain associated with breathing or motion of the chest wall? If so, it may involve the lung or the lining of the lung, the pleura. If the pain is persistent, bothersome and localized, further study is in order.

Possible causes of the pain include diseases of the colon, the lung, the spleen and the diaphragm. Another is a cancer of the tail or end of the pancreas, although this is an unusual tumor and not high on our list of possibilities. We use a computerized-tomographic (CT) scan of the abdomen to look for pancreatic cancer. How long should we wait before ordering such a study? We have no definite rules.

What is important for you to know and to tell your doctor are the answers to these questions: 1) Does the pain persist for some days? 2) Is it consistent each day; does it wax and wane? 3) Could a direct cause exist—bumping into a door the night before or bleeding hemorrhoids? 4) Is it associated with anything else that you do? With this information, you and your doctor must consider how aggressively to pursue the cause. Keeping a diary will help. What is your own personal threshold for pain? It may vary with what is happening in your life.

Finding a cause for persistent and unexplained pain may be difficult. Pain, whether vague or definite, localized or general, persistent or intermittent, may defy initial diagnostic studies. The pain may persist even after negative results for X-rays, CT scans, blood studies, ECGs, heart catheterization for heart function and an angiogram (injection of dye into the coronary arteries to evaluate them). Consultation with a neurologist and/or a neurosurgeon may give a clue. Other specialists may help. What if no cause is found? What if treatment by pain medications for relief is leading to addiction? The next step is referral to a pain clinic where experts try local anesthetic blocks, sympathetic nervous system, nerve or ganglion blocks or other methods to decrease pain perception.

Remember, there is much we do not know. Sometimes diseases defy an exact diagnosis, at least early in their course. It may be necessary to repeat diagnostic studies, such as a CT scan, every few months to see if any new findings could explain your pain. Dr. Gawande says most doctors believe that pain is due to an injury or an abnormality. This dates back to René Descartes who wrote over three centuries ago that pain is purely a physical phenomenon. Dr. Beecher observed during World War II that severity of pain and pain medication required were not closely related to severity of injury. Then in 1965 Melzack and Wall theorized that pain signals go through a gate-control mechanism in the spinal cord before getting to the brain, a process that can decrease or increase the perception of pain. New information suggests that pain is not a passive signal felt in the brain but generated by the brain itself in "neuromodules" with or without signals from elsewhere in the body. A neuromodule is not a separate or specific part of the brain but rather a network. Patients with pain where no cause can be found are not imagining their pain but rather experiencing a circuit problem in the brain. Treatment centers on drugs that quiet down these circuits. Anti-epileptic drugs help some such patients. (Chapters 8 and 23)

Doctors are taught to strive to make a diagnosis, to find the specific exact cause for your problem—whether a duodenal ulcer, cancer of the lung or a heart attack. Determination of treatment and the possibility of cure require a specific diagnosis. If no specific disease or cause is found initially for your symptoms, given time they may go away by themselves. In the meanwhile, what about the symptoms that brought you to the doctor—a cough, fever, or pain? You would like treatment and should receive it.

Years ago doctors carried a bag of medicines with them when they made house calls. They would give you something for what seemed to ail you. Pharmacies were not readily available and over-the-counter medicines were not common. I remember comments by my parents that, if you went to a particular doctor, he would always give you a bunch of pills. In those days antibiotics were not available. Cures may not have been possible but treatment for symptoms was always given.

Some say that doctors now are too scientific and don't care enough. This should not get in the way of trying to relieve and comfort.

In our zeal to make a diagnosis, we can overdo. An elderly aunt of my mother's had some unusual complaints. I recommended that she be admitted to a hospital to get to the bottom of her problem. She came into the hospital on the medicine service and was immediately put through intense diagnostic studies. She was wheeled from this lab to that. Usually an active woman, she was now always in bed or on a cart going somewhere for studies. After three days of this she developed blood clots in her leg. One went to her lung—a pulmonary embolus—and killed her. No one ever did determine what was wrong with her.

STOICAL PEOPLE—PAIN CLINIC

20. Why does a little pain bother me a lot? How can I get pain relief?

The amount of pain that bothers you is called your pain threshold and is different for everyone. Generally, women tolerate pain fairly well, perhaps because they have more experience with it due to menstrual cramps and childbirth. Young males have less experience unless they have had injuries. Recent surveys by Men's *Health Magazine* and CNN showed that men with severe chest pain are less likely than women to see a doctor or go to an emergency ward. Their reluctance may reflect stoicism, confidence that they are fine or fear that they are not. But it may not be safe to ignore pain and try to carry on.

The perception of pain—how bad it seems or how much it bothers you—is also very closely related to how you feel about yourself. Are you lonely or depressed? Do you feel sorry for yourself? Bothersome pain should lead you to see a doctor for tests to determine the cause. Your doctor can prescribe pain medication beginning with non-narcotic agents and going on to narcotics such as codeine, demerol or oxycontin only if necessary and then for a short time. More powerful narcotics such as morphine are reserved for short-term use in a hospital or for terminally ill patients in a hospice. For patients with pain from metastatic cancer the threat of addiction is not a problem.

What is a pain clinic or pain center?

Persistent pain is a common health problem. It is estimated that fifty million Americans have chronic pain lasting over six months. Pain should be checked as the fifth vital sign along with pulse, blood pressure, temperature and respiratory rate.

Many hospitals now have pain centers where the medical staff has expertise in the study and relief of pain, a specialty called algology. Algologists may be anesthesiologists, psychiatrists, psychologists, neurologists, physical therapists, and neurosurgeons, all working together. With many advances in pain control, many doctors recommend that it be called pain medicine, not just pain management.

The many different methods of therapy in use include medications, epidural steroid injections along the spinal cord, implantable devices that give drugs intermittently, biofeedback, physical therapy, psychological interventions, nerve blocks, intrathecal or spinal, pumps, and spinal cord stimulators. Better posture may play a part. Occupational and behavioral factors may come into play.

Acupuncture is used for a number of painful conditions. Kim recommends it for treatment of arthritis; headaches; facial pain; post-herpetic neuralgia; painful forefoot (Morton's neuroma); pain with malignancy; childbirth; menstrual pain and cramps; painful surgical scars and fractured bones; phantom limb pain; pain from healed bone fractures; and neck, elbow and lower back pain. Multimodal pain management strategies include education about surgery in advance of an operation, nonopioid analgesics, local anesthetic techniques, opioids and alternative nonpharmacologic therapies and consultation. At some hospitals, pain management teams visit patients and distribute pain management brochures.

For more information contact: American Academy of Pain Management, 209-533-9744 or *www.aapainmanage.org*; American Chronic Pain Association 916-632-0922, *www.theacpa.org*; American Pain Foundation 888-615-7246, *www.painfoundation.org*.

PROGNOSIS

21. What does the future hold for me after treatment of a disease?

You should ask your doctor and receive a reply. Remember, however, that no doctor has a crystal ball. All your doctor can do is to give you an educated guess, drawing upon experiences with similar patients or the medical literature. If you have a certain kind of cancer of the lung that is removed completely and all lymph nodes do not contain tumor and the cancer has not spread to other organs in distant metastases, then you have a 65% statistical chance of being alive and free of tumor in five years. However, for you the tumor may return sooner, later, or never. You are not a statistic.

People are told on occasion they have only a short time to live. I believe patients should always be told the truth. However, no patient should be given a death sentence. Your doctor cannot know how long you will live. You may want as accurate a prediction as your doctor can make so that you can make plans. You may wish to sell your business, retire, take an extended vacation or stay home with your family but you should always be given hope for the future. Miracles happen. Wonderful things occur because of a positive attitude, faith, and enthusiasm for life and those around you. Don't give up. (Chapter 17 "Faith, Hope and a Positive Attitude."

Chronic illness, crippling diseases and other problems may prevent you from being fully active. You can enjoy other aspects of life—family, friends, music, literature and other interests. I urge my patients: Don't ever give up, and don't let anyone count you out. When the end approaches you can hold your head high and say "I did what I could do."

PRIVACY

22. Does everyone have to know what is wrong with me? Whatever happened to confidentiality?

P roblems with confidentiality arise with third-party payers, insurance carriers, and managed care groups that require access to your medical record. Concerns about patient privacy also go along with the use of electronic medical records and patient data transfer by computer. As reviewed by Portman, this information may be available to hackers or others not entitled to it. The DHHS described a need for federal legislation as both real and urgent. Their recommendations to the U.S. Congress should be enacted. As described by Portman, they would prevent holders of individually identifiable health information from using or disclosing it without the patient's consent. Disclosures would be limited to minimal information. An employer would not be able to use health information for personnel decisions. The DHHS calls for security measures, consumer control, accountability and penalties for noncompliance. This recommended legislation tries to balance the need to protect patient privacy rights in health information with the need to insure availability of patient data for socially beneficial purposes.

Medical record and patient confidentiality bills were introduced in two Senate bills and two House bills. They would require your authorization for release of health information and safeguards to prevent unintentional disclosure, and would provide for criminal penalties for violation. Unfortunately, the deadline for passage expired when Congress bowed to pressure from police, district attorneys and the insurance industry. Police can obtain your medical records from hospitals and doctors offices without a court order. Patients have avoided treatment because of fear of disclosure.

The federal Health Insurance Portability and Accountability Act of 1996 dealt with protection of the privacy of your medical information. In 2003 federally mandated privacy rules went into effect for health insurers, health providers and health-care clearing houses. Strict guidelines were set for release of patient health information. Fearing civil and criminal penalties, hospitals perhaps over-reacted. For example, when you go into a hospital as a patient and register as a member of a church or synagogue, they will not let the priest, minister or rabbi know so they can call on you. Many clergy and patients have complained about this.

Here are some rules that provide protection: information from a patient's medical records cannot be disclosed to an employer without specific authorization by the patient; patients can review and request corrections of errors in their medical records; researchers cannot use names, addresses or social security numbers of patients in a disease outbreak; drugstores cannot give your name to drug companies.

Genetic test results must also be protected. Some states are protecting you but Congress must act. Health plans and insurers must not be allowed access to your genetic information or the ability to prohibit enrollment on the basis of such information. We must prevent insurers and employers from requiring genetic tests. Many industries are opposed to such prohibition.

Public health review, or surveillance as it is called, is an important part of disease control. Epidemiologists need to identify, study and document epidemics, sexually transmitted diseases, the frequency of infectious disease outbreaks, food poisoning occurrences, cases of tuberculosis, health status of workers, cancer registries, the need for quarantine and many public health issues. The question is: Should the studies name individuals or just groups? In some cases the protection of public health may require some limitations on privacy. Thus, although medical privacy is a fundamental value, it is not an absolute, as noted by Bayer and Fairchild.

NEW DISEASES

23. There always seems to be a new virus. Where do all of these new diseases come from? Are some chronic diseases caused by infection? What is "mad cow" disease and where did it come from? What is foot and mouth disease?

Infectious diseases are the leading cause of death in the world and the third leading cause of death in the U.S. In response to the growing problem, the Centers for Disease Prevention and Control (CDCP) track epidemics and public health threats around the world, through their Epidemic

Intelligence Service. In its own survey, the *Harvard Health Letter* notes the emergence of more than 30 new infectious diseases in the past 20 years. Ten diseases thought to be suppressed have resurfaced. Contributing factors include global warming, environmental degradation, and international travel.

Many bacteria have developed resistance to antibiotics, an increasing hazard. Tuberculosis, malaria and streptococcus pneumonia now appear in resistant forms. Infectious diseases of wildlife are reservoirs of pathogens. One problem with diseases worldwide is the cost of vaccinations, a problem addressed by Bill Gates' foundation with a donation of a billion dollars to WHO.

New diseases may come from mutations, or spontaneous changes in the DNA of gene structure, in viruses and bacteria. Bacteria and viruses can acquire human genes which make them more dangerous, as happened with tuberculosis. Some diseases with no known cause previously have now been found to be due to bacteria, among them Whipple's disease of the digestive tract, ulcer disease and stomach cancer. In 1967 the Surgeon General of the U.S. said that "the time has come to close the book on infectious diseases." This is no longer true. Kreiswirth said "The World Health Organization and global society have to be concerned now about the threat of an increase in infectious diseases." There will always be new diseases.

Infectious diseases are a threat to increasing numbers of patients with immunity diminished by chemotherapy, organ transplants, diabetes, the effects of surgery and human immunodeficiency virus (HIV) infections. In HIV infections, the virus attacks the body's immune system, particularly the T cells that control acquired immunity, and produces the acquired immunodeficiency syndrome or AIDS. Victims become susceptible to opportunistic infections or malignancies, causing wasting and death. The virus was thought to be confined to African monkeys until it was transmitted to humans by bites, transfer of mucous substances or other contact. Among humans it is transmitted by blood, blood-contaminated needles and sexual contact. The pandemic of HIV infection requires development of a vaccine, which may be forthcoming, but in the meantime the best defense is preventive measures, like education about safe sexual practices. As pointed out by Nathanson and Auerbach, it is necessary to realize "The full potential of prevention science to help stem the HIV/AIDS epidemic in the U.S. and around the world."

The herpes simplex virus type 2 is also sexually transmitted. Attempted development of antibodies and vaccines so far has not been effective in treating this problem.

Other new viruses have caused transient epidemics in Africa. From a reservoir in shrews, rodents and chimpanzees, the Ebola virus surfaced in Congo and Sudan in 1976 and re-occurred in Uganda in 2000 and Gabon in 2001. One of the most virulent diseases in man, it causes vomiting, diarrhea and internal and external bleeding after transmission by body fluids—mucous, saliva and blood. Rift valley fever spread by mosquitoes has spread from Africa to Saudi Arabia and Yemen. A fatal illness called the New World Arenavirus has come to the U.S. from Africa. Now human diseases such as measles, polio and scabies may threaten great apes.

A new virus, the Nipah virus, was identified in Malaysia and spread from pigs and bats to people. A new parahaemoloyticus vibrio has been found in raw oysters. The West Nile virus now active in the eastern U.S. came from the Middle East. A new tick borne disease, Chaffeensis, was found in Connecticut. The other more common tick-borne problem is Lyme Disease, discovered 25 years ago by Dr. Allen Steere. Opinions vary as to how common it is for it may be confused with chronic fatigue, mental illness or fibromyalgia. One injection of the antibiotic doxycycline will prevent the disease if given within three days of the tick bite. Ticks also may carry viruses for encephalitis. The influenza virus from birds is a threat.

Some infections find their source in bad food. The consumption of undercooked beef, fresh cheese and eggs has led to E. Coli infections. A similar link exists between campylobacter infection and raw poultry, meat and unpasteurized milk. Contaminated food and water have caused outbreaks of Hepatitis A, which produces diarrhea, nausea, fatigue and jaundice. It is highly contagious, sometimes spreading from sick food handlers to food and so called deli-belly. Children should be vaccinated where outbreaks have occurred. A Listeria organism causing gastroenteritis comes from corn. Salmonella infection in the intestine may come from infected cattle. Close confinement of pigs and chickens promotes infection with resistant organisms. Cute chicks and ducklings given to children may transmit salmonella infection.

Another new virus, parvovirus B19, produces the glowing rash of "Fifth Disease." It is self limited. A small parasite causes the infection cryptosporidiosis, marked by protracted outbreaks of diarrhea, vomiting and abdominal cramps. Resistant to chlorine, the parasite sometimes gets into swimming pools through fecal contamination by swimmers with the disease.

In Latin America a "kissing bug" (a pink bollworm moth) carries a parasite that transmits the deadly chagas disease. Other diseases such as meningococcal meningitis from Neisseria meningitidis are less common but well known. These have been called emerging infectious diseases.

The severe acute respiratory distress syndrome (SARS) is a new respiratory infection originating in the Guandong Province of China in late 2002 and spreading throughout Southeast Asia, Europe and North America. This highly virulent and contagious disease produces respiratory failure and death in ten percent of patients. Ventilatory support is the only treatment at present. The cause seems to be a new coronavirus, transmitted by sputum, and perhaps by stool.

We have no clue as to the origin of hepatitis C infection, previously called non-A, non-B hepatitis, now spreading worldwide. We know of no animal reservoir. The main routes of transmission are tainted blood transfusions and dirty needles. Called "the silent killer," this virus damages the liver, often after many years. It is estimated four million Americans may be unknowingly infected. For many of them nothing bad will happen but twenty to thirty percent will develop cirrhosis of the liver and some may develop liver cancer or liver failure. If not infected now, it is unlikely that you will be in the future. Since 1992 blood screening has succeeded in eliminating the use of hepatitis C-contaminated blood in transfusions. A reduction in drugs and needle use also help contain the epidemic. Aggressive 24 week therapy with interferon-alfa-2b will get rid of the virus. This must be done before late effects develop. Vaccines are being developed. Meanwhile yet another new hepatitis virus may have emerged.

For additional information about the hepatitis C virus, contact the CDCP, Hepatitis Hotline, 888-443-7233, or www.cdc.gov/ncidod/diseases/hepatitis.

The most common sexually transmitted infection now is the papilloma virus, transmissive even if condoms are used. It is estimated that ten million young American woman have active infections. The virus may produce no symptoms but does produce cancer of the cervix. That is why all sexually active women over the age of 18 should have a pap smear with virus testing at least once a year, and, if the virus is present, every 4-6 months. Some forms of the virus target the skin of the hands and feet and lining of the mouth.

A new scientific technique called the polymerase chain reaction (PCR) allows the identification of new diseases by detecting small fragments of bacterial DNA in the blood of sick patients. This can indicate not only the presence of an infection but its cause. In many infections the bacteria or virus cannot be grown in culture and identified. PCR helps with such identification. Infectious disease experts at the CDCP are working with a special pathogen laboratory, the Unexplained Illness working group in California to identify new infectious diseases. Seventy known enterovirus strains have been found. This has led to many exciting contributions.

Are some chronic diseases caused by infection?

For years, we thought duodenal and gastric ulcers were caused by stress with too much stomach acid. Now we know that the cause is the bacterium Helicobacter pylori, a spiral bacterium in the stomach. The ulcers can be treated with antibiotics and vaccines are being developed. Whipple's disease, which prevents normal absorption of nutrients from the small intestine, is caused by bacteria. Many cancers are caused by infectious agents, particularly viruses. Chlamydia pneumoniae organisms have been found in arteriosclerotic placques in the aorta. Infection elsewhere in the body is associated with blockage of coronary arteries. Patients with chlamydia infections are more likely to have strokes and, possibly, multiple sclerosis. A study is underway to see if antibiotics will help. A Borna disease virus could be involved with schizophrenia, autism, panic disorders, chronic fatigue syndrome and bipolar disease. Herpes simplex viruses have been implicated in Alzheimer's disease and schizophrenia. Infection may be the cause of other chronic diseases.

Some diseases have been around for a while but until only recently have gone unnamed. Fibromyalgia, first investigated by rheumatologists in the 1970s but not named until 1990, produces persistent muscle pain in most of the body and sometimes severe fatigue, diarrhea, insomnia, abdominal bloating, headache and bladder irritability. Groopman indicates nearly six million Americans may have this disease. In the past many Fibromyalgia patients would have been called hypochondriacs. The cause may be increased sensory perception and unusual sensitivity to pain. Rooks has developed a program of exercise, flexibility and strength training for treatment at the Beth Israel Deaconess Hospital in Boston, and many patients have responded favorably.

Diseases that may be on the way out include poliomyelitis, guinea-worm disease in Africa, measles, lymphatic filariasis in Africa, Asia and South America, river blindness in Africa, blinding trachoma, leprosy, hepatitis B, maternal-neonatal tetanus and iodine deficiency disorders. Small pox seems to be gone.

Anthrax gave us a scare in the U.S. recently as a possible bioterrorism agent. A safe vaccine is being given to U.S. troops. For inhalational anthrax, an early diagnosis and new drugs—triple antibiotics—may save lives.

What is mad cow disease?

Bovine spongiform encephalopathy (BSE) or mad-cow disease, is a chronic, progressive and fatal disease in cattle caused not by a virus, bacteria, parasite or fungus but by a radically different new infectious agent, a prion, an abnormal or misfolded protein that damages the brain. Untreatable, incurable and ultimately fatal, the disease gets its name from the strange behavior of infected cattle. Symptoms include loss of movement of the rear legs so that the cattle can no longer stand up. They lose weight and die in two weeks to six months. The disease spreads from animal to animal by feeding cattle with infected animal parts, particularly meat and bone meal (MBM). A very small amount of infected material will transmit the disease. Since 1986 180,000 infected cattle have been found in the UK and smaller numbers in other countries in Europe but BSE has not been identified in the United States. The USDA and the beef industry have what seems to be adequate surveillance and controls to prevent or control its development in the US. The US cattle industry used much less animal based feed than did their counterparts in Europe and the UK and now uses none.

When people eat contaminated beef they may develop the human equivalent of the disease, called new variant Creutzfeld-Jakob disease (nvCJD), a fatal or incurable disease in humans that may take 10 years to develop. The disease results in progressive rapid dementia, muscle and balance problems, and inability to walk. So far the disease has killed 187 people in the UK, 3 in France and 1 in Ireland. Beef sales plummeted abroad but while you should limit your intake of beef in this country for a number of health reasons so far the threat of BSE or nvCJD is not one of them. For comparison each year in the U.S. 323,000 people go to a hospital because of bacteria contaminated food and 5,000 of them die. The AMA, FDA, USDA and DHHS are all carrying out safeguards for Americans. If you travel abroad, be careful about eating beef brains or cuts containing spinal cord from cattle, like the popular T-bone steak No one can be sure where BSE came from. A similar disease occurs in some wild animals. A similar disease in sheep called scrapie is not transmitted to humans.

Another prion disease is Fatal Familial Insomnia (FFI), an incurable genetic disease that usually begins between the ages of 40 and 60, with slight insomnia. At the end victims cannot sleep at all. It is a strange disease.

What is foot and mouth disease?

The very infectious picorna virus is the cause of this widespread disease of cattle, pigs, sheep and goats (cloven hoofed animals), the most contagious disease known. Inhaling ten virus particles carried by the wind can transmit the disease. In young animals the outcome can be fatal with cardiac arrest. Most adult animals recover but produce less meat and milk. The only effective control is to kill all the animals in a herd if it develops in one of them. Thousands of animals were slaughtered during the recent epidemic in England. So far, the disease has not reached the U.S. due to the vigilance of the USDA and Immigration authorities.

RISK VERSUS BENEFIT

24. What is meant by risk versus benefit?

Every treatment whether it be a medicine, an operation or treatment has some risk. You could have a reaction to the medicine. You could lose your hair from chemotherapy. Chemotherapy and x-ray therapy for cancer may damage your bone marrow so that you don't have enough blood cells to fight infection. There are many potential complications of operations. Some can occur after any operation, such as bleeding, a wound infection, a heart problem, a blood clot in the legs going to the lungs, a stroke and other events. In addition, there are complications occurring after specific operations, such as a clot forming in a bypass graft or compression of the trachea (windpipe) causing trouble breathing after a thyroidectomy. Some of these complications could kill you. Also, you may have a disease that makes a treatment or an operation very risky.

Thus, we try to estimate the risk to you to have a treatment or an operation as compared with how much benefit you will receive. In emergency situations where your problem is life threatening you may accept a higher risk. If your medical problem is not urgent such as an inguinal hernia, gallstones or some other benign condition then the risk should be low before you agree to have it corrected. For cancer, the risk must be balanced against what your doctors believe can be accomplished. If a cancer involves an organ which can be removed completely (the lung, colon, stomach) this is the best cancer treatment unless the tumor has spread elsewhere. Sometimes this can't be determined without an operation. Risk versus benefit is something you can discuss with your doctor.

PSYCHIATRIST

25. Why was I referred to a psychiatrist?

Your doctor referred you to a professional doctor to counsel you, help you or treat you for problems of life adjustment such as depression, anxiety, agoraphobia and many other conditions. Psychiatrists also treat patients with severe mental disorders called psychoses, like schizophrenia, manic-depressive disorders and others, but they treat many more patients with problems of life adjustment.

Psychiatrists can do much for patients with severe mental illness or psychoses to allow them to function to some extent in society. Help is available for patients with psychosomatic illnesses in which emotions bring on physical or functional problems and with psychosocial illnesses in which emotions alter behavior. A generalized anxiety disorder, said to be the most common of all mental disorders, is treatable by biofeedback, cognitive-behavioral therapy, medication, psychotherapy or a combination of these. Depression, also common, is very treatable when diagnosed. It should not be thought of as a weakness. Depression is common in elderly people and should be treated.

All diseases, however, have some psychological aspects, and it is my impression that the greatest contribution of psychiatry is to help us adjust to our problems and environment so that we may live happier, healthier and more productive lives. My wife and I sought out psychiatrists for our children, as did I for my own need to stop smoking cigarettes. You should not feel bad if your doctor suggests psychiatric help to benefit you. Think about it, talk with your doctor about it, ask questions and determine what concerns you. It does not mean a label has been put on you. It does not mean you have a mental illness.

Of course, some psychiatrists do like to put labels on people. If some patients are labile, getting high emotionally and then low or depressed, some psychiatrists may be too quick to call them manic-depressives. A true manic-depressive, however, has a psychosis, a persistent and serious mental illness. In contrast, for many of us our moods go up and down only on occasion, and as a matter of personality. Resist the use of a label for you without a definite and exact reason for that label.

FOOD PROBLEMS

26. What are the differences among food intolerance, food allergies, and food poisoning?

You may have had abdominal pain, cramps, vomiting, gas and/or diarrhea shortly after eating ice cream, shellfish, frog legs or other favorite foods. This was not a case of a food allergy but rather of *food intolerance*. Your gastrointestinal tract did not tolerate the food or something with it, in it or on it.

Food intolerance is caused by the body's inability to metabolize certain foods, like lactose in milk and saffrose in beans, but the cause of any particular case is often unknown. Milk products, citrus fruits, spicy foods and fatty foods may cause trouble. In the event of an attack it is important thing to record exactly what you ate and to avoid it in future. Could it have been contaminated? Was it washed thoroughly? If you wish to experiment and can tolerate it, try eating the food alone to learn whether it causes trouble again. Milk is a good candidate for this kind of trial. Lactose intolerance to milk may turn out to have been temporary.

Like food intolerance, a food allergy may produce vomiting, diarrhea, and cramps. In addition, however, it produces allergic manifestations of hives, swollen lips, swollen tongue, mouth and throat. In response to a protein in certain foods, the body's immune system releases antibodies that attach to immune cells, or mast cells, which then release chemicals such as histamine causing an allergic reaction. Other possible reactions include itchy skin and itchy lips or throat.

Most seriously, an episode of food allergy can lead to an anaphylactic reaction or anaphylactic shock. This is a sudden, severe and potentially life-threatening reaction with swelling of the tongue and throat and difficulty in breathing, with wheezing as in asthma, or bronchospasm. It can occur in minutes or seconds after ingestion of the responsible agent. Treatment requires prompt injection of epinephrine to relax the breathing tubes and contract dilated blood vessels. If you ever have hives, feel faint, choke or wheeze after eating something, see a doctor or an emergency facility right away and take precautions for the future. If you are not sure what caused your reaction, an allergist may give you a skin or blood test to help determine it. The diagnosis is dependent on elimination diets, skin testing and antibody assays (for serum—specific IgE antibodies, by a radioallergosorbent test).

According to the Harvard Health Letter, the causes of most allergic reactions are cow's milk, eggs, fish, shellfish, peanuts, soy protein, legumes, wheat, and tree nuts like walnuts and cashews. By school age most children "grow out" of allergies to food, except for allergies to seafood and nuts, which may be lifelong, but adults can develop allergies to foods that have not bothered them before. Exercise after eating can also trigger an allergic reaction.

Peanut allergy is a growing problem in this country, and processing may play a role. In the U.S. most peanuts are dry roasted. In China, where peanut allergies occur less often, peanuts are boiled or fried. It is not enough for people with this allergy to avoid peanuts *per se*. They must be on the alert for the hidden use of peanuts in other foods, carefully checking labels of baked goods, baking mixes, pastries, battered and breaded foods, breakfast cereals, candy and chocolates, Chinese, Thai and Vietnamese foods, ice cream, margarine, vegetable fats/oils, snack chips, soups, soup mixes and snacks. Children with a family history of allergy should avoid all peanut products until age three. A vaccine is under study.

The only treatment for a food allergy is avoidance of the food. Those who have anaphylactic reactions should carry an Emergency Epinephrine (EPI) Pen or ANA kit with them, ready for use at the first sign of an anaphylactic reaction. Patients with allergies to foods, antibiotics and other substances should wear a bracelet, necklace or medallion with personal medical identification, available at American Medical Identification, PO Box 925517, Houston, TX, 77292-5617; 1-800-363-5985. For more information about food allergy contact the Food Allergy and Anaphylaxis Network at 800-929-4040 or *www.foodallergy.org*, the Academy of Allergy, Asthma and Immunology at 1-800-822-2762 or *www.aaaai.org* and/or the National Institutes of Allergy and Infectious Diseases for the food allergies fact sheet: *www.niaid.nih.gov/factsheets/food.htm*. For a list of foods recalled due to possible contamination with allergens—*www.safetyalerts.com/rcls/category/alrgy.htm*.

What is food poisoning?

I once thought I had frog leg intolerance because of severe abdominal cramps and diarrhea after eating frog legs on two occasions. I learned later the frogs had eaten an herbicide sprayed around the pond where I had caught them. The chemical was the culprit; normal frog legs later caused no problem. It was a case of food poisoning and not food intolerance.

The General Accounting Office estimates that 85% of food poisoning cases come from fruits, vegetables, seafood and cheese. Symptoms usually appear 12 to 24 hours after an incident of food poisoning, although reaction to a toxin may occur within three to six hours. Food-borne illness fall into three basic categories: 1) intoxication/poisoning, with the production of toxins in the food by bacteria, 2) consumption of the bacteria, viruses or parasites, 3) and toxic effect upon the nervous system, with the occurrence of neurological symptoms. Wash fruits and vegetables well to remove traces of insecticides or other poisons that can cause toxic reactions.

In the *Harvard Men's Health Watch*, health officials estimate 30 million Americans contract food-borne infections each year and perhaps as many as 9,000 die. See Chapter 23 for some of the leading pathogens. Others include *Closteria* in chopped meat, and staphylococci in custards and mayonnaise. *Trichomonas* may be present in pork and fungi, molds and insects in fruits, spices and grains. Parasites such as the ascaris worm, flat worms, pin worms, tape worms and others in the G.I. tract can be big problems.

The vast majority of foods are not tested for toxins or bacteria but adequate cooking will kill many of these agents and make the food safe. Meat, beef as well as pork, should be well cooked as should eggs. A rare steak or roast beef may cause problems. Proper food handling should decrease, if not eliminate, disease from food. There is no excuse for sloppy food handling.

The Harvard *Men's Health Watch* recommends some "low-tech prevention":

- Shop at reputable markets, check expiration dates, never buy cracked eggs, get pasteurized fruit drinks, etc.
- If concern about pesticides leads you to organic produce, remember it does not protect you from infection. You must still wash food well before cooking.
- Keep your kitchen and instruments scrupulously clean.
- Cook meat and poultry thoroughly. Never leave previously frozen poultry, meat or fish at room temperature for over 30 minutes when thawed out.
- Avoid rare and undercooked foods.

Be careful with leftovers—don't keep them after four to five days.

Outbreaks of food poisoning should be reported to your city, county and state health departments. States have milk boards to assure a safe milk supply and food protection. At least a dozen federal agencies are involved in keeping food safe, including the FDA, CDC and the EPA

Is irradiation of food safe?

The FDA says irradiation of food is safe, with no hazard to those who cook or eat the food. It also will kill all the organisms previously mentioned that may be in contaminated food. All irradiated foods will be labeled as such but you have no reason to avoid them. I am convinced of the safety of irradiation and recommend it.

Section C

Emergencies

CALLING 911—WAITS IN EMERGENCY ROOMS.

27. When should I call 911?

That is a difficult question. Use of the 911 systems for non-emergency conditions is widespread. True emergency conditions, such as time-dependent illnesses in which a patient may get into trouble during the prehospital period, represent only about 5% of all calls to 911 centers. Urgent conditions represent another 20 to 25%. The remaining 75% include inappropriate calls that may cause ambulances and EMTs to be unavailable for true emergencies. One should call 911 when it is a necessity and not a convenience. Please see the table for specific suggestions. Many areas are developing alternative methods of handling the overwhelming number of 911 calls for non-emergent problems. This is being implemented in St. Louis with the Emergency Medical Priority Dispatch System developed by Clauson, et al., in Salt Lake City. The system allows operators at 911 to question the patient about the problem and decide on a priority, a first step toward improving emergency medical service operations.

The FDC has announced it will allow local areas to use a 311 public access number for non-emergency calls, to relieve the overburdened 911 system. The need for 311 indicates success of the 911 system for a universally recognized access point for emergency medical services. The use of 311 for non-emergency conditions may help patients get the health care advice they need 24 hours a day.

Alternative transport systems are also being developed, to prevent the use of 911 as a taxi service. In San Diego, for example, Ambucabs transport non-emergency patients to medical providers. The dilemma is that we encourage patients to seek medical attention early for a number of possibly acute events for which we can help them. Limiting that opportunity could be a problem. At present, however, overuse of the 911 system and emergency facilities outweighs the difficulty of evaluation. When true emergencies wait because the EMS system is serving as a taxi service, we have a situation that requires urgent attention.

Some medical insurers or HMOs, like Kaiser Permanente, have a health plan emergency number. The person answering may be thousands of miles away but can give advice. Health plans now want to oversee your emergency services. This concerns many doctors and may undermine the 911 system. Medical decisions about what is an emergency should not be in the hands of a dispatcher.

Who should decide? This has recently been reviewed by Gambill.

Table

When to Call

It is appropriate to call 911 if you have an emergency which does not allow you to travel to a hospital in a private car or by taxi or you are by yourself and unable to drive. Call 911 if you think treatment by paramedics is needed before you can get to a hospital. Specific circumstances are:

- An accident with injuries
- Severe sudden chest pain
- Severe difficulty breathing
- Uncontrollable bleeding
- A fall with severe hip pain and the inability to get up. If you are lying on your back and your foot on the painful side is pointed out from your body, you probably have a broken hip
- Convulsions—unconsciousness
- Uncontrollable vomiting and/or diarrhea
- Severe pain in the chest after vomiting
- A stroke and inability to walk or get around
- Any problem where you would have to be transported to a hospital on a stretcher

Waits in emergency rooms. When I go to a hospital emergency room for a health problem, why do I have to wait so long?

Perhaps you wait because your problem is not really an emergency. When I worked in an emergency ward, I once saw a patient at 3 a.m. complaining of a bad headache, which he had had for two weeks. Unable to sleep he had come to the emergency ward for a checkup. Right after him waited four true emergencies: three patients with severe burns and one with a stab wound of the heart. For non-emergency health problems like the headache, call your doctor. Don't use an emergency ward as your primary care doctor or as a primary care clinic. Emergency wards are staffed and equipped for true emergencies. They should not take care of health problems that are not emergencies.

The difficulty we all have is identifying a true emergency. How does a patient with chest pain know that it is heartburn and not a heart attack? How does a doctor know unless he sees the patient? Something that has been bothering you for some days and has not increased in severity is not likely to be an emergency. Shapiro lists appropriate indications for use of an emergency department as:

(1) severe acute conditions within the past 72 hours;
(2) fever above 102°F for over 48 hours;
(3) postoperative complications;
(4) acute onset of a problem with inability to be evaluated promptly;
(5) transport by ground or air ambulance to an emergency facility;
(6) severe exacerbation of prior chronic problems.

If you belong to an HMO, be sure to find out which emergency wards you may go to for care. Otherwise, if you go to a different emergency ward, they may be forced to send you to one under contract with your HMO.

Under federal law, if you go to an emergency facility, you must be examined and treated, you cannot be turned away. States have attempted to define emergencies such as one passed recently by the Missouri State legislature and contained in the Managed Care Reform Legislation quoted by Fred Peterson:

> An emergency medical condition is defined as the sudden and at the time unexpected onset of a health condition that manifests itself by symptoms of sufficient severity that would lead a prudent lay person, possessing an average knowledge of health and medicine, to believe that immediate medical care is required.

Such an approach may affect mostly the Medicaid population because they may believe they have no resources or places to go for health care other than an ER. O'Grady quoted by Shapiro says, that, patients who do not share costs for emergency department expenses make more ER visits than do patients who must co-pay for service with a health insurance plan. A statewide voluntary program to increase access to primary physicians has decreased the use of emergency facilities.

Another problem for emergency facilities relates to alcohol abuse. Drunks are frequently brought to emergency wards and are kept there for 23 hours until they sober up and can be discharged or taken to jail wherever they belong. This is a misuse of hospital emergency facilities.

We have no easy answer as to what is a necessary visit to an emergency ward and what is not. I believe it is better to err on the side of being evaluated and getting care rather than not going at all. Some people believe ER charges for non-urgent care should be reduced. If you go to an emergency ward for a sprained ankle or a sore throat, charges of $200 to $300 may seem unnecessarily high. However, an emergency ward is a very high cost facility because of the need for specialized and excellent physicians and nurses on call, or awake and working in rotation 24 hours a day.

Section D

Women's and Men's Health Issues

WOMEN'S HEALTH

28. A. What are the health problems occurring mostly in women?

H ealth problems specific to women include cancers of the cervix, uterus, and ovaries; premenstrual tension; endometriosis; uterine bleeding; menopause; and pregnancy and delivery. Cancer of the breast is much more frequent in women as is osteoporosis, a thinning of bone with aging that occurs particularly after the menopause. Diseases occurring more frequently in women than in men, accounting for 75 per cent of cases, include multiple sclerosis, rheumatoid arthritis, scleroderma, lupus erythematosus and thyroiditis. The effects of pregnancy, estrogen and prolactin may be involved in these autoimmune diseases in which some cells in the body attack other healthy cells. More information is available at the American Autoimmune Related Diseases Association (AARDA) *www.aarda.org* or 810-776-3900.

Women are vulnerable to pain problems and at higher risk for migraines, arthritis, fibromyalgia, temperomandibular disorders, and pelvic and abdominal pain. Drug metabolism may be different in men and women. The FDA now requires all drug trials to include enough women to detect any differences in toxicity or affects of the agent. Under treatment is more common in women.

As reported in *Healthy Woman, Healthy Lives,* The Harvard Nurses Health Study of more than 120,000 women for 25 years yielded the following lessons: Don't smoke, watch your weight, exercise, eat right, and take a daily multivitamin. Women live longer than men for reasons that are not clear. Lifestyle enters into it.

National Women's Health

The NIH, under pressure from women Senators, created the Office of Research on Women's Health in 1990. They develop research programs on women's health and study whether treatments are more or less effective in women than in men. For more information: Office of Research on Women's Health. www4.od.nih.gov/orwh and the Society for Women's Health Research— *www.womens-health.org.*, 1828 L Street, N.W., Suite 625, Washington, DC 20036, 202-223-8224. Another source is the National Women's Health Information Center is at 200 Independence Avenue, SW, Washington, DC, 20201, 1-800-994-WOMAN (1-800-994-9662) 1-888-220-5466 (TDD), *http://www.4woman.gov.*

What are the most common cancers in women?

The most common cancers in women are cancers of the lung and bronchus, breast, colon, rectum, uterine lining, cervix, ovaries, urinary bladder, pancreas and thyroid gland; non-Hodgkin's lymphoma; and melanoma. Cancer of the lung was less frequent until women took up smoking under heavy solicitation in cigarette advertising. Cancer of the colon also occurs frequently in women.

Most of you are aware of the importance of early detection of breast cancer. It allows treatment before the tumor has spread to lymph nodes underneath the arm or to other places in the body where it can lie dormant for many years only to reappear sometime later in bones, lungs, brain, or elsewhere.

Self-examination of the breasts should be done by you on the same day each month. The Susan G. Komen Breast Foundation recommends the following routine. **In the shower:** Raise one arm and place your hand on the back of your head. Slowly and methodically move the pads of your fingertips over the breast in a circular pattern. Don't forget to feel in the armpit area. Repeat on the other side. **Before a mirror:** With your arms resting at your side, look for changes in the shape of your breasts, swelling, dimpling or indentations in the skin, or changes in the nipple. Then raise your arms over your head and look again. Finally, place the palms of your hands on your hips and press down so that your chest muscles flex. Again, look for changes in the breasts and nipples. **Lying down:** Lie down with a pillow under your right shoulder and your right arm behind your head. Using the pads of your fingertips, make the same circular pattern of your right breast as you did in the shower. Don't forget to feel the armpit and the chest area from the collarbone to below the breast. Repeat, using firmer pressure. Squeeze the nipple gently to see if there is any discharge. Repeat the procedure on the left breast. Report any unusual findings or changes to your physician immediately.

Although breast self-examination is important, mammography remains the single most effective method of early detection of breast cancer. A mammogram will find a smaller nodule than anyone can feel. Richard C. Muckerman II recommends a mammogram for a woman at age 35 to establish a baseline and then every other year after age 40. After age 50, he recommends a yearly mammogram. Women at high risk should have one each year beginning at age 40; those with no risk factors can begin at 45-50. The American Cancer Society (ACS) and National Cancer Institute (NCI) generally agree with these guidelines. In its brochure "8 Tips for Good Mammograms," the ACS stresses the importance of getting the mammogram at a facility with a lot of experience and expert doctors.

Much has appeared in the press recently about problems with mammography. Some people have suggested that early diagnosis of breast cancer by mammography does not lengthen lives. In Lancet on January 8, 2000, a group in the Netherlands claimed an absence of scientific support for breast cancer screening by mammography, a claim that has led to much discussion. I believe, however, as do almost all medical experts in the U.S., that mammograms are of great value. Mammography detects breast cancer about 1.7 years before a woman can detect a lump. When breast cancer is found early, the five year survival rate is about 96%. The cure rate for breast cancer is getting better and many believe that mammography is helping. An imperfect tool, it is the best available. The Federal Preventive Services Task Force and the National Cancer Institute strongly support mammography.

A cancer can be missed because it may look like a "snowball in a blizzard." Overall mammograms miss about 30% of breast cancers, and this has resulted in malpractice suits for "errors of diagnosis." Thus, some radiologists do not want to read mammograms because of the risk. On the other hand, many suspicious findings turn out to be benign. Cancer is suggested but not found, and the outcome may be an unnecessary biopsy. A new technology, a digital mammography system, may help by supplementing the use of x-ray film.

Information for women about problems of breast cancer is available from the American Cancer Society (ACS) at 1-800-ACS-2345 or their website *www.cancer.org.* and from the National Comprehensive Cancer Network (NCCN) (1-888-909-NCCN or www.nccn.org). The Midwest Breast Care Center in St. Louis describe the signs and symptoms of breast cancer, which include: a mass or thickening in the breast; asymmetry of the breasts; a change from normal, prominent veins on one side; unexplained redness or bruising; shiny skin and large pores called a peau d'orange [skin like that of an orange]); ulcerations; dimpling; puckering; retraction of skin or of the nipple; nipple scaling, crusting, erosion, or discharge, especially if bloody or straw-colored; changes in the surface characteristics of moles or scars; and any change in the breasts that lasts longer than a menstrual cycle.

What are risk factors and options for treatment of breast cancer?

Risk of breast cancer is increased in women with a family history of the disease. Inherited mutations of the BRCA1 and BRCA2 genes can cause both breast and ovarian cancers, often at earlier ages. In gene-positive women the risk is about 50-50, compared with 11-12% for all women. For women with these genes, removal of the tubes and ovaries reduces the risk of breast cancer and related gynecologic cancer.

Women with breast cancer in one breast have a greater risk of cancer in the remaining breast. Preventive measures include removing the breast tissue on the other side, Tamoxifen drug therapy, prophylactic ovary removal or a combination of therapies. Tamoxifen (Nolvadex) is standard for women with estrogen sensitive tumors. A five-year course reduces the risk of recurrence. A switch then to exemestane (Aromasin) (blocks estrogen production) will continue to reduce risk of recurrence. This drug may, however, worsen osteoporosis.

The breast cancer risk rises with weight gain but falls with an active lifestyle. Women who took oral contraceptives (OC) before 1975 are also at increased risk. The original birth control pill, Enovid, developed in 1960 and used through the 1970s, contained ten times the amount of estrogen and progestin needed for contraception, a high dosage that led to many complications and fatalities from blood clots and other problems. Increased levels of estrogen may contribute to development of breast cancer.

The current OC contains a safer level of hormones and is not associated with significantly increased risk of breast cancer. The trade-off is that OCs reduce the risk of ovarian cancer. The American College of Obstetricians and Gynecologists, however, recommends that smokers over age 35 or women with diabetes, high blood pressure or heart problems use an alternative method.

Treatment of breast cancer now gives women some options. A modified radical mastectomy removes the breast and the lymph nodes under the arm but leaves the muscles of the chest wall. A breast reconstruction can be done at the same time. Removal of the chest wall muscles, as was done in the original radical mastectomy, is unnecessary. Recently, breast conservation operations have been done with a biopsy to confirm the cancer and local removal by lumpectomy, preserving the breast and sampling the lymph nodes under the arm. This is followed by x-ray therapy to the breast and adjuvant or drug therapy to decrease the risk of spread. The results of these operations are similar. Some women wish to get rid of the offending organ and some want to save the breast. It is up to the patient. Fisher and other experts in a 20 year study say, "Lumpectomy followed by breast irradiation continues to be appropriate therapy for women with breast cancer, provided the margins of the lumpectomy are free of tumor and an acceptable cosmetic result can be obtained". A study in Italy indicates also that breast-conserving surgery is the treatment of choice for women with relatively small breast cancers. If breast cancer returns, much can be done. For more information, contact the following organizations—

American Cancer Society, 1599 Clifton Road, NE, Atlanta, GA 30329, 1-800-ACS-2345, *http://www.cancer.org.*—supplies publications, statistics, news, programs and research on prevention and early detection and treatment of cancer. **Breast Cancer Research Foundation**, 654 Madison Avenue, Suite 1209, New York, NY 10021, 646-497-2600, 1-866-FIND-A-CURE (toll free), *http://www.bcrfcure.org*— dedicated to the prevention and cure of breast cancer through support for clinical and genetic research. **Cancer Care, Inc.,** National Office, 275 Seventh Avenue, New York, NY 10001, 212-712-8080-1-800-813-HOPE (1-800-813-4673) *http://www.cancercare.org*—offers free professional counseling, education, information, referrals and financial assistance. **National Alliance of Breast Cancer Organizations (NABCO)**, 9 East 37th Street, 10th Floor, New York, NY 10016, 1-888-80-NABCO (1-888-806-2226), *http://www.nabco.org*—offers breast cancer information, education, resources, news and publications nationwide. **NCI**, Cancer Information Service, 6116 Executive Boulevard—MSC 8322, Room 3036A, Bethesda, MD 20892-8322, 1-800-4-CANCER (1-800-422-6237), 1-800-332-8615 (TTY), *http://www.cancer.gov*—provides facts about cancer prevention and treatment, statistics, resources, support and literature. **The Susan G. Komen Breast Cancer Foundation**, 5005 LBJ Freeway, Suite 250, Dallas, TX 75244, 1-800-I'M-AWARE (1-800-462-9273—national breast care helpline), *http://www.komen.org*—strives to eradicate breast cancer by advancing research, education, screening and treatment.

What should I take for premenstrual stress (PMS) and discomfort?

Before taking anything see your primary care physician or gynecologist. You may have a correctable or treatable problem like endometriosis. A baseline history and pelvic examination are in your best interest.

Prozac has been given for PMS and for depression. It takes weeks to help with depression but can diminish PMS symptoms in a few hours. Other antidepressant drugs include Wellbutrin, Zyban, Zoloft, Luvox and Paxil. They are used to treat severe PMS symptoms and true depression, as well as to alter personality to overcome shyness, low self esteem, and pessimism. Calcium supplements like TUMS also may help. Kramer points out that Sarafem, a new medication from Eli Lilly and Company is really basically Prozac with perhaps some slightly different ingredients and a different name.

What has happened to hormone replacement therapy (HRT)?

For years HRT was commonly prescribed for post-menopausal women despite many uncertainties about its effects. Was it all good? What else did it do? Recently, a landmark NIH study, costing $100 million and carried out by the Women's Health Initiative with 16,608 women, was halted three years early upon the discovery that the risks of taking estrogen plus progestin for more than four years outweighed the benefits. Women on hormones had fewer fractures and colon cancers, but more heart attacks, breast cancer, blood clots, strokes and gallbladder trouble. Other studies found increased breast cancers with HRT, even with short-term use. Postmenopausal women with a family history of breast cancer or other risk factors should be careful about taking hormone replacement therapy. If you are at increased risk of heart disease or stroke, look for alternatives to HRT.

The drug studied, Prempro by Wyeth, now offers the following caveats: No woman should go on such hormones to protect against heart disease, women taking HRT to protect against osteoporosis should consider other drugs, for relief of menopausal symptoms like hot flashes use the smallest dose for the shortest time. Many similar drugs are available.

Some authorities have criticized the NIH study for including women who were too old. It has left many uncertainties and unanswered questions. In a much shorter study of HRT on coronary heart disease in women with established coronary artery disease, the Heart and Estrogen/Progestin Study (HERS) found no difference in heart disease after 48 weeks. It also found relief of post-menopausal flushing and consequent improvement in the quality of life.

HRT is the most effective treatment for menopausal symptoms, hot flashes, night sweats, sexual dysfunction and vaginal dryness and for some women may be worth the risks. These symptoms usually resolve in a few years so long-term use is not needed. According to Margery Gass, M.D., "The message is not that all women should stop hormones but that each woman should consider exactly why she's on HRT and how she might accomplish her health goals in another way."

Tamoxifen, a drug opposing the action of estrogen in certain tissues, is successful in helping to treat hormone-responsive breast cancer. Women at high risk for breast cancer, halve their risk of developing it by taking Tamoxifen or a related drug Raloxifen. They are selective estrogen receptor modulators (SERMs). However, they stimulate endometrial cells lining the uterus and increase the risk of endometrial cancer.

Raloxifen, Tamoxifen, and estrogens increase somewhat the risk of blood clots in veins of the legs. If you have had problems with blood clots, it is best to avoid these drugs. Raloxifen is associated with an increase in hot flashes and leg pain but this is not reported to be a big problem. Raloxifen is associated with increased bone density in the vertebrae and hips in postmenopausal women with osteoporosis and with reduced occurrence of vertebral fractures and possible reduced likelihood of hip fractures, although this has not yet been clearly demonstrated. (Chapter 9)

Estrogen therapy has been associated with a decrease in atherosclerosis, blockage by plaques in the vessels and cardiovascular disease in women. Some believe, however, that this has not been proven by randomized controlled trials. This may be a direct effect of estrogen on blood vessels. However, estrogens increase the risk of breast, ovarian and endometrial cancers. Whether the new SERMs drugs will help protect blood vessels in older women has not been studied.

Investigators are hoping to develop the perfect SERM which will take care of all these problems. Ipriflavone, a synthetic isoflavone, does not prevent bone loss and may be hazardous. Use of conjugated equine estrogen after hysterectomy increases risk of stroke, decreases hip fractures and does not affect heart disease. A new class of drugs, aromatase inhibitors (exemestane—Aromasin), reduces the amount of estrogen produced in the body by blocking the action of aromatase, an enzyme that helps convert androgen into estrogen in post-menopausal women. It seems to have the same good effect as Tamoxifen without bad effects on the uterus.

Should every woman have an obstetrician and gynecologist?

Every woman should see a gynecologist from time to time. Gynecologists and obstetricians are now considered by many to be primary health-care providers for women. They are experts at examining pelvic organs and obtaining Pap smears to check for cervical cancer. They can help with abnormal menstrual periods, excessive menses or prolonged flow, along with problems of ovulation and conception. *In vitro* fertilization and other interventions require such expertise. Women beyond the age of 50 should have a pelvic examination each year, with observation of the vagina and cervix and palpation of the uterus, tubes and ovaries. Vaginal bleeding in postmenopausal women requires attention. With pregnancy, it is very important to consult an obstetrician about prenatal care.

How do I prevent cervical cancer?

The best way to decrease the chance of its occurrence is to have a yearly checkup and a Pap smear for changes in cells suggesting premalignancy, although some now believe that if a woman's Pap smears have always been negative, she may discontinue them after the age of 65. When precancerous cells are found in a Pap smear, removal of the cervix is required by an operation or laser treatment.

Regular testing also should be done for the human papillomavirus (HPV), a major risk factor for cervical cancer infecting about 20% of adults. Aggressive screening for HPV has reduced the number of cervical cancer cases in the last 40 years. Screening for HPV and a PAP test every two years appears to save additional years of life compared to figures for PAP tests alone. The most recent HPV diagnostic test is called the Hybrid Capture II HPV DNA assay by the Digene Company. It costs about $60, a Pap smear from $20 to $40.

HPV infection may produce no symptoms. It is sexually transmitted, so easily that condoms may not totally prevent transmission. Promising vaccines for HPV are being tested. In a large study, an HPV type 16 vaccine developed by two women, Laura Koutsky and Kathrin Jansen, reduced the incidence of both HPV-16 infection and related neoplasia, or cell changes preceding cancer. Drugs inside the vagina, or vaginal microbicides, may kill the virus.

Other agents that may contribute to cervical cancer are yeast infections, Herpes, *Chlamydia* and *Trichomonas bacteria*. A very real association exists between cervical cancer and chlamydia trachomatis infection. That and other infections such as gonorrhea can produce pelvic inflammatory disease, or infection of the fallopian tubes and ovaries, and infertility. For more information—The Gynecologic Cancer Foundation, 401 N. Mich Avenue, Chicago, IL, 60611, 312-644-6610, *www.wcn.org/gof.*

Is there a way to prevent cancer of the ovaries?

The only way to remove the risk of ovarian cancer is to remove the ovaries, not a recommendation for otherwise normal women with no family history of ovarian cancer. The disease is not common enough to justify removing the ovaries (an oophorectomy). Menopausal hormonal therapy increases the risk of ovarian cancer, particularly if estrogen alone is used for a long time. Short term HRT did not increase risk. The symptoms are non-specific such as bloating, constipation and heartburn. A blood test for ovarian cancer, in clinical trials, measures a protein called osteopontin or a protein expression panel,

What are Herpes Simplex infections?

Two strains of the herpes simplex virus cause these infections, each with different symptoms. HSV-1, usually transmitted by saliva, produces cold sores around the mouth. HSV-2 or genital herpes, which is sexually transmitted, can produce sores on the vagina, cervix, penis and scrotum. Diagnosis can be made by viral culture of a lesion. A blood test can also help (POCKit rapid test, Herpeselect ELISA kit and Herpeselect Immunoblot kit).

The virus never goes away although, after its first occurrence, it can lie dormant for years, and then recur, possibly in response to stress. Antiviral agents may keep the disease under control and decrease the possibility of transmission to another person, but can never cure it. These drugs are Acyclovir, Famciclovir and Valacyclovir. A vaccine has now shown efficacy against the herpes in women who are seronegative for HSV—1 and 2 but not in men. Condom use offers significant protection against HSV-2 infection in women.

What are the current methods of contraception?

The current oral contraceptive does not pose the health risks associated with its forerunner, as noted earlier. A contraceptive patch is available as well. Now new methods to eliminate or stop a pregnancy shortly after sexual intercourse may take the place of the contraceptive pill. The morning-after pills are two .75 mg. tablets of levon orgestrol (brand name Plan B) taken separately or together as soon as possible and at least within 72 hours of intercourse. The pills are 85% effective in preventing pregnancy and are safe. The FDA was asked to make them an over-the-counter drug not requiring a prescription. Political pressure from the present administration is believed to have prevented this.

Other methods of contraception such as condoms and vasectomy have become more popular. Unlike the contraceptive and morning-after pills, condoms offer some protection against sexually transmitted diseases,

What are the alternatives to hysterectomy?

We now have alternatives to hysterectomy for uterine fibroids. Radiologists can inject particles in the uterine artery, thus blocking the blood supply to the fibroids and making them shrink. Fibroids also shrink after injections of a Gonadotropin Releasing Hormone agonist that block the production of estrogen, essential to fibroid growth. Fibroids can also be removed by an operation, a myomectomy, without removal of the uterus.

Heavy menstrual bleeding can be controlled by endometrial ablation, or removal of the lining of the uterus, in the absence of other abnormalities like polyps and hormonal imbalance. This is not for women who wish to have more children. For some problems, hysterectomy may be needed such as for prolapse, or falling down or out, of the uterus. For some women, a hysterectomy, removal of the uterus and cervix, may be preferred, particularly for abnormal uterine bleeding. Cancer of the cervix does not always require a hysterectomy. Cancer of the uterus does require a hysterectomy.

Table

Alternatives for Menopausal Symptoms

Depression—Selective serotonin reuptake inhibitors (SSRIs) like Paxil are effective and nontoxic antidepressants.

Hot flashes, night sweats—SSRIs may help, paroxetine controlled release or clonidine (Catapres), a Prozac like drug (Effexor, vitamin E) estrogens. Avoid caffeine, alcohol and spicy foods.

Sexual function—Over the counter lubrication, moisturizers, topical estrogen creams, tablets or rings may be helpful.

Alternative therapies—Studies show a significant decrease in hot flashes for women who consume Soy and Black Cohosh, phytoestrogens, or plants producing effects like those of estrogen.

Estrogen—progestin—Use a very low dose or for a short period.

CEE—conjugated equine estrogen and 17B-estradiol are equally affective for hot flashes but not for chronic disease prevention in postmenopausal women.

MEN'S HEALTH

28. B. What is benign prostatic hypertrophy? How should prostate cancer be diagnosed and treated? Is there a male menopause with a need for hormone replacement? What are other male medical problems?

The prostate gland is a walnut-sized organ lying just below the bladder and surrounding the urethra, the tube from the bladder through the penis. Tiny at birth, the prostate gland begins to enlarge at puberty and produces the fluid that accompanies sperm during sexual ejaculation. Many men in their 60s and most men in their 70-80s show symptoms of a swollen prostate gland known as benign prostatic hypertrophy (BPH). The reason for the continuing enlargement is not known.

As the prostate gland enlarges, it presses against the urethra slowing or interrupting the flow of urine and causing a strong and frequent urge to urinate despite little urine in the bladder. One symptom is nocturia, or having to get up in the night to urinate, although nocturia can be a symptom of other health problems as well. Another BPH symptom is dribbling at the end of urination

Eventually the enlarged prostate gland may totally obstruct the urethra causing inability to void. This is an emergency requiring insertion of a tube, or catheter, into the bladder. Depending on severity of symptoms, an operation may be done through the penis to remove the inner obstructing portion of the gland: a transurethral postatectomy or a transurethral resection of the prostate (TURP). Laser surgery can also be done. Drugs like Proscar will shrink the gland. Drugs like Flomax, Cardura or Hytrin help by relaxing the prostate muscles. Finasteride also helps by inhibiting the enzyme 5 alpha-reductase, which is involved in growth of the prostate gland. Finasteride has been associated with cancer of the breast in some men but the relationship is not clear.

Infections or inflammation of the prostate can also occur. Prostate gland cancer is a problem in older men. Beginning at age 40 or 50, if you are at high risk, you should have a yearly blood test and rectal exam of the prostate for nodules or lumps. The blood test screens for prostate specific antigen (PSA) but a positive PSA only suggests, and does not prove, cancer. The PSA also helps in determining the stage of development of the cancer. For instance, Stage B cancer occurs in several places within the prostate. In Stage C, it has spread throughout the prostate and possibly to nearby tissue or the bladders. A PSA below 20-25 indicates a low risk of spread, one above 50 a high risk of extensive disease. PSA is also a guide to treatment.

The exact diagnosis requires a biopsy of the gland through the rectum. The pathologist who examines the biopsy specimen and makes the diagnosis of cancer can grade the tumor as low grade or high grade—an aggressive tumor. Then the question is how best to treat it.

Originally, a radical prostatectomy was recommended but it can lead to loss of urine control and sexual function. Alternatives such as external beam or interstitial beam radiation therapy may be as good without the complications. The cancer may be localized in the gland and grow slowly. Watchful waiting may be appropriate particularly in older men with other health problems. Urologists tend to recommend radical prostatectomy and radiation oncologists tend to recommend radiation therapy. The outcome is not very different for these treatments. After a radical prostatectomy the PSA should immediately fall to 0. After radiotherapy the PSA will also fall but slowly.

The other treatment for prostate cancer that has spread to bone or adjoining structures is getting rid of androgens by orchiectomy, or removing the testicles. This often relieves symptoms and results in less pain.

Other factors may influence the prostate. Exercise may lower the risk of both BPH and prostate cancer. Diet may also influence prostate cancer. Dietary fat is a major nutritional contributor to occurrence of the disease. Selenium supplements decreased prostate cancer in a study in Arizona but most authorities believe that a healthy diet contains enough selenium without supplements. Other possibly protective substances include Vitamin E, calcium, vitamin C and fructose, found in fruit. Daily aspirin may also help decrease occurrence of prostate cancer.

Is there a male menopause? Are hormones needed?

In some men, testosterone levels remain high throughout life. In most, they decline slightly after age 40. At age 70, the average male's testosterone levels are only 30% below the peak and remain in a normal range in 75% of older men. Thus, while sexual activity tends to diminish over the years, there is no real male menopause or andropause as it is called by some.

Impotence is more frequently due to atherosclerosis, diabetes, hypertension, medications, and psychological disorders, not testosterone deficiency. Testosterone replacement therapy is usually unnecessary and fairly ineffective. Untested, it is a vast uncontrolled experiment, in the view of many people. Could it become as controversial as estrogen therapy for women?

The first drug for impotence therapy was sildenafil (Viagra). The best summary from a study by Goldstein et al is that "oral sildenafil is an effective, well tolerated treatment for men with erectile dysfunction". Now there are other drugs for this purpose, such as Levitra (vardenafir) and Cialis (tadalafil). All of these drugs act by relaxing blood vessels and muscles in the penis allowing increased blood flow to produce an erection. They involve some mild side-effects and are not recommended for patients with heart trouble, hypertension, liver disease and kidney disease. They may also interfere with other drugs.

What about other male problems?

Penis problems include phimosis, tightening of the foreskin. Circumcision provides protection against penile human papilloma virus infection, which puts female partners at risk for cervical cancer. It is more hygienic and decreases the possibility of cancer of the penis. Other male problems include torsion of the testicles and testicular cancer.

For further information:

The AMA—Complete Guide to Men's Health $34.95, phone 1-800-621-8335, fax 1-312-4646-5600, *www.amapress.com*.
Harvard Men's Health Watch—$32/year, monthly, phone 1-800-829-3341, *harvardmen@palmcoastd.com*, Harvard Health Publications, PO Box 420173, Palm Coast, FL 32142-1073.

Section E

Operations

SURGEONS—SURGERY

29. Are the terms "surgery" and "operation" interchangeable? What is minimal surgery? Why are there differences around the country in how often some operations are done?

Surgery is a discipline or specialty in medicine where therapy consists of an operation. Surgeons perform operations but surgery and operations are not synonymous. Operations are procedures whereas surgery is a form of therapy which is a part of the overall body of medicine. The terms "surgery" and "surgeries" have become slang expressions used by many who should know better. Kollef et al described surgical procedures in a recent article in the journal *Chest* and then wrote that: "Eleven surgeries involved the thoracic aorta." We surgeons believe it is more appropriate and correct to say: "Eleven operations involved the thoracic aorta." "Surgeries" as a term for operations is incorrect.

The Concise Columbia Encyclopedia defines surgery: "as the branch of medicine concerned with diagnosis and treatment of injuries and pathologic conditions requiring manual or instrumental operative procedures." In the American Century Dictionary surgery is defined as: "Medical treatment by incision or manipulation as opposed to drugs. A surgeon is a medical practitioner qualified in surgery." They go on to define surgery as the operating room. This is also a slang expression which has sneaked into usage and is not appropriate. How can surgery be synonymous with the operating room when a surgeon is a medical practitioner qualified in surgery? That would be the same as saying that a surgeon is a medical practitioner qualified in the operating room, which is ridiculous. Technicians, nurses and others may be qualified in the operating room but here again they are qualified to participate in operations. No one is qualified in the operating room unless they are architects who design operating rooms. One dictionary definition has an additional category: the treatment of other than human disease by methods analogous to those of a surgeon, i.e. tree surgery.

Other slang expressions are to "surgerize" (how awful!) or "do surgery," "have surgery," and "perform surgery." The Charlie Brown comic strip shows Snoopy the dog wearing a cap, mask and gloves asking the question "Am I going to do surgery or have surgery?" then greatly relieved to find he was going to do surgery rather than have it. Here again a slang expression is used for what should have been called an operation or procedure. Unfortunately, the incorrect use of words for a prolonged period of time becomes accepted usage.

Secretaries, nurses and lay personnel may say: "The doctor is in surgery." The correct statement is: "The doctor or surgeon is in the operating room." Surgeons do operations in operating rooms, or theaters in England. Surgeons do not do surgery in surgery. The only place where the word surgery denotes a place is in England where a physician refers to his office as his "surgery."

When asked how long I have been in surgery I reply "for 44 years." I entered the discipline in 1954 when I became an intern in surgery at the Massachusetts General Hospital. I became a surgeon when I completed my residency in 1962 and was certified by the ABS.

Patients or families of patients may seek to determine the experience of a surgeon by asking "How many of these surgeries have you done?" I don't mind the question but I abhor the terminology. An appropriate question would be: "How many of these operations have you done?" This question requires a response and I am happy to describe my experience to a patient or the patient's family.

Thus, a pet peeve for many of us in the field of surgery, particularly those with literary or editorial responsibilities, is the use of the word surgery as a synonym for operation. I am not overly pedantic. Catherine Allen wrote "Surgery is what a surgeon practices. An operation is what a surgeon performs." There is no such word as "surgeries."

What is minimal surgery?

Minimal surgery means operations done by minimally invasive techniques. A large incision in the chest, abdomen or elsewhere may no longer be necessary. In a so-called keyhole operation, the surgeon makes several small incisions measuring several centimeters or about 1-2 inches and carries out the operation with a miniaturized video camera and special long instruments. The surgeon no longer sees directly or touches any part of the patient's body but does the operation by guiding the instruments from a television monitor. This equipment was developed in the 1970s and 1980s. Minimal operations are a great advance for patients. Their impact on your system is much less. The small incisions heal easily. You have less pain, recover faster, and can often safely leave the hospital one to two days after the operation.

Surgeons who do such operations must have special training and experience. If the surgeon encounters a complication like bleeding, it may be necessary to quickly make a large standard incision to deal with the problem but this should happen infrequently. Operations in the abdomen done most commonly by minimal techniques, or laparoscopy, include cholecystectomy, appendectomy, hernia repair, colectomy and splenectomy. Certain lung problems, including a pneumothorax or lung biopsy, can be treated by use of these techniques, in a thoracoscopy. Some heart operations, such as coronary artery bypass grafts, can be done in this way without the need for a heart-lung machine. Joint problems can be diagnosed and repaired by arthroscopy. This field is advancing and changing rapidly. It is a great benefit for you.

Why are there differences around the country in how often some operations are done?

Where you live can determine what operation you might have. In an extensive study based on 1996 Medicare data published in a Dartmouth Atlas of Health Care Series and reviewed by Vergano and DeBarros in USA TODAY, a map showed the rate of various operations across the U.S. Partial mastectomy or lumpectomy for breast cancer, rather than removal of the entire breast, was done most commonly in New York, New England and California. Leg amputations were done more frequently in Texas and the south, possibly because of the frequency of diabetes and lack of foot care for Hispanics. Back surgery was done more frequently in the Northwest and mountain states. Louisiana claimed the highest operation rate of all, reflecting perhaps consumption of rich foods, smoking and vascular disease. Besides that, Louisiana did not reimburse indigent patients for medicines but did pay for operations. Next on the list came Texas, Alabama, Palm Springs, California and some communities in Pennsylvania and Michigan. The study found the lowest operation rate in Hawaii, a ranking some ascribe to free preventive care for the elderly. The most frequent kinds of operations are: 1) lumpectomy for breast cancer; 2) prostatectomy; 3) angioplasty, or dilating a narrowed blood vessel,—not really an operation; 4) lower extremity revascularizations; 5) carotid endarterectomy; 6) back operations; 7) thigh fracture repair; 8) hip replacement; 9) leg amputation and 10) heart valve replacement.

Not all differences from one community to another 300 miles away are due to disease frequency. Other factors enter in, such as honest disagreements among doctors about what is best for you. Vascular surgeons believe that removing a significant arteriosclerotic plaque producing narrowing of a carotid artery, a carotid endarterectomy, will decrease the likelihood of stroke. Some neurologists disagree. As noted earlier, urologists most often recommend prostatectomy for prostate cancer whereas radiation therapists recommend radiation therapy. Surgeons are more aggressive. Many internists are conservative, some too conservative in preventing operations that would improve their patients' quality of life. Some physicians prefer certain operations to the point of blind loyalty. If more diagnostic studies like angiograms are done, more operations will be done. The map also reflects examples of inadequate science, some patients' ignorance of their options and inequities due to disparities in care. A breast cancer patient in a rural area may find it difficult to have a lumpectomy, for instance, since it requires postoperative radiation therapy that may not be readily available there.

If told you need an operation, it is important for you to ask why. What will happen if you don't have it done? What are your options? A second opinion may help, perhaps by a physician in another community. Don't accept everything told you unquestioningly. Ask questions and seek information. The differences in frequency of various operations around the country will decrease if the right questions are asked.

OPERATIONS

30. I have been told I should have an operation. What questions should I ask the surgeon? Do some surgeons do unnecessary operations?

If you are facing an operation, the most important question to ask is: Do I need it? You should go on to ask: Why do I need it? What will happen if I don't have it done? Will the problem get worse? Will it threaten my life or kill me? What are my risks? What are my chances of dying? What are the complications? How much will it cost? Will my insurance cover it? A good surgeon, discussing an operation with you, will answer these and other questions before you ask them.

Operations can be emergency, urgent or elective procedures. An emergency operation is performed for a life-threatening condition like a ruptured blood vessel, or a ruptured abdominal aneurysm; a blood clot on your brain resulting from an injury; acute appendicitis; a perforated ulcer; or a bowel obstruction. An urgent operation might be the term for removal of a cancer that could grow and spread if not attended to. Examples of an elective operation would include removal of gallstones that have bothered you or repair of an inguinal hernia that is not incarcerated, sticking out and not reducible, or strangulated, pinching off circulation to the bowel in the hernia sac. For an elective operation that should be done soon but not this week, you have time for another question: Should I get a second opinion?

Perhaps you have a condition that bothers you but lets you get along. Your doctor recommends an operation. You must decide whether the condition bothers you enough to encounter the discomfort and potential risks of an operation. The relationship between risk and potential benefit becomes very important for you (Chapter 24).

Suppose you have gallstones. If an attack of right upper abdominal pain led to their discovery but the pain has now disappeared, should you have an operation? Giving an honest response, your surgeon would note that the attack and the presence of gallstones indicate more attacks in the future even though we don't know when. The stones may drop down into the bile ducts and cause a block leading to jaundice and/or infection. Before you have a bad attack or complications, it is best to remove the gallbladder and stones if your health is otherwise good. This can be done safely by the new technique laparoscopy. Ask the surgeon about his experience with this operation, how many he has done, and how frequently. If he is skilled at performing this procedure, and if your health is good, the risk of your dying should be less than 1 in 200-300 operations.

What are unnecessary operations?

An operation should be done only to correct an abnormality, but in the past some operations were done more often than necessary. Years ago it was believed that all children should have a tonsillectomy and an adenoidectomy before they went to school. Now these operations are done only after repeated attacks of tonsillitis. In the past, women with fibroid tumors of the uterus, recurrent uterine bleeding or severe menstrual bleeding would undergo hysterectomies. Now this operation is done much less often. Fibroid tumors will shrink after menopause; hormones can control abnormal bleeding. A dilatation and curettage (D&C) should be done, however, to check for uterine cancer.

Other operations that have become no longer necessary include mastoidectomies in children with chronic ear infections, now treated with antibiotics, and thyroidectomies to remove overactive thyroids, now controlled by radioactive agents and drugs. Operations for peptic ulcer disease are rarely warranted now that we know the cause usually to be bacteria in the stomach (*Helicobacter pylori*). Other questions about operations are covered in Chapter 29 and 31 and questions about second opinions in Chapter 6.

Honest differences of opinion may arise between primary care doctors and surgeons. Surgeons tend to be more aggressive, particularly if they believe an operation will safely control symptoms or other problems. Internists may be more conservative and not recommend an operation in the belief that a patient can get along without it. Some internists believe that surgeons operate too quickly and without sufficient indication of need.

Sometimes patients suffer along with chronic conditions that could be easily repaired by an operation. My mother-in-law developed a hiatal hernia, a protrusion of the stomach up into the chest, with reflux esophagitis and narrowing of her esophagus, in her 50s. She could eat only baby food and liquids and often had severe substernal chest pain when acid from the stomach came up into her esophagus. Her internist recommended that she put up with this condition, take antacids and other medications, and she followed this advice.

I first met her when she was in her late 60s, and, although I had often done the operation to correct this problem—safe and easy for patients in good health—

I thought she would not have been up to it at that time. She suffered with this problem until her death at age 94. The failure to explore the option of surgery at the outset of her suffering points up the excessive caution of some doctors.

QUESTIONS TO ASK A SURGEON BEFORE YOU HAVE AN OPERATION

(A good surgeon will have answered these questions before you ask.)

1. Why must I or should I have this operation?
2. What will happen to me if I don't have it done? Will the problem get worse?
3. What are the risks? What is the potential mortality?
4. What complications can develop and how often do they happen?
5. How long before I can back to work? How long is the recovery?
6. Are there other ways to treat this condition without an operation?
7. How many of these operations have you done in the past year? What is your success rate?
8. What happened to people who have not had this operation?
9. Should I get a second opinion?
10. Will my insurance pay for it?
11. Does my insurance require a second opinion?
12. What are your qualifications? Are you board certified? In what specialty? Are you a fellow of the ACS?
13. At which hospitals do you work?
14. Have you ever had a malpractice judgment against you or been disciplined by a state board or hospital?

Board Certified—Call 1-866-275-2267.
Fellow of the ACS—Call 1-800-621-4111.

31. What Is N.P.O. after midnight? Why do operations frequently start late? What is Same Day Surgery? How should I prepare for an operation?

Nil por os (NPO—nothing by mouth) after midnight is the instruction for patients having an operation the next day with sedation or a general anesthetic. It is critical for the stomach to be empty of food and drink. An anesthetic lessens or abolishes the reflexes protecting the larynx, trachea and lungs from the passage of stomach contents into the windpipe, aspiration. If it occurs, it is like drowning. Aspiration of food into the windpipe may cause a cardiac arrest, instant death, lung damage and later death or disability from lung failure.

It is safe to take a light meal like tea and toast up to six hours before operation. Liquids (water, black coffee, soda or fruit juice without pulp) may be taken up to two hours before. If a patient has eaten or drunk more than that, the operation should be canceled and re-scheduled. If the need for an emergency operation arises after a patient's meal, a skilled anesthesiologist can put a tube in the windpipe with the patient awake to protect against aspiration. The patient would then be anesthetized and later would remember only some discomfort from the tube insertion.

Studies to be sure your general health is good enough to have an anesthetic and an operation safely should be done the day before the operation if not earlier. For most patients this checkup includes an EKG, a chest x-ray, a urinalysis (to be sure the bladder or kidneys are free of infection or diabetes) and blood studies to rule out anemia and to evaluate kidney, liver and blood function. Preparation is made for blood transfusions from the blood bank, should you need them. If you wish to provide your own blood for an elective operation this must be arranged some weeks in advance. Your surgeon and his office can help with this.

We have a new phenomenon called "same-day surgery"—a silly expression, but one in common use. All operations are done on the same day they are scheduled. What else could it be: "some other day surgery," "next day surgery" or "all in one day surgery?" What is meant is that the patient comes to the hospital early in the morning and is prepared for operation that morning or afternoon, on the same day. In the past, patients came into the hospital the night before for preoperative preparation. The patient was frequently given sleeping medication and was taken to the operating room early the next morning. Now the patient may visit the hospital the day before for tests and for an appointment with the anesthesiologist to review the safety of a general anesthetic and a history of any allergies. The patient then goes home to sleep (hopefully) and comes back at the crack of dawn: An arrival time of 5:00 am for an operation scheduled for 7:30am is not unusual.

What brought about this change? Insurance carriers believe spending the night before operation in the hospital is a wasteful expense unless active treatment is given. Medicare began to pay, not for days in the hospital and services rendered, but by disease, in standard amounts as calculated for the disease related group (DRG). Hospitals shortened the stay and eliminated the leisurely night before. Is the practice safe? Surgeons and anesthesiologists believe it is. Is it better? Only you the patient knows. You must weigh the difference between sleeping at home in familiar surroundings but with the anxiety that goes with an early morning trip to the hospital versus a sedated rest in a hospital bed. If active therapy such as intravenous medication is required the night before operation, admission to the hospital will be allowed, although your insurance carrier may not pay the hospital for that night. It is common now for patients having major heart or lung operations to come to the hospital on the morning of operation. Minimal surgical procedures such as laparoscopic cholecystectomy allow the patient to go home shortly after the procedure, if not the same day, at least the following day.

The Operating Room Schedule

Operations are scheduled one after another, beginning usually at 7:30 or 8:00 am with others "to follow". Generally speaking, "to follow operations" have reasonable estimated starting times. However, emergencies take precedence, including treatment of severe accident injuries, transplantation when an organ becomes available and other crises. Thus, an emergency may "bump" or delay your operation until much later in the day or even until the next day; an elective operation which was to start at 10 am may not be done until 6 pm or even later. Fortunately, the "same day surgery" suites allow your family to stay with you until you are taken into the operating room.

When I worked in a teaching hospital with many emergencies, I tried to avoid scheduling to-follow operations. It isn't pleasant for a patient to lie in a hospital bed from 6 am until 6pm awaiting an operation with no food or drink by mouth. If you are tired, thirsty and hungry and it is late in the day, ask to be rescheduled as the first operation on a day in the future and go home. Your operating room team may be tired also.

A unique system of communication with families during operations was developed at the last hospital where I was active, St. Louis University Hospital, by Velma Willman, the wife of the Chief of Surgery there. A waiting room for the families of patients adjoined the operating room. It offered the usual amenities of coffee, snacks, comfortable chairs, reading material and television. Most importantly, the waiting room was staffed by a volunteer who would periodically call the operating room for progress reports. How was the operation progressing? When would they be finished, etc.? Thus, a family did not wait for hours and wonder what was happening. The first time I was asked to give a progress report to the volunteer and family, I was taken aback. I had never done that before but I quickly learned to appreciate this service and used it routinely to volunteer messages for families during long operations. I recommend it to you and your hospital.

How should I prepare for an operation?

Stern provides a checklist before you go into the hospital. 1) Do you want a second opinion? 2) You must meet your surgeon ahead of time. Is your surgeon Board Certified, with residency at a first-rate hospital and extensive experience with the operation you are to have? 3) What is the experience of the hospital with the operation you will have? How often is it performed and what is the success rate? The results of operations are better in hospitals where they are done frequently.

Tell the anesthesiologist everything about you—allergies, reactions, and previous health problems. Don't be a docile patient who accepts whatever; never hesitate to ask questions. Ask who will be in charge of your care at each stage. Do not sign advanced directives or operative permits until you understand them. Pack a list of phone numbers you want in an emergency. Keep accurate records. Plan for your recovery before you go in. Pack all your medications so the hospital will know what you take. Take creature comforts, photos of family, etc., but no cash or jewelry. If you are having an operation on one side of your body, mark the location with a pen before you go to the operating room, to make sure the operation will be done on the correct side. When my son had to have varicose veins removed in one of his legs, he insisted on being awake in the operating room until he could point out to the surgeon, "It is this leg." Make arrangements in advance for going home. Will you need help, a visiting nurse, meals on wheels? Most hospitals have social workers to help. For information write to the U.S. Agency for Health Care Policy and Research, AHCPR Clearing House, PO Box 8546, Dept. P, Silver Spring, MD 20907 for their booklets on 1) Questions to ask your surgeon; 2) Pain relief after surgery; 3) Preventing bed sores. For hospital experience write to the Joint Commission of Accreditation of Healthcare Organizations, 1 Renaissance Boulevard, Dept. P, Oakbrook Terrace, IL 60181 or the American Hospital Association and the Picker Institute *www.amphi.com/eyeonpatient.*

Section F

About Doctors

PRIVATE PRACTICE

32. What is the difference between doctors in private practice and academic or full-time doctors? Should doctors be allowed to advertise? How should doctors be paid or reimbursed?

Medical care in the U.S. developed with independent and often single physicians in offices who saw patients and charged fees for the care given, in a fee for service practice. Continuing to the present day, private practice allows the doctor and the patient to have a private arrangement for care. Doctors know their patients and vice-versa.

Years ago, most doctors were generalists with little formal education. Medical schools were proprietary-owned or run by doctors in practice who charged students for attendance at lectures. Early in the 20th century, the Flexner study and report, supported by the Rockefeller Foundation, recommended major reforms in medical education in the U.S. Many proprietary schools closed, with the opening of the major medical schools of today. In a major provision, this reform mandated a salary for the faculty both in the basic sciences—anatomy, physiology, biochemistry, etc.—and in the clinical disciplines—medicine, surgery, pediatrics, etc. The faculty members were called full-time or academic doctors in contrast to private practitioners. Almost all medical schools adopted some form of this system.

Now it is recognized that since medical schools lack the means to pay for clinical faculty salaries, academic doctors must collect fees from their patients. Thus, medical school clinical departments are large group practices much like private practice. The difference is that they teach and do research in addition to their practices. Medical schools do not pay faculty for teaching alone. In addition to full-time faculty many physicians in private practice teach medical students and residents in the hospital. They have a part time faculty appointment and are called volunteer faculty.

How should doctors be paid or reimbursed?

For many years, doctors were paid a fee-for-service, based upon "usual, customary or reasonable" fees for the service provided. Office visits cost so much, operations cost so much and there was general agreement about the fees. Many patients could not pay anything, so wealthy patients were charged a bit more (the Robin Hood system). Abuses and new technology and drugs led to escalating health care costs.

In the 1980s, reports focused on the need to control physician charges. A group at Harvard led by William Hsiao developed a Resource-Based Relative Value Scale (RBRVS) as a way to pay for physician services based on an evaluation of various services and procedures (S/PS) performed. S/Ps are determined by the Physicians Current Procedural Terminology (CPT-4). The factors used are: 1) time for the S/P; 2) pre S/P and post S/P time; 3) intensivity/unit time for performing an S/P; 4) practice costs including malpractice insurance; 5) cost of post-graduate training required to become a specialist. The Physician Payment Review Committee, a congressional advisory panel, recommended such a program to Congress and the HCFA adopted this fee schedule for Medicare in 1992. Physician payments now conform to the schedule. Some doctors are paid more, like primary care doctors in rural areas, and others, like surgeons, less. HMOs and insurance companies have adopted such fee schedules, which tend to control increases in health care costs but leave many doctors frustrated and angry enough to sue carriers or retire early. Many doctors believe Medicare does not compensate them adequately, and Medicaid fees are sometimes so low the doctors cannot afford to care for such patients. If your doctor accepts Medicare fees, Medicare pays the doctor, and he or she can't bill you for more. If you are on Medicare, before you seek care find out if your doctor accepts Medicare fees.

Physicians may be reimbursed by fee-for-service methods, including relative-value programs of Medicare; by salary if doctors are employed; or through capitation in which they receive a fixed amount per patient no matter what the need. Cleary found that patients are often unaware of how doctors are compensated and may not want to know, even though the kind of compensation may influence care. HMOs may give financial bonuses to doctors for giving less care or may withhold money for later payment to keep doctors from doing too much. Some HMOs pay a doctor a salary but withhold a small percentage until the end of the year and upon completion of goals like high immunization rates, positive membership feedback and restriction of expenses. Other chains or HMOs provide financial incentives to doctors to increase revenue by more laboratory studies and x-rays.

Should doctors be allowed to advertise?

For years, doctors did not advertise. They were professionals, not businesses. The AMA banned it. We all thought it was wrong to advertise. Then in 1982 the FTC ruled organized medicine was in restraint of trade not to allow advertising. This agency called us a trade, not a profession, an opinion backed by the Supreme Court. Plastic surgeons began to advertise tummy tucks, liposuction, face lifts, breast augmentation or "lifts" for sagging breasts and so on. Pictures of surgeons and their prices now appear in ads. I think it is deplorable. The only advertising I ever permitted was a listing of my name under cardiothoracic surgeons in the phone book yellow pages.

Laser eye centers and ophthalmologists not only advertise but are in a price war. So much each month for each eye, the ads read; see better, look better, feel better. Do not pick an eye doctor on the basis of price but rather for experience and results. Remember things can go wrong, and your vision could get worse. As for me, I am content to wear my glasses.

Some reputable practitioners will only do two laser eye operations in an hour but they can take as little as 10 to 15 minutes. At roughly $1000 an eye and four in an hour, a doctor could bring in $32,000 a day with two hours for lunch. This is disgusting. There is a Surgical Eyes Foundation which could give you information at *www.surgicaleyes.org*. I cannot vouch for what they provide but they seem to be concerned with quality.

Why is there so much dissatisfaction among doctors?

Managed care is a major reason. HMOs have changed many aspects of doctors' care for you. As noted earlier reimbursement has decreased. Instructions to doctors remove their freedom to do what is best for you (chapter 53). Other factors include a malpractice crisis (chapter 36), too much paper work, and loss of independence with doctors forced to act as double agents—for patients and for the insurer, courts, etc. Many doctors are retiring early, leaving their practices, moving to other states and limiting their practices. The solution requires better discipline in the health care system (chapter 53).

COVER-UPS

33. Do doctors cover up for each other? Is that true that doctors will not testify against each other in court?

Good doctors do not cover up for other doctors. On the other hand, they usually do not publicly discuss your care by another doctor nor do they criticize that care, for a very good reason. They did not see you, review your history, examine you, review your lab reports and x-rays, treat you or operate on you. Another doctor is not aware of the circumstances of your illness or medical problem.

Be wary of the doctor who, although not involved in your care, has strong opinions about what took place or what should have been done. I call this "the reckless courage of the noncombatant." Doctors are reluctant to comment on what others have done because they do not know the exact circumstances your doctor was dealing with. I am reluctant to comment upon an operation carried out by another surgeon because I was not on the scene in the operating room. Findings at operations make all the difference in what procedure(s) should or can be carried out. First-hand observation is essential to judgment. Also, there are honest differences of opinion about operations and when they should be done.

Is it true that doctors will not testify against each other? What is a "hired gun?"

No, that is not true. Doctors will testify against other doctors in certain circumstances. I have testified against doctors when I found what I thought was evidence of medical negligence that led to serious medical problems or death. I have advised attorneys as to whether there is evidence of negligence. Other doctors will do the same.

A few doctors act as "hired guns," serving as paid expert witnesses for patients. I hear a national registry of such doctors is available to attorneys specializing in malpractice. From my own observation, many such doctors are older, retired, can't make a living as a doctor in their specialty but can make big money testifying in malpractice cases. The fees can be huge. A minimum is $100 to $200 an hour up to $500 to $1,000 an hour for reviewing records and writing opinions plus extra money for travel, depositions, and court appearances to testify before a jury. I have also testified for doctors against such "hired guns." A "hired gun" would testify that "if I was there, I would have done this or that." If you weren't there, how do you know what you would have done? Things happen fast in an operating room. New situations confront us. The problem may not be what we expected. The operative note in the patient's record is a brief description, a synopsis. It is not a 50-page article about every stitch and every drop of blood.

Our legal system is a good one in many ways but has weaknesses. Some attorneys no longer seem interested in determining what is right, what is moral, what is ethical, what is "the truth," but rather what can they convince a "lay" jury of peers to think about the situation. Have they forgotten truth? Is truth dependant upon the powers of persuasion and a contest with opposing lawyers? It sometimes seems so. Doctors are actively trying to make some sense out of the malpractice problem so that malpractice insurance would cost less and they would not have to charge patients as much. They also would like to limit the judgments, ending the practice of giving huge amounts simply out of sympathy (Chapter 36). The high cost of malpractice insurance is driving many doctors to retire.

DIAGNOSIS

34. How accurate is the diagnosis of my illness?

The diagnosis of your illness may be made in several ways. The first part is the medical history of what is bothering you and of how it has progressed. Next, the physical examination may confirm the presence of a lump, a bump, a bulge or an enlargement. The medical history and the examination are not diagnoses, however. For most diseases, the diagnosis can be confirmed by x-rays and/or blood studies, urinalysis and other laboratory tests.

For example, diabetes mellitus can be suspected from your symptoms and confirmed by the presence of sugar in your urine, an elevated blood sugar and an abnormal glucose tolerance test. Kidney failure or liver disease can be determined by blood studies. Heart disease can be found by an examination, electrocardiogram and/or cardiac catheterization, a coronary arteriogram, or angiogram, and certain blood studies. Vascular disease is found by the detection of symptoms like absence of pulse and weakness in the legs or hands, by doppler ultrasound blood vessel studies and by arteriography. Problems of the brain are identified by a skull x-ray, arteriography, and MRI and PET scanning.

Radiologic studies such as a mammogram show only anatomic abnormalities: a shadow by chest x-ray, a torn cartilage by MRI, or uptake of a radioactive compound suggesting a malignancy by PET scan. X-ray studies with dye will show anatomic abnormalities in the gallbladder, with a cholecystogram; the kidneys, with an intravenous pyelogram or IVP; the spinal cord, with a myelogram; the stomach, with an upper GI series or a barium swallow; and the colon, with a lower GI series or barium enema. An ultrasound of the abdomen will show gallstones or fluid or a mass. Again, these studies are not diagnoses.

A diagnosis requires looking at the abnormality by endoscopy: by looking into the esophagus or stomach by esophagoscopy and gastroscopy, the pancreas by endoscopic retrograde cholangiopancreatoscopy, the colon by colonoscopy and the urinary bladder by cystoscopy.

Suggestion of malignancy must be confirmed by a biopsy, obtaining a small sample of tissue by piercing the skin with a needle, making an incision or doing an exploratory operation. The tissue is cut in a very thin slice, stained and inspected under a microscope. The appearance of the cells allows the pathologist to diagnose the presence or absence of cancer and, if present, its type. If the diagnosis of a potential cancer is uncertain, then more tissue must be obtained. Cancer treatment is not begun until the diagnosis is certain. Pathologists frequently seek second opinions themselves in the event of uncertainty. The Armed Forces Institute of Pathology (AFIP) in Washington D.C. is considered the best and final place to resolve doubt about a diagnosis. The diagnosis of cancer is often easy from a biopsy. If it is difficult, the pathologist will often send the slides to the AFIP.

Is the diagnosis ever wrong?

If appropriate studies are done little uncertainty should exist. Almost all well-established diagnoses are correct. However, there are no absolutes in human biology. While errors are very infrequent, we cannot say always or never. And some illnesses have no manifestations that can be confirmed by diagnostic studies. Discuss the accuracy of the diagnosis with your physician or surgeon.

The diagnosis may be certain and sufficient to make a recommendation for you about therapy. We do not proceed with procedures or therapy that might be difficult or uncomfortable or devastating for you without being absolutely sure what we are dealing with. If you are doubtful, however, request a second opinion.

35. Are all doctors pill pushers? Are antibiotics used too much?

Critics say that some doctors are pill pushers.* Every time you see them they give you one or more prescriptions. This is an easy way out for doctors, recalling the old joke "take two aspirins and call me in the morning." Perhaps your doctor thinks you would be disappointed if you did not receive a prescription during an office visit. You might think the doctor can't do anything for you or does not even believe you are sick.

Tell your doctor you came to see him because something bothers you. You would like help; you did not come just to get a prescription. You may seek an opinion as to whether your problem is serious, dangerous or merits study. Many patients make office visits for conditions that will take care of themselves, but they do not know that at the time or before the visit. If something bothers you, see your doctor. Don't wait; your problem could be serious. If you believe you need medication, tell your doctor that also.

You may have heard about a new drug. A drug company ad may suggest you ask your doctor whether you should be taking the drug instead of something else. (Where should I get medical information? Chapter 56) In making a decision about treatment, whether medicine or an operation, you must consider safety, applicability, evidence from trials, and a possible need for further studies. Discuss these topics with your doctor. A prescribed medicine will come with an insert describing uses and side effects. Be sure to read it.

Are antibiotics used too much?

Most doctors believe antibiotics are used too much, particularly for colds, the flu and gastroenteritis caused not by bacteria but by viruses. Antibiotics will not help with viruses. Sinus infections may be viral or bacterial, but coughing and bronchitis are almost always viral. Some patients insist on getting antibiotics if they are sick with fever, loss of appetite, and muscle aches and pains even though the cause may be viral. Widespread use of antibiotics has produced resistance to them in bacteria. Frequently found in intensive care units, these resistant organisms can cause serious illnesses.

Bacteria also can become resistant through the widespread use of antibiotics in farm animals to promote growth. It is very important to cook pork, beef and fowl thoroughly; fatal gastroenteritis has been caused by bacteria contaminating chickens and pigs. The World Health Organization advises ending antibiotic use in livestock. Alternatives are being sought.

---

* Other derisive nicknames for doctors include Dr. Doublits because, if one dose of a medicine doesn't work, they ask you to double the dose, and Dr. Addanother (prescription).

The Nutrition Action Newsletter included these guidelines in a consumer' guide to antibiotics: Don't expect or demand antibiotics from your doctor; take the full course of antibiotic treatment; don't save antibiotics for later use or share with others; let your doctor know about side effects, which can be severe.

Interest is growing in what is called the new medicine. Treatment includes self-awareness of stresses and strains. The new medicine holds that relaxation, meditation and a healthy lifestyle with proper nutrition, weight control and exercise may be more helpful than medicine (Chapter 65).

MALPRACTICE

36. What is malpractice? What if something went wrong but I am okay? What is defensive medicine? What is a frivolous lawsuit? What are punitive damages? Why didn't the doctor tell me this might happen after the operation? Is there a solution to the present malpractice crisis?

Medical malpractice is defined as negligence in the care of a patient below the level of practice in the community, resulting in injury, damage, or loss. First, negligence must have occurred; something clearly was done wrong and led to a problem, complication, or a poor result. Secondly, the care must be below the level of practice or standard in the community in which the doctor worked. Community standards vary. The standard in the mountain tourist town of Branson, Missouri, doesn't compare to that of a large urban academic medical center like St. Louis. Some medical leaders have tried to develop a national standard of care but some states do not want one. Unfortunately, bad results will happen after an operation or treatment, but, without negligence and substandard care, a bad result or complication is not malpractice.

Medical negligence may arise from:

1. Deficiencies in experience, education, and skill to do certain procedures or carry out certain treatments.
2. Inadequate supervision of students, interns or residents.
3. Medical record documentation not satisfactory, considered inadequate or even inappropriate.
4. Communication failures, particularly with informed consent to operate.
5. Inadequate quality control, such as office systems and delays in treatment.

What if something went wrong but I ended up being okay?

Even if there is negligence (How do you know?), but no complications for you, why are you suing? You may want money, you may be angry, or you may want to get the doctor. If you have not suffered any injury, however, you do not have a valid claim for medical malpractice.

Many malpractice lawsuits are frivolous. We are a litigious society. People sue about everything and anything, and lawyers make a living accordingly. Juries have given huge awards, sometimes millions of dollars. Juries may feel sorry for patients. Insurance companies will pay for the awards anyway. Many doctors, scared of lawsuits, practice defensive medicine. During my career all our property and savings were in my wife's name so that a judgment against me would not wipe us out. That meant I couldn't fall out with my wife, either.

Costs of malpractice insurance are very high. Twelve states have malpractice premium crises. All doctors should have insurance but it is so expensive that it is driving many doctors from practice or making them drop certain high risk activities, such as obstetrics. Lawyers use billboards and ads in the yellow pages to advertise: "Malpractice? See us. We get results! Aggressive personalized representation. Call now!" Froma Harrop wrote recently about greedy lawyers who are driving doctors out of business. The lawyers would say these are "bad doctors," but while bad doctors may cause some problems, more frequently problems are the result of predictable complications. The best of doctors cannot prevent some bad results, and a few honest errors occur. If doctors are driven from practice, the public does not benefit. Some controls are needed, particularly for excessive awards.

Some doctors have been arrested and charged with murder by a prosecuting attorney in the Los Angeles area when a patient did poorly or died. I know of several cases where capable physicians were charged with murder when a patient they saw or helped died. Only massive support from the medical community convinced the judge to throw the cases out.

The AMA Voice expresses concern that "Liability insurance rates are soaring, hurting both physicians and patients." The answer is that patients must insist on reform to help their doctors. Doctors have little influence on legislatures. Lawyers have a lot of influence. Many legislators are lawyers. Insurance companies are doing well.

Our colleagues in Risk Management at St. Louis University Hospital measured the frequency of claims for non-negligent injuries. Behind some claims were unusual anatomies of certain patients, poor results not due to errors, and common complications of treatment and operations. Other causes included rare drug reactions, unforeseeable accidents, some underlying problem in an instrument or equipment, and emergency circumstances. Psycho-social factors enter into some lawsuits as do unrealistic expectations; physical and emotional pain and suffering; negative attitudes about hospitals and doctors; poor communication with the doctor; pressure to file a malpractice suit from family members and lawyers; fraud, or greed; and finally, family and individual dysfunction with loss of wage-earning capacity, medical bills, and other financial drains. The three C's for physicians for a better relationship with you and a decrease in the likelihood of frivolous suits are: communication, concern for you as a patient, and competence.

I have heard that some doctors practice defensive medicine to avoid lawsuits. What is defensive medicine?

An example provides the best explanation. Suppose you have sprained your ankle. A doctor examines you and believes your injury is just a sprain, with no broken bones. Unless he gets an x-ray of your ankle, however, he can't be positive. If you do not have an x-ray and later find that you have a painful ankle and a fracture, you may sue the doctor for not getting an x-ray. So, he gets an x-ray. A doctor thinks he must do other diagnostic procedures, treatments, and referrals to specialists so that patients cannot sue in the future for not discovering or treating a problem, or for delays in treatment. Medicine is not an exact science. We cannot be sure about many things. Doctors do not know who will sue. A number of lawsuits, threats of lawsuits and trivial lawsuits lead to defensive medicine. Doctors can't take chances so they take measures to protect themselves.

What is a frivolous or nuisance lawsuit?

This is a patient's lawsuit based on nothing more than a minor complication or anger at the doctor or feelings of neglect or depression. A good attorney will try to calm the patient down or explain that the facts do not support a claim of malpractice. If pressed by the patient and/or family, the attorney should find a competent and trustworthy physician to review the medical record and the situation and provide advice about proceeding. I have done this for several attorneys with problems in areas I felt competent. Some lawyers may proceed with lawsuits no matter what the merits. I suppose they think they will get some money out of it by a settlement from the doctor and/or his insurance company. Most of us fight such suits until the end rather than settle and pay such attorneys and patients.

What are punitive damages?

In a liability trial whether it be a suit against a doctor for alleged malpractice or against General Motors for an injury resulting from a problem in car design, the jury may award compensation for medical and other expenses plus punitive damages. An example of this was a verdict against General Motors of $4.9 Billion.

This was $107.6 Million in compensation to six people in a crash and car fire and $4.8 Billion in punitive damages. This amount may be reduced on appeal. Glaberson in the New York Times quotes David Leebron, Dean of the Columbia Law School "The system awards punitive damages not out of concern for the plaintiff but out of concern about the defendants conduct". This huge award against GM was meant to punish them. Excessive punitive damages and malpractice awards have led to a national movement for court reform. Some states put a cap on punitive damages of $250,000 in medical malpractice. The 12 states with malpractice crises also need a cap on awards. Is it fair to allow punitive damages based on the outrage of a jury? Many recent headlines concern mistakes in medicine—like a heart-lung transplant of the wrong blood type for a young Mexican girl at Duke University Hospital.

Why didn't the doctor tell me this might happen after the operation?

The question is "were you warned satisfactorily about potential risks of an operation or a treatment, and the potential benefits?" Did you ask any questions of your doctor? How much did you want to know preoperatively? Your doctor should tell you about the risk of dying, the possibility of general complications, and the risks versus the benefit of the procedure. It is standard practice for surgeons to convey that information. Remember, before an operation you must sign a form consenting to it and anything related to it and on the same form, you must indicate you had been informed about risks, benefits, and problems of the operation. If you believe you have not been properly informed, don't sign the form and don't have the operation. It is as simple as that.

Most of us do not go into great detail about everything that could happen during treatment or an operation. If you are having an operation requiring a general or spinal anesthetic, we give you a general warning about the possibility of death but may not specify all possible causes such as (1) a heart attack, an arrhythmia, or a cardiac arrest that would kill you on the spot; (2) a stroke, (3) a severe allergic reaction, (4) a wound infection (5) a wound separation (dehiscence), (6) blood clots in your legs that go to your lungs, (7) bleeding into your wound. These complications may occur after any operation. Specific complications occur after certain operations.

Some possible complications after an operation are extremely rare. For example, certain patients develop insufficiency of the adrenal glands, a condition so rare it is not even listed in some textbooks. It can happen, however. Is this something your doctor must tell you? No. Your doctor can't tell you every single, little thing that might happen after an operation. You have to go on generalities. In a recent article in JAMA, Bulgardes, et al., indicated "virtually every course of medical action is associated with some associated risk to the patient, and discussing such a risk is an obligation of the physician." General risks should be discussed. Do you want to know what the chances are of your dying during the operation or afterward in the postoperative period? I would tell the patient that the risk of that happening in one hundred patients is about 5%. We will try to make it zero but that is not possible. Things can happen that we have no control over. A detailed list of every possible problem is not necessary.

Is there a solution to the present malpractice crisis? What are some approaches to alleviate malpractice problems?

When things occur in hospitals that should not have occurred, the approach in the past was to "deny and defend". Now some doctors believe it is better to say, "I am sorry." They develop an honesty policy: to admit errors and propose settlements for injuries or lost days of work. Doctors may avoid getting sued by offering an apology. Paternalism by doctors is being replaced by telling the patient the whole story: What went wrong and why.

The Medical Malpractice Prevention Alert suggests nine ways to stop complaints before they occur: 1) Return phone calls; 2) don't keep patients waiting; 3) be open and honest, especially when you don't know the answer; 4) eliminate bad listening habits; 5) learn something personal about each patient; 6) get patients actively involved in their own care; 7) be more medically suspicious; 8) don't avoid the unhappy patients; 9) survey your patient to see if your methods are working.

CAN DO—MUST DO

37. If a doctor can do something for me, must he do it? What is the technological imperative?

If you are an Alzheimer's patient at the end of life, unable to know family or surroundings, you may develop other medical problems. An example is a perforated duodenal ulcer, an emergency that can be treated successfully in normal people by an operation. Because we can do it, must we do it? I can, therefore I must? I think it depends on the circumstances. If you were such a patient and could give informed consent, you might not want an operation. Would your family insist that you have one? I hope not.

I have reviewed many such cases when the patient seems to need an emergency operation but afterward is labeled, "do not resuscitate (DNR)." Why can't such a patient be made "DNR" pre-operatively and not put through a painful procedure. If patients know and enjoy their relationships with their family, their surroundings, and their God, then it is a different matter. I am writing about patients who are not in control or are in a chronic vegetative state. "I can, therefore I must" has been called "The Technological Imperative in Health Care" by Fuchs. Barger-Lux and Heaney, point out the distortion or if a doctor values things or operations over people. They cite Moser who attributes the driving power of technology in health care to a concept of the "intellectual imperative" which underlies pursuit of new ideas. In the past, insurance companies were more willing to pay for diagnostic and technical procedures like operations than for office visits to doctors.

As a resident in training to become a surgeon, I participated in a weekly conference called the morbidity and mortality (M & M) conference. At this meeting, all deaths and complications of our patients were reviewed in detail. This is an excellent example of quality assurance or control carried out voluntarily by surgeons as a continuous teaching and learning experience. The central theme was: How could we have done better? The emphasis was on how to prevent complications and to keep patients alive. Death was the enemy, and we worked hard to prevent it. For a young surgeon it is important to know that if you operate on a patient, the patient should survive and leave the hospital alive. Otherwise perhaps you should not have done the operation. This goal can become an obsession, however, so that patients are kept alive longer than is appropriate (Chapter 46) and End of Life Decisions (Chapter 49-50).

The technological imperative contributes to the high cost of health care. More diagnostic studies may be done than are necessary. Should everyone beyond the age of 50-60 have colonoscopy? Colonoscopists say yes. I say no, if you have no family history of colon cancer or polyps and your stool contains no blood. Examples abound of overused laboratory studies and diagnostic procedures, treatment programs and operations. The questions are: Do I need this? Why? What is the rationale or justification for it? This should slow down application of the technological imperative: "I can do this for you, therefore I will do it."

FRAUD—ABUSE

38. What are fraud and abuse laws? Are there really dishonest doctors?

The cost of Medicare in 1964 was $500 million, now it is tens of billions. A minor provision in the original bill prohibited false statements to obtain benefits. A series of amendments since then have created complex laws on fraud and abuse. The original misdemeanors have become felonies with fines and imprisonment. Sage describes the vagaries of fraud and abuse law as underlying tensions in the health care system, with conflicts between the Government's roles as purchaser of health care and as its regulator and between the goals of protecting the financial integrity of Medicare and protecting patient welfare.

Kick-backs, self referrals, and inducements to influence the purchase or sale of health care services or goods are illegal. Penalties are so severe that everyone is scared, leading to some silly consequences. A St. Louis hospital provided an annual or birthday chest x-ray, laboratory studies and a stress test EKG for doctors on its medical staff. This is good medical practice and the hospital expected nothing from the doctors. The program was stopped, however, because of worry over fraud and abuse.

During my career, we took care of fellow physicians and their families without charging a fee, a practice called professional courtesy authorized by the oath of Hippocrates in ancient Greece. I was proud to care for colleagues and their families and would mark their accounts—insurance only. If they had insurance, I would accept it but sent no other bill. That practice is now illegal. What kind of monster has the government created?

Some doctors may manipulate reimbursement rules for your benefit so you receive care your doctor thinks you need but your health plan does not allow.

Are there really dishonest doctors?

Probably so but not many. Some doctors may have been dishonest in their patients' care but they are very rare. I have never known one. A few doctors have submitted false claims for services they did not provide, like diagnostic tests or have inflated claims. This is infrequent and such doctors have been tracked down and punished.

Medicare officials have complained about fraud by doctors and hospitals but most problems come from companies that pay claims, Medicare Contractors. The GAO said, "Deceptions and improprieties become a way of doing business at some companies as employees taught one another how to cheat the government and cover up their mistakes." In 1998, Blue Cross and Blue Shield of Illinois paid $4 million in criminal fines and $140 million in settlement to the government. If some doctors are dishonest, they are small players in the perpetration of fraud.

It is said some doctors employed by hospitals or health systems are told to see patients more frequently to increase revenue. They may instruct the doctors to see fee-for-service patients every month or frequently whether they need it or not. The doctors are to see capitated patients, under plans that pay flat fees for all care, as infrequently as possible. Honest doctors condemn such practices.

Ethics is now being taught in all medical schools and integrity in medicine is stressed. Dishonesty in research occurs infrequently. An investigator may manipulate results of a research study or make up results to make the study seem important. Fraud in research is eventually discovered when other laboratories cannot confirm these results. It is then dealt with severely.

REFERRAL TO A SPECIALIST.

39. What is the basis for referral to a specialist? Is it an old boys' or girls' network? Why was I referred to a woman urologist to have my prostate gland checked?

A good primary care doctor will get to know specialists to whom he can refer his patients for care. Your doctor and the specialists may be on the same hospital staff. They get to know each other and learn they can work together for your care. Your doctor will not refer you to someone who is incompetent; that would not be in your best interest and would reflect badly on your doctor's judgment. Your doctor does not want to refer you to someone he or she does not know, and especially not to someone whose results are unknown.

It may seem to you referrals are based on old boys' or girls' networks or clubs but that is not true even if your doctor and specialists may be friends, colleagues, medical school or college classmates, or play golf together. These relationships reflect friendship and trust. It is much easier for your doctor to ask a specialist who is a friend and colleague for an opinion about your medical problem. Frequently in the medical staff lounge over lunch or a cup of coffee, a physician would ask me what I would do with a problem. All of us communicate freely in that way. Your name does not come into the conversation unless you are being referred to that specialist. If the medical care you require is not available in your community, you may be referred to a medical center in a large city and to a specialist not known to your doctor but with a reputation in the field. You may ask your doctor why he has referred you to a certain specialist. What is his or her reputation?

If you belong to an HMO, you must see their specialists. Generally, they are competent and you can trust them. However, if you must be hospitalized, you must go to the hospital where they work. Your doctor may not be on its staff and therefore would be unable to see you.

Why was I referred to a woman urologist to have my prostate gland checked?

Women perform well in any specialty of medicine and in the operative disciplines. I remember a few years ago when one of my female residents in general surgery expressed an interest in orthopedic surgery and another in urology. While I was a bit mystified as to why they would choose those specialties, I helped them and they have done well. However, just as women over the years have hesitated to see male gynecologists or male breast surgeons, men may be uncomfortable about seeing a female urologist for a rectal/prostate exam. This is a cultural problem. If it bothers you, state your feelings to your doctor before the referral is made.

Many women are much more comfortable now with a woman gynecologist and obstetrician, and many female residents are entering that specialty. Also, many women with breast cancer are more comfortable with a woman surgeon. Many departments of surgery have a female surgeon who specializes in breast cancer. I believe this is a healthy phenomenon. A woman better understands the importance of the breast to another woman than does a man.

COCKTAIL PARTY CONSULTATIONS

40. What are informal or curbside consultations?

These can take place at a cocktail party between you and a doctor or between doctors in a hospital, medical staff lounge, or cafeteria. Informal consultations can produce information but cannot give the final answer on care. They are a common practice. On the way to the parking garage, George calls out to Tom, "I have a patient with this disease. What do you think? Where should I go? Have you had any similar experiences?" Such conversations may help the patient.

I frequently went to the x-ray department, got out the x-ray studies of a patient of mine and reviewed them in detail with a radiologist. We discussed the possibilities and what might be done. Sometimes the radiologist suggested additional studies. If I needed help with a patient I would call a colleague and describe the problem and get advice. I was an expert in chest surgery but I sought help from cardiologists, pulmonologists, radiologists and others.

At a cocktail party or a reception or a dinner you may say "Doctor, I hate to bother you but what do you think about my problem?" Don't be embarrassed to do this. Doctors love to talk about medicine and therapy. It is their life. They love to be authoritarian, particularly if they can help, so go ahead and ask them. Just be sure it is private between you and the doctor. Such conversations should not be used by you as the basis for your health decisions. They are for information only. See your doctor.

BEDSIDE MANNERS

41. Why aren't doctors taught bedside manners? Are there concerned and caring doctors with a good bedside manner? Why do doctors talk to my husband and my family about my illness but not to me? What is empathy?

We should produce good doctors and doctors who are good.

Joseph E. O'Donnell, MD
Ideas for Medical Education
Acad Med 1998; 73-74

Yes, we have many good doctors, and you should be able to find one. A question I am asked is: "My doctor seems to be good but he has a terrible bedside manner. He is curt, abrupt and never spends much time with me. Why is that?" To that question, I have another question: "How do you know he is a good doctor?" Many of us believe it is impossible to be a good doctor or a good surgeon without being a good person. Concern for you as a person and as a patient is part of the healing process. Many doctors may be extremely capable scientifically. They may be very knowledgeable about disease and its treatment. However, something in their background has not allowed them to communicate with patients or to let patients know they are concerned about their well being. Caring and concern are part of being a doctor.

The selection criteria for admission to medical school emphasize an excellent college grade point average; courses in physics, chemistry, and biology, among other subjects; and high scores on a daunting standardized test called the MCAT, or Medical College Admissions Test. The admissions process also includes a personal interview and a statement by the student about why he or she is interested in medicine. The future doctor must be bright, capable and competitive. How about caring? How about concern for sick people? These attributes have not been part of the formula. How would you measure it if it is to be considered? Some pre-medical students learn to say the right things. In an interview, students may say "I want to help people." The remark may not be facetious or dishonest; they may actually want to help people. However, the other criteria so overwhelm the criterion of caring that it is lost in the shuffle.

When I was at Yale, my wife took a course on compassion at the Yale Divinity School under Professor Henri Nouwen, a well-known Priest-scholar. Assigned to do a project, my wife decided to ask the Admissions Committee of the Yale School of Medicine how they measured compassion in selecting future students. Nouwen agreed that merely asking the committee this question would accomplish as much as getting any answers from them. It would make them think about compassion in students.

This is now changing. Courses in medical schools are adding exercises in communication, the humanities and caring, which should be part of being a good doctor. Howard Spiro at Yale Medical School developed a program in the Humanities in Medicine for students and faculty that included these lectures: "Medicine, Ethics and the Third Reich," "Hygeia Revisited: Lessons to Comfort," "When a patient wants to die," "The Human Encounters in Medicine" and "Meeting the Challenge of Alternative Medicine."

Formerly, the first two years of medical school were devoted to the sciences, with intense courses in anatomy, biochemistry, physiology, pathology, pharmacology, and the neurosciences. Students took no courses with patients. Many of us wondered what this exclusive focus on science had to do with being a doctor. The information was important. Good doctors must be well versed in science. It would have been worthwhile, however, to also have some programs devoted to becoming a doctor. During the first two years some basic scientists or MDs would suggest eventual clinical importance of their subjects. Many, however, were PhD's who had never practiced medicine. While good teachers and investigators, they could not relate their areas of expertise to the care of patients.

The current emphasis on people skills and better communication will produce more thoughtful and caring physicians. Medicine has gone through an intense period of scientific development, and these changes will only accelerate. It is encouraging to see at the same time a return to emphasis on humanitarian concerns and ethical considerations.

An oath written by the Harvard Medical School Class of 1997 combines the classical oaths, the Hippocratic Oath, Maimonides prayer and the 1948 Declaration of Geneva: "Now being admitted to the profession of medicine or dentistry, I solemnly pledge myself to the service of humanity. I will practice medicine with conscience and dignity. I will hold in confidence all that my patient confides in me. I will strive to promote the honor and integrity of the medical profession. I will give respect and gratitude to my deserving teachers, ever mindful of my continuing role as both a student and a teacher. In the service of patients I will promote the health and well being of myself and my colleagues. I will treat all in need without bias and with openness of spirit. I will maintain the utmost respect for the dignity of all people. Even under threat, I will not use my knowledge contrary to the laws of humanity. And above all, the health and life of my patient will be my first consideration. These promises I make freely and upon my honor."

A movement in medical education now emphasizes professionalism. In *Time to Heal—American Medical Education from the Turn of the Century to the Era of Managed Care,* Ludmerer recommends courses on what it is to be a professional. He notes complaints from the public that doctors "are impersonal, self serving, and greedy". If true, these complaints apply to a small number of doctors but reflect on all of us.

Some medical schools employ chaplains. At the Yale School of Medicine, the chaplain is Allen C. Mermann, an M.D. and ordained minister who practiced pediatrics for 27 years, then earned a Master of Divinity at Yale Divinity School and became Chaplain for the Medical School. He believes his work has little to do with formal religion but everything to do with helping students understand what it means to be a good doctor. As reported by Carolyn Battista, Dr. Mermann once said: "Students want to become caring, compassionate physicians but they worry about losing compassion as they train in hectic hospital settings where the patient may seem less a person than the subject of clinical laboratory reports." Dr. Mermann aims to help students keep on caring. Dr. Bernard Jaffe points out the values of respect, integrity, honesty, commitment, concern for others, and responsibility cannot necessarily be taught in medical school or in a residency program. They should be part of growing up for those who wish to become physicians.

For those who are already physicians, continuing medical education programs now seek to enhance their personal awareness and improve their effectiveness in patient care. One proposed program comprises four core topics for reflection and discussion: physicians' beliefs and attitudes, physicians' feelings and emotional responses in patient care, challenging clinical situations and physician self care. Journals and books for doctors now contain articles about caring, with lessons doctors can learn from their patients. A little generosity creates a lot of good will.

Patients who feel ignored are more likely to file lawsuits against doctors. It is too bad that the possibility of litigation is the cause but doctors are being taught to listen and to let patients know they are listening. Hospitals in St. Louis developed a course for doctors emphasizing the importance of communication with patients, with patient-centered interviewing. The doctor, after knocking at the door of the patient's room, is to enter and ask open-ended questions: "What do you want to talk about? What do you come to see me about?" Florence Shinkle described the technique in wonderful detail in the *Post-Dispatch* for August 26, 1998. She points out that HMOs stand in the way of popularization. Under their pay-per-patient reimbursement plan for doctors, the more patients the doctor sees, the more money he makes. Asked to see a large number of patients, doctors are unable to spend very much time with each one of them. Shinkle quotes a doctor joke in which a patient says, "Doctor, please help me. I think I am invisible." The doctor says, "Next, please." Communication patterns indicate patient satisfaction with primary care physicians at its highest when the subject is the individual patient and covers personal habits, entire background and problems, rather than just biomedical aspects of the illness.

For an article in *Academic Medicine,* Frederic W. Hafferty, who teaches behavioral science at the University of Minnesota/Duluth School of Medicine, asked his mother and her friends to write about their concerns, problems, and positive experiences in their relationships with doctors. One woman said, "What do I look for in a doctor? I want a person with whom I can communicate freely and easily without intimidation because of his special knowledge. I want an excellent technician/a perfectionist who will treat me as an important patient, not someone on a conveyor belt who is hurried along." The women warned future physicians about being too cheerful; it may be a distancing maneuver by the doctor. A caring touch was important to them and sometimes they felt like hugging their doctor in appreciation. Their biggest concerns were barriers they experienced in obtaining test results and related information. Unreturned phone calls were common; untold hours were spent by phones in hopes of calls from doctors that never came. Many medical students would benefit from learning from elderly, or even not-so-elderly, patients about what they expect from their doctors, what they appreciate, and what is worthwhile for them.

Stephen A. Schmidt on the faculty at Loyola University in Chicago suffers from a gastrointestinal disease called Crohn's disease. Addressing doctors in the JAMA section titled "A piece of my mind," he says "when you come into my hospital room, you need to know the facts of my life . . ."

"there is information not contained in my hospital chart
I am 40 years married with four children and four grandchildren
I have led a chronic illness group for 12 years
I have been hospitalized more than a dozen times for partial bowel
    obstruction
I am chronically ill, and am seeking healing, not cure
my disease has narrowed my life, constricted it
I can no longer eat fresh salads or drink a glass of wine
I hate rounds held outside my room, that do not include nurses,
    my wife, my children, my pastor or even me . . . rounds done
    over me, around me, but not with me this body seems battered,
    old vulnerable, tired . . . but still me
I live by waiting in the eternal "advent season" of doctors' offices
I am emotional . . . a fully functioning feeling person
I am afraid of the NG tube, sometimes wrapped in my mouth,
    clogged
I fear surgery, each time, I have lost confidence in my body
I seek meaning in suffering
I am slowly coming to believe meaning is what we bring to suffering,
    not what we gain from it, I believe deeply that I need to engage
    suffering.

When you come into my room, you need to sustain hope
You need to know I believe love wins over hate, hope over despair,
    life over death
I pray and believe prayer heals, I hope against hope—and bear my
    rage about my disease
I am angry and sad, support my hope."

Concerned and caring doctors will show you that interest and care are important. They will greet you in a friendly way and give you the feeling that all of their attention is on what concerns you and how they might help. I always sat down close to the patient so we could talk on the same level. I always talked to the patient before asking the nurse to help the patient undress while I left the room. When I returned to examine the patient, the nurse stayed in the room. After the examination, I asked the patient to dress and again I left the room. I returned to summarize the visit and answer questions. This need not take an hour. It can be done in 10 to 15 minutes without rushing unless the health problem is difficult or complex.

Francis Weld Peabody in a lecture to Harvard Medical students and the public in 1926 concluded, "The secret of the care of the patient is in caring for the patient." This well-known quotation should be a hallmark for all physicians; caring for patients requires we care about our patients. Peabody also said, "Treatment of a disease may be entirely impersonal; care of a patient must be completely personal."

A colleague and friend, Dr. John Ashmore, Jr., reviews in a medical context the books of three writers on etiquette: Emily Post's *Etiquette* and her heirs— Letitia Baldrige *Revision and Expansion of the Amy Vanderbilt Complete Book of Etiquette* and Judith Martin's *Miss Manners Guide to Excruciatingly Correct Behavior.* "Doctors should avoid presumed omnipotence," says Miss Manners. "Its consequences are like the arrogance of an automobile mechanic." She rails against making patients wait for physician services and asks that physicians warn the patient of any delay in the same way airlines do. In these books, Ashmore finds the word "kindness" significant in all definitions of proper behavior. Elizabeth L. Post, in the preface of her grandmother-in-law's book, defines etiquette as "a code of behavior based on kindness and consideration." Ashmore concludes, "In all encounters with patients that involve family, we would do well to remember that age-old maternal admonition, 'Mind your manners'."

Why do doctors talk to my husband and my family about my illness but not to me?

Some families tell the doctor, "Don't tell her what it is or how bad it is." This may be sound advice particularly for elderly patients when telling them of a dire disease or prognosis could eliminate any will they have to live. Patients should always be encouraged and given hope no matter what the problem.

There are no rules for this, only common sense. Some patients want to know the details of their illness and what is in store for them. Other patients do not. For patients who cannot understand or don't want to know the seriousness of their condition, careful encouragement is needed. Patients should not be given a death sentence with no hope for the future. Some patients told me "Don't tell me I have cancer," so I didn't. I told them they had a tumor or growth which must be removed. This they accepted. The word cancer is a terrible devastating word for many concerned patients.

What is empathy?

Empathy is described in the medical dictionary as intellectual and sometimes emotional identification with another's feelings. Sympathy, on the other hand, is the feeling an individual has in the close sharing of another's experience or feelings—commonly sad, painful, or unpleasant feelings. Compassion is sympathetic consciousness of others' distress together with a desire to alleviate it. Until recent times none of these expressions had appeared in a medical school curriculum. Now, all medical schools use them in considering communication with patients.

In their article "The Importance of Empathy as An Interviewing Skill in Medicine," Bellet and Maloney describe empathy as the capacity to understand what another person is experiencing from within the other person's frame of reference, i.e., the capacity to place one's self in another's shoes. "The essence of empathic interaction is accurate understanding of another person's feelings." This should be the foundation of a physician-patient relationship. It is important for doctors to understand not only the patient's disease but also the patient's experiences and feelings about the disease and related problems. Reassurance and patient-parent education are not necessarily part of empathy. A hasty remark meant to reassure a patient and his/her parents, if it is a child, may actually increase anxiety and concern.

Some of the distinctions pointed out by Spiro are "Empathy is a feeling I might be you" or "I am you". It is more than just an intellectual identification". Empathy must be accompanied by feeling. Sympathy brings compassion, "I want to help you," but empathy brings emotion. In care of patients, physicians must balance empathy and equanimity, or an evenness of mind especially under stress. The physician must be able to study and treat the patient objectively, carry out an operation if necessary, and attend to other matters requiring some detachment from the emotional problems of the patient.

The importance of empathy is now recognized by many medical schools, as in Spiro's *A Program for Humanities in Medicine* at Yale. *Empathy and the Practice of Medicine—Beyond Pills and the Scalpel*, published by Spiro and colleagues, should be required reading for medical students before their internship. In the Introduction, Spiro states: "Some considered praise of empathy a criticism of science but that is a mistake. Medical practice is not an either/or situation. There are no dichotomies: clinicians need science and emotion, reason and intuition, technology and narratives, equanimity and empathy." Writing in the 1980's about physician-patient relationships, Bellet and Maloney found that in the previous five years 85% of the patients in their study changed doctors or were thinking of changing them, many because of the physicians' poor communication skills. Bellet and Maloney believe if physicians have not learned empathy in their training as medical students and residents, they may be ineffective in patient care.

A study of communication during routine office visits recommended that surgeons develop skills to enhance patient education and counseling and to understand the influences of surgical communications on patients behavioral, psychological, and biomedical outcomes. Surgeons infrequently expressed empathy toward patients and kept social conversation brief. Sarr and Warshaw point out "What to a surgeon is just a routine breast biopsy for an abnormality of a women's breast determined by mammography carries for the patient terrifying concerns of cancer, mutilation and death . . . . For a patient with a simple inguinal hernia it means pain, time lost from work, and inconvenience for the family, and perhaps decreased income." Surgeons must remember these effects upon patients of what to a surgeon may seem a simple clinical or technical problem.

An empathic approach to patient care in today's world takes time. Physicians are paid per patient rather than per hour. Visiting with patients about their feelings, concerns, anxiety, illness, and basis of their illness takes time but is very important. Hopefully, the empathic approach will not be lost in managed care.

42. What is alternative, complementary or integrative medicine? Is it for me? Will doctors be taught these new things?

Alternative medicine uses methods to prevent and treat disease that are not established scientifically or taught widely in medical schools or used in U.S hospitals. For the most part medical schools teach allopathic medicine, called conventional, traditional, or orthodox medicine, a system of treatment producing effects on the body different from those produced by disease. Focused on treating symptoms, the allopathic system is the opposite of the homeopathic system, which seeks to treat the whole individual instead of the disease. This definition may not help much. I will provide other information to help you understand differences between allopathic and alternative, complementary or integrative medicine.

Also sometimes called herbal medicine, alternative medicine is much more than that. Because of its popularity and extensive use, many medical schools now offer courses about it, and academic health centers recognize the merit of some of its applications. Future doctors will be quite familiar with alternative medicine. The *Journal of the American Medical Association (JAMA)* and its *Archives Journals* devote yearly issues to complementary, alternative, unconventional or integrative medicine. James Whorton chronicles it in *Nature Cures: The History of Alternative Medicine in America,* Oxford Press, NY 2002.

Alternative medicine takes many different forms, as shown in Table 1. *The Practitioners Guide to Integrative Therapies* describes 59 types of treatments by alternative approaches, including Reiki, an ancient Tibetan healing system; Shiatsu, a Japanese form of massage; a macrobiotic diet of only whole grains, vegetables and seeds; and Feng Shui, the ancient Chinese belief that arrangement of objects in the home influence the owner's fortunes.

It is estimated that $14 billion a year is spent in the U.S. for alternative therapy and that it is used by one in three Americans and some doctors. Why is it so popular? First, it is part of the culture of much of the world. Home remedies have always been popular, as reviewed by Sangiorgio: as chicken soup for a cold, pineapple for overindulgence, cranberry juice for urinary tract infections, ginger for nausea, oatmeal or baking soda for itchy skin, a hot bath for insomnia, yogurt for yeast infections or water for a hangover. My family knows I always recommend gargling warm salt water for a sore throat and laryngitis.

Second, conventional medicine can do little about ailments like a cold or the flu other than relieve symptoms, and it may be able to provide little relief for chronic problems like back pain, sprains, headache and arthritis. Third, use of some dietary supplements, herbs, vitamins and other agents is thought to produce a healthy lifestyle and ways to stay healthy.

Plants have long provided effective medicines, like the active ingredient from willow bark, salicin, similar to aspirin; digitalis for the heart from the foxglove plant; and many others. Now, however, many herbs without known effective ingredients have become popular. The word natural ingredient does not mean safety. You must learn what herbs can and cannot do. The list of herbs used for medicines is long and includes some associated with many problems and deaths. (Tables II and III) If you are taking any of these be sure your doctor knows. Many of these may conflict with conventional or prescription drugs.

A new federal requirement may help you. Dietary supplements must include a new information panel to provide a list of ingredients and the quantities, including herbal products. The FDA provides information about dietary supplements and gives warnings about available substances that cause trouble at *http://vm/gfsan.fda.gov/~dms/*. *A Physicians Reference to Botanical Medicines* and *Complete German Commission E Monographs—Therapeutic Guides to Herbal Medicines* can be obtained from Integrative Medicine Communications, 43 Bowdoin St., Boston, MA 02114, 1-800-217-1938. Medical Economics Co., Montvale, NJ, publishes *A Physicians Desk Reference (PDR)* for herbal medicines and nutritional supplements (order from PDR, PO Box 10689, Des Moines, IA 50380-0689).

Public health officials believe herbal remedies and dietary supplements should be regulated. The Dietary Supplement Health and Educational Act (DSHEA) in 1994 allowed manufacturers to sell supplements with review by the FDA for safety only and to put information about benefits on the label. Many believe this is a terrible law, promoting market growth but failing to protect you. The manufacturers do not have to report adverse reactions to the FDA. They should be required to turn over any reports about harm to consumers. Industry seems to have fought against safety.

The popularity of alternative medicine has led to the publication of many magazines and books on the subject. A leading example is the best-selling *Spontaneous Healing* by Andrew Weil, M.D., also the author of *Eight Weeks to Optimum Health* and *Eating Well for Optimum Health*. A graduate of the Harvard Medical School who has studied herbal and alternative medicine extensively, Weil believes, and I agree, that alternative medicine should be integrated with traditional medicine. He makes no grandiose claims, offering sound advice and sensible views, always supported with evidence. Weil is practical: "If I am hit by a car," he says, "don't take me to an herb doctor. I want to go to a modern emergency ward". He advocates eating plenty of fruits and vegetables, taking vitamins, cutting down on fats, maintaining good oral health, getting enough rest, drinking lots of water and avoiding indiscriminate use of antibiotics to strengthen your immune system. For anti-oxidants, he describes what they do, where they are found in natural foods and when supplements can help. I agree with Weil's recommendations for a healthy, healing diet. They are sensible and consistent with other nutrition experts' advice.

Weil notes that doctors occupy the position in our society occupied by shamans and priests in earlier cultures. He believes patients want shamans: someone to listen and help them achieve mental comfort and serenity as well as treat their disease. Some doctors don't do this well. Weil believes medical education and doctors have focused on disease rather than on healing. He says conventional medicine does well in managing injuries, handling emergencies, treating infections and replacing damaged joints. He also says conventional medicine can't do much for viral infections, most chronic degenerative diseases, most forms of allergy or autoimmune diseases and many cancers, and for these problems he recommends combining traditional medicine with integrated medicine. He describes strategies used by patients who have had spontaneous healing and makes sound suggestions for managing cardiovascular, digestive, and other diseases. Weil emphasizes the importance of meditation. With his approval, I include at the end of this chapter the appendix from his book *Spontaneous Healing* under the title "Finding practitioners, supplies and information."

Dr. Jeremy Geffen, an oncologist, writes in *The Journey through Cancer* that his clinic tries to address the emotional and spiritual needs of his patients along with traditional therapy.

In *The New York Times Guide to Alternative Health,* Jane E. Brody and Denise Grady cover scientifically proven therapies, herbal medicine and prescription drug interactions, unregulated supplements, promising remedies and dangerous frauds and scams.

In *Perfect Health* Deepak Chopra, MD, a prolific writer and a guru of alternative medicine, focuses on Ayurveda of India, an ancient holistic system of medicine. As with all these advocates, he has his own center, Chopra Center for Well Being in LaJolla, California. By and large, fruits and vegetables are favored; calories and fats, proteins and carbohydrates are not mentioned.

Why have courses in alternative medicine been latecomers to medical schools? The major reason has been lack of scientific evidence for its effectiveness. Evidence for such treatments is anecdotal, not rigorously scientific. Practitioners of alternative medicine were called herb doctors, and chiropractic and similar forms of treatment were thought akin to witchcraft.

In traditional medicine we believe a new agent or treatment should be studied by a trial in patients who volunteer to receive the active agent or a placebo, a harmless pill or treatment thought not to influence the problem and therefore able to serve as a control. No one knows the active agent from the placebo until results are recorded and the code is broken. This is called a randomized, double-blind clinical trial, the gold standard for evaluation of treatments. But how do you do a randomized, double-blind study of—to take one example—acupuncture? You either put in needles or you don't. How do you control the study?

Many alternative medicines may make you feel better but that does not prove that they are effective. If you take a medicine and feel better, it may be due to the medicine, or to spontaneous relief, or to your belief that it helps (the placebo effect). The placebo effect of a positive attitude towards a medicine can be powerful and good. (Chapters 17 and 55) Moreover, if 100 people say an alternative medicine helped them, you do not know how many people did not get relief.

Some people believe that if an alternative medicine helps, take it and don't worry about scientific studies. Some therapies, herbals and botanicals, however, may be harmful, toxic, fatal, or at the very least, worthless, (Table III) unchecked by standards or controls on purity as with drugs approved by the FDA. The amount of active ingredients in the products available varies greatly. Are there active ingredients in St. John's wort or ginseng? No one knows. What you buy at the health store may or may not contain any active ingredients. Internet marketing of herbal products may make misleading claims about the quality of ingredients. Many believe internet sales should be regulated.

A randomized controlled trial of a commercial garlic preparation found it had no effect on blood lipoproteins (cholesterol and triglycerides) and did not seem to offer protection against high cholesterol, despite claims to the contrary. In a good randomized trial Gingko did not help memory. In a 1998 trial published in JAMA, the Asian herb Garcinia cambogia did not help produce weight loss.

The FDA has received thousands of reports of adverse events with ginkgo, St. John's wort, ginseng and many other herbs and believes that many go unreported. Ephedra, now banned as is the ephedra drug Metabolife, has caused more than 172 deaths and thousands of strokes and heart attacks. Some herbs can cause cancer. The Chinese herb Aristolochia Fangchi is associated with urinary tract cancers and kidney failure.

Alternative medicines may cause problems if you have an operation with an anesthetic. St. John's wort intensifies anesthesia, gingko biloba and ginseng increase blood pressure and heart rate, and feverfew reduces blood platelets during anesthesia and operation. Interactions of herbal medicines with regular medicines can be a big problem. Tell your doctors what you are taking. Bring the bottles with you to the hospital. The best thing to do is to stop taking these herbal medicines two to three weeks before an operation.

Creatine has no proven value for athletes even though Mark McGwire took it. Congress has banned drugs used by athletes to build muscles like Verve, Thunder, Invigorate and Serenity, which produce a central nervous system depressant. But overall the lack of regulation of herbal medicines is a problem. They should be controlled by the FDA like any medicine. Nutritional companies are estimated to have contributed 10.9 million dollars to candidates for election over the last five years, with President George W. Bush, and Senators Orrin Hatch and Tom Harkin among the recipients. Of course they are not going to push to regulate these companies but how can they sit idly by when people die?

Natural products, functional foods, dietary supplements and herbal remedies are a big business. This, and the advertising claims, may lead public health officials and the FDA to look into such claims. Be careful about them. Ask what the evidence is. How do the manufacturers know an herb helps a certain problem? I recently received an advertising booklet about herbal medicines suggesting herbs could save your life, help your sex life, treat arthritis, help with menopause, help your heart and assure many other wonderful benefits. The brochure contained not a single reference to a study to indicate the herb was effective. No evidence backed up the claims. Advisors were named who approved of claims but provided no evidence for their approval. Why is this? I can only believe that, with no evidence to support the claims, they are not based on anything other than advertising and perhaps experiences of a few people.

I ordered an alternative medicine book claiming 88 new breakthrough cures for serious illness to see if it provided any evidence for the claims. It did not. The *Art of Better Living* offers to help you "discover the secret to stay young indefinitely" by using Secretagogues in a nasal spray to increase the human growth hormone. It goes on to say, "The statements in this publication have not been evaluated by the FDA". In other words, it did no controlled studies. From an ad for *Eat and Heal:* "Bananas can calm a chronic cough, strawberries can help reduce stress and calm anxiety" and so on.

The doctor in *Ask the Doctor—Answers to your Health Questions* seems to be a naturopathic physician; his credentials are not given. He recommends IHP— inositil hexophosphate found in fiber for anticancer and immune enhancing effects, citing studies that show it prevents certain cancers in rats and mice. No studies in humans were described. The book gives no address for readers who seek more information.

In contrast to many herbal remedies, acupuncture is much more established as worthwhile treatment. Considered a complementary medicine, acupuncture causes the release of pain-blocking brain and spinal opioid peptides such as beta endorphins, enkephalin and dynorphin. I have seen it used successfully for anesthesia for operations in China. It has been documented to be effective for relief of chronic pain like arthritis, headaches, facial pain, post-herpetic neuralgia, neck, elbow and low back pain, childbirth, pain of malignancy, phantom limb pain and others as described by Dr. Jung Sook Kim. George Ulett, a professor of psychiatry, uses the technique without needles but with neuroelectric acupuncture stimulation by EKG type electrodes over various sites for anxiety, depression and fibromyalgia. *Integrative Medicine Communications* published a review "Alternative Medical Therapies for Pain" (1-800-217-1938). Adverse events can occur with acupuncture but are infrequent when used by an experienced therapist.

A number of recent studies have been done of chiropractic. From personal experience I know this therapy can help provide relief for pains, sprains and other related problems, but there is a limit to what can be helped. Spinal manipulation, for example, did not help tension-type headaches or childhood asthma and had limited effects on low back pain. Acupuncture can be useful as adjunctive therapy for pain relief.

The use of magnets for sprains, arthritis, painful joints and low back pain has become popular. A number of athletes believe it keeps them going. It is thought magnets may increase blood flow to an area or block pain fibers through an electromagnetic field, and considerable anecdotal evidence indicates that they help. Copper wrist bands or bracelets are also used. One of the few objective randomized double-blind studies of magnets, published in JAMA, found they had no effect on patients with chronic low back pain. The most effective diagnostic use for magnets is magnetic resonance imaging—MRI.

Homeopathy is a form of therapy with two main principles: (1) "Like cures like." Thus, you would be given a treatment which produces symptoms similar to those that you have when you went to see the homeopathic doctor; (2) "Minimal dilution." That is, use the lowest amount of medication or treatment that induces a response. Few homeopathic practitioners are active now, and this form of therapy has no validity.

Some doctors have been concerned about the possibility of malpractice with referrals to alternative medicine practitioners. Medical malpractice problems with alternative medicine have not been explored but any injury is usually slight except for death from consumption of Ephedra and other dangerous herbs. Many doctors use complementary medical therapies themselves.

Many magazines periodically review what is happening in the field of alternative medicine. Andrew Weil, M.D., editor of the quarterly *Integrative Medicine*, devotes it to integrating conventional and alternative medicine (Elsevier Science, P.O. Box 882, New York, NY, 1-888-437-4636). It is a peer-reviewed journal, with all articles submitted for publication reviewed by a panel of experts. Wallace Sampson, M.D., the editor of the semi-annual *The Scientific Review of Alternative Medicine*, (Prometheus Books, Amherst, New York, 1-800-421-0351) describes it as the first peer-reviewed journal exclusively devoted to applying tests to the claims of alternative medicine. According to Stephanie Stapleton of *AMA News*, this journal "hopes to weed out the plausible from the fraudulent among alternative medicine therapies now enjoying the surge of popularity." The purpose of *The Integrative Medicine Consult* is to inform physicians about alternative therapy, reviewing mind/body healing, phytomedicinals, homeopathy, nutrition, chiropractic, acupuncture, and other therapies that lie outside of traditional medical practice. The address is 43 Bowdown Street, Boston, MA 02114 (617-720-4080). Another journal is *Alternative Therapies in Health and Medicine*, edited by Dossey and Riley (Innovision Communications, 169 Saxony Road, Suite 104, Ecinatas, CA 92024). Over 20 journals now focus on the subject Alternative Therapies.

Many cancer patients seek alternative medicines either as primary treatment for incurable cancers or as an adjunct to conventional therapy, out of fear of the disease or depression or distress. The New York doctor Nicholas Gonzalez in New York treats cancer patients with diet, supplements, and coffee enemas. He has been denounced by spokesmen for traditional medicine but patients go to him. Soon his method will be submitted to a legitimate trial.

Books and magazines I receive with material I cannot evaluate include *Fat Blocker Foods, The Doctors Handbook of Foods that Heal, New Foods for Healing, Never Feel Tired Again,* and *Miracle Medicines* (all from Prevention Health Books, 33 East Minor Street, Emmaus, PA 18098). Who knows? Perhaps we can live forever.

Problems with alternative medicine have been described by Angell and Kassirer, former Editors of the *New England Journal of Medicine* (Table IV). Andrew Weil would not accept all of these as problems but because of this list he believes complementary or integrative medicine must be combined with conventional medicine. Some internists now practice with naturopaths forming an integrative medicine practice. Attached is information on finding practitioners from Weil's book, information sites on holistic health and those recommended by JAMA. A rise in Integrative Medicine Clinics is described in Weil's *Self-Healing* (Jan. 2004) with addresses of many of them across the country. To study alternative medicine, the NIH established an office of alternative medicine, designated by Congress as the National Center for Complementary and Alternative Medicine (NCCAM). They will carry out trials of herbal agents currently in use.

This office has sparked controversy. Some alternative medicine proponents believe it was set up to put them out of business. Some scientists believe studies previously done by the NCCAM have not been as rigorous scientifically as conventional studies require. The director, Dr. Stephen Straus, is a recognized scientist who will bring legitimacy to the office and pursue good studies to "separate remedies from snake oil". The other institutes of the NIH will work with Straus to determine whether common therapies used by are worthwhile. An example is a combined study with the NCI of a substance derived from shark cartilage for cancer treatment

Table I

Complementary, Integrative or Alternative Medicine

Homeopathy
Holistic medicine
Mind-body medicine
Osteopathy
Herbal medicine
Acupuncture-Moxibustion—shiatsu ysubo jinshin iyutsu—Acupressure
Traditional Chinese medicine and herbs
Ayurvedic Medicine
Maharishi—Ayurveda (expensive)
Yoga—Pranayama, Abhyanga
Rosoayana, Panchakarma
Environmental medicine

Body work, postural or massage therapy—Alexander, Feldenkrais, Trager, Rolfing, Shiatsu Methods
Biofeedback
Hypnotherapy
Religious healing
Therapeutic touch—healing touch, reiki, jin shin Jyutsu, Johrei
Chiropractic
Aromatherapy
Light therapy
Naturopathic medicine
Qigong
Curanderism
Voodoo
Applied Kinesiology
Craniosacral therapy
Gerson diet therapy
Biorhythms
Mesmerism
American Indian Native Healing
Magnets
Hyperbaric oxygen
Chelation therapy
Colon therapy/colonics
Hallelujah Diet
Reflexology
Reiki
Shamanism
Tai Chi
Yoga
Therapeutic touch
LaStone Therapy

Table II

Echinacea—may bolster the immune system—can cause allergic reactions.
Fever few—migraine prevention—anticoagulation—bleeding.
Ginkgo Biloba—relaxes arteries, memory enhancer, may help dementia—internal bleeding.
Ginseng—does not seem effective for anything—may cause nervousness, insomnia, indigestion.
St. John's Wort—for depression (studies have found it ineffective)—see your doctor—it interferes with cancer drugs and other medications.

Saw Palmetto—prostate—? effective.

Chaparral—may cause liver damage.

Comfrey—may be related to liver cancer.

Ephedra (Ma Huang)—dangerous, cause strokes, heart attacks and death.—
   Now banned (172 deaths, thousands of illnesses)

Germander—damages the liver.

Indian snake root

Ma huang—liver damage.

Lobelia

DHEA—no evidence it fights aging—? increased cancer risk.

Rombucha

Penny royal—may cause miscarriages—cardiac arrest—kidney failure.

Yohimbe—may cause hypertension.

Dieters Teas—can cause diarrhea, vomiting, fainting and heart damage.

Sassafras—is probably not good for anything

Licorice root—results in potassium loss.

Evening primrose oil—headache, GI disturbances.

Senna

Shark Cartilage—? for cancer

Wild yam

Tumeric

Snakevine—for new antibiotics.

Dong Quai—immune system.

Flax seed—delays absorption of medicines.

Kava Kava—increases effects of alcohol—South Pacific—to relieve anxiety, may
   produce sedation,—liver damage, increase symptoms of Parkinsonism.

High doses of vitamin E—bleeding

High doses of vitamin A, D, C, iron and selenium can cause trouble.

Valerian root—said to be a relaxant.

Chomper—a laxative which may cause cardiac arrest.

Bilberry—England—anti-oxidant.

Black Cohosn

Chamomile

Gotu Kola

Grape Seed

Green tea

Hawthorn

Horse chestnut

Milk Thistle—Argentina—cirrhosis, hepatitis C.

Willow bark—may help low back pain.—linked to Reyes syndrome and GI
   irritation.

Garcinia cambogia—does not help obesity.

Co-enzyme Q10—may be an antioxidant
Glucosamine sulfate/chondroitin—of some help for osteoarthritis.
Garlic—a little reduction in cholesterol.
Daffodils—United Kingdom—Reminyl
Senna pods—Egypt
Yew twigs—Taxol—chemotherapy for breast cancer.
Chili peppers—China—Zostrix—arthritis
Aspergillus Cerrens—Pakistan
Capsaicin
Ipecac root
Cinchona bark—Quinaglute Dura-tabs—heart irregularities
Beauveria nirea—a fungus—Sandimmune—organ transplant rejection
Bluebell—England, Wales—leprosy
Gypsy mushroom—blocks herpes simplex
Pigs and cow testes—male sex drive
Snake venom—multiple sclerosis.
Male urine—menopause, osteoporosis.
Mistletoe—France
Bitter orange—undermines prescription drugs—increases blood pressure.
Aloe vera—may produce diarrhea.
Burdock

Table III

Herbs with potentially harmful or toxic effects or interactions with other medicines include:

Garlic—interacts with aspirin and blood thinners
Chaparral—may cause liver damage
Chomper—a herbal laxative
Comfrey—may cause cancer
Ephedra (ma huang)—kills patients with heart or thyroid problems and causes heart attacks and stroke (banned now)
Germander—Sleeping Buddha—a sleeping potion
Herbal Fen-Phen—weight loss, withdrawn from the market— caused heart problems
Indian snakeroot
Rombucha
Lobelia
Pennyroyal
Wormwood
Yohimbe

Aristolochic Acid

Ginger—interacts with aspirin and blood thinners

St. Johns Wort—may interfere with Coumadin as may gingko biloba and ginseng

Kava kava—may interact with Xanax—bad in pregnancy

Ginkgo—interacts with aspirin and blood thinners

There are many others—see Table II.

Table IV

Problems with Alternative Medicine

1. Many not scientifically tested.
2. Anecdotal evidence—or theory.
3. Not reported in peer-reviewed journals.
4. Ignores biologic mechanisms
5. Probably most untested dietary supplements are:
   a. herbal remedies that are harmless
   b. are used by healthy people
   c. are used by people who have common and minor problems.
6. Use could delay getting effective treatment.
7. Contamination—toxicity may occur.
8. They may or may not have active ingredients. Some ginseng preparations contained no ginseng.
9. Some herbs sold with no knowledge of action.

From Angell and Kassirer, New England Journal of Medicine 1998;339:839-841.

APPENDIX:

Finding practitioners, supplies and information

(Reprinted with permission of Dr. Andrew Weil)

Acupuncture:

American Academy of Medical Acupuncture
5820 Wilshire Boulevard, Suite 500
Los Angeles, California 90036
213-937-5514

Biofeedback

Biofeedback Certification Institute of America
10200 West 44th Avenue, Suite 304
Wheat Ridge, Colorado 80033
303-420-2902

Cranial Therapy

Cranial Academy
8606 Allisonville Road, Suite 130
Indianapolis, Indiana 46250
317-594-0411

Feldenkrais Work

The Feldenkrais Guild
PO Box 489
Albany, Oregon 97321
800-775-2118

Guided Imagery™ Therapy

Academy for Guided Imagery
PO Box 2070
Mill Valley, California 94942
415-389-9324

Herbal Medicine

American Herbalists Guild
PO Box 1683
Soquel, California 95073
408-464-2441

Herb Research Foundation
1007 Pearl Street, Suite 200
Boulder, Colorad 80302
303-449-2265

Holistic Medicine

American Holistic Medical Association
4101 Lake Boone Trail, Suite 201
Raleigh, North Carolina 27607
919-787-5146

Homeopathy

National Center for Homeopathy
801 North Fairfax Street, Suite 306
Alexandria, Virginia 22314
703-548-7790

Hypnotherapy

American Society of Clinical Hypnosis
2250 East Devon AVenue, Suite 336
Des Plaines, Illinois 60018-4534
708-297-3317

Milton H. Erikson Society of Psychotherapy and Hypnosis
PO Box 1390
Madison Square Station
New York, New York 10159
212-628-0287

Naturopathy
American Association of Naturopathic Physicians
2366 Eastlake Avenue East, Suite 322
Seattle, Washington 98102
206-323-7610

Osteopathic Manipulative Therapy

American Academy of Osteopathy
3500 De Pauw Boulevard, Suite 1080
Indianapolis, Indiana 46268
317-879-1881

Rolfing

Rolf Institute
205 Canyon Boulevard
Boulder, Colorado 80306
303-449-5903

Traditional Chinese Medicine

The American Foundation of Traditional Chinese Medicine
505 Beach Street
San Francisco, California 94133
415-776-0502

Institute for Traditional Medicine
2017 Southeast Hawthorne
Portland, Oregon 97214
503-233-4907

Trager Work

The Trager Institute
33 Millwood
Mill Valley, California 94941
415-388-2688

For those interested in holistic health or integrative medicine—following is a list of resources:

American Holistic Medical Association, 6728 Old McLean Village Dr, McLean, VA 22101; 703-556-9728/8245 (*holistmed@aol.com*).
American Association of Naturopathic Physicians, 2366 Eastlake Avenue East, Suite 322, Seattle, WA 98102-206-323-7610.
Integrative Pharmacy, PO Box 1603, Newburgh, NY 12551-9965.
Alternative Therapies in Health and Medicine, PO Box 627, Holmes, PA 19043; 1-800-345-8112.
Scientific Review of Alternative Medicine, W. Sampson Editor, Stanford University—1-800-421-0351.
Herbal Gram (quarterly publication of the American Botanical Council and the Herb Research Foundation) PO Box 201660, Austin, TX 78720; 1-512-331-8868.

The Integrative Medicine Consult. Integrative Medicine Communications, Boston, MA 1-617-720-4080.

Physician Desk Reference (PDR) for Nonprescription Drugs and Dietary Supplements. Med Economics CO, Montvale, NJ.

PDR Companion Guide, Med Economics Co, Montvale, NJ.

Murray MT. Natural Alternatives to Over-the Counter and Prescription Drugs. New York, NY William Morrow and Co. 1994.

Balch JF, Balch P. Prescription for Nutritional Healing. 2nd Ed. Garden City, NY Avery Publishing Group, 1997.

Fact: Focus on Alternative and Complementary Therapies. E. Ernst, Editor. Nurnberg Germany Verlag Perfusion GMbH 1996.

Alternative Medicine: An Objective Assessment. JAMA, AMA, Chicago, IL 1999.

Natural Medicines Comprehensive Database. Jellin JM, et al. Editors. Pharmacists Letter/Prescribers Letter, Stockton, CA 1999.

Alternative Medicine and Ethics. Humber JM, Almader RF, editors. Humante Press, Totowa, NJ 1998.

Fundamentals of Complementary and Alternative Medicine. Mare S, Micossi, editors. New York, Churchill Livingstone 1996.

Spontaneous Healing, Andrew Weil, Fawcett Columbine, New York 1995.

Physicians Desk Reference for Nutritional Supplements.

FDA—*www.fda.gov* or vm.cfsan.fda.gov/-dms/aems.

American Holistic Health Association—*www.healthynet/ahha*

American Botanical Council—*www.herbalgram.org*

Ask Dr. Weil—*www.drweil.com*

The Alternative Medicine Homepage—*www.pitt.edu/~*cbc/altem.html

National Center for Complementary and Alternative Medicine—*www.nccam.nih.gov*

Alternative Health News Online—*www.altmedicine.com*

The Alternative Medicine Foundation—*www.amfoundation.org*

The University of Texas Center for Alternative Medicine Research—*www.sph.uth.tmc.edu/utcam/default.htm*

Center for Complementary and Alternative Medicine—www-camra.ucdavis.edu/

Phytochemical and Ethnobotanical Databases—*www.ars-grin.gov/duke/*

US National Institutes of Health Office of Alternative Medicine—*http://altmed.od.nih.gov/*

Quackwatch—*www.quackwatch.com/*

FDA Guide to Choosing Medical Treatments—*www.fda.gov//oashi/aids/fdaguide.html*

Fact Sheets on Alternative Medicine—*http://cpmcnet.columbia.edu/dept/rosenthal/factsheets.html*

MEDICATIONS—PHARMACISTS—COSTS

43. Who can help me understand all these medications I am taking? Is my druggist—my pharmacist—my ally? Are there problems with combinations of drugs. Is the internet safe for drugs? Do doctors get kickbacks from drug companies? Why do medicines cost so much? Is there a way to decrease my pill bill? Will Medicare help with the new legislation? Why do medicines cost less in other countries? What are generic drugs? Should prescription drugs be advertised?

Many people have told me of concerns about their medicines. Take all of them with you when you see your doctor so they can be reviewed. You can also take them to your pharmacist for review. A good pharmacist knows medicines and drugs better than many doctors. That is their business. I rely on my pharmacist for advice and review of what I take.

Stick with one pharmacist and drug store so that they can get to know the medications you take and can be sure they do not conflict with one another other or cause toxicity. They can review doses with you. Reputable pharmacies give out printed descriptions of the drugs dispensed, listing side effects like low blood pressure (hypotension) and internal bleeding. They will check with your doctor for any problems. Drug interactions, especially antibiotic interactions with other drugs, occur frequently, and good pharmacists know about them. Significant drug interactions, described in the *Harvard Health Letter* (April 2004), include Warfarin (Coumadin) with antibiotics, ACE inhibitors with NSAIDS, Digoxin with azithromycin, clarithromycin and erythromycin, potassium supplements with potassium sparing diuretics, the azole antifungals and statins, and erectile dysfunction drugs and nitrates. Drug interactions are also described in *Consumer Reports on Health,* January of 2002.

If you get prescriptions from different doctors, take them all to the same drug store. I knew patients who were taking several kinds of the same or slightly different medicines all at once because they went to a different pharmacist each time. Be sure your doctor and pharmacist know about all your allergies to drugs. A new drug may be similar to a drug you are allergic to with a different name. If you think you are having an allergic reaction, stop taking the drug and call your doctor.

In a brochure titled "How to take your medications safely," Schweiger describes five common problems: 1) not considering drug interactions; 2) not reading the directions; 3) changing the dose yourself; 4) taking drugs leftover in your medicine cabinet; 5) not keeping drugs in an airtight container in a cool dry place—the medicine cabinet in an occasionally steamy bathroom is not the best place to store medications. The brochure is available at the Institute for Safe Medical Practices, 3000 W. Street Rd, Warminster, PA 18974. *www.ismp.org.*

The Society of Critical Care Medicine, doctors who specialize in caring for you in ICUs, sponsor a small book by pharmacists called *The Injectable Drug Reference.* It describes drugs that can be given by injection under your skin (SC-subcutaneous), into a muscle (IM-intramuscular), or into a vein (IV-intravenous). A drug-injected IV will have an immediate effect but will not last as long as the other injections. The book describes methods of administration, doses, what to look for as the drug is given (monitoring) and, most importantly, what other drugs are compatible or incompatible with the injected drug. The use of this book by nurses and doctors should increase the safety of medications, particularly in ICUs.

Lucian Leape, et al, recently reported in JAMA a much lower rate of adverse drug events with a pharmacist on rounds as a member of the team in a medical ICU. Also, reviews of medication orders by pharmacists and pharmacist consultations reduce errors and costs.

Accidental misuse of drugs is a problem. Eastman of AARP lists "9 crucial questions to ask your doctor or pharmacist:

1) What is the name of the drug and what is it for?
2) Is a generic version available?
3) How and when do I take the drug and for how long?
4) Will this drug work safely with other drugs and supplements I take? What about alcohol?
5) Are any tests required with this medicine to check liver or kidney function?
6) What are the potential side effects?
7) Can I get a refill? When?
8) How do I store this medicine?
9) Where can I find written information about this medicine?

On occasion, a drug approved initially by the FDA is found after extensive use to produce complications that were not apparent in the initial controlled trials. Long-term or more widespread use could bring out these problems. Such may have been the case with Vioxx (rofecoxib), a coxib belonging to a subclass of non-steriodal anti-inflammatory drugs (NSAIDs) that selectively inhibit Cyclooxygenase-2 (COX-2). This acute pain medication was voluntarily pulled from the market in the fall of 2004 by its manufacturer, Merck & Co, because it caused heart attacks in a number of patients. The FDA subsequently estimated that Vioxx has caused over 27,000 heart attacks, some of them fatal. Within a month after the withdrawal, Merck's stock price had declined precipitously, from $45 to the $20s.

Merck and the FDA have been criticized because they knew that the drug caused trouble some years ago, perhaps as early as 2000, and did not promptly withdraw it. In April 2005 the FDA did not wait for a manufacturer to move but took the initiative in asking Pfizer Inc to pull its COX-2 painkiller, Bextra, upon reports that it poses a risk of potentially lethal skin reactions. Partly because of costs connected with the withdrawal, Pfizer reported a drop of 87 percent in quarterly earnings.

Are there problems with combinations of drugs?

A classic example is fen-phen for weight loss, combining Fen or fenfluramine, which is harmless and has been prescribed for years, and Phen or phentermine, which has never been associated with health problems. In the 1990s, doctors began prescribing these two agents together even though they had never been tested or approved together by the FDA. Use of fen-phen produced severe heart valve defects. After that finding by the Mayo Clinic, the FDA pushed for fen-phen to be removed from the market. The FDA, however, has no control over "off-label" prescribing, the practice in question of using of a drug in combination or alone for diseases or purposes different from what they were originally approved for. Many people think the FDA should receive more oversight of such problems as well as a larger budget; in 1996 alone the agency received 193,336 voluntary reports of drug problems. Over 3,000 lawsuits were filed in the wake of fen-phen; and one verdict against the drug company, under appeal, amounted to $23 million. Who is at fault? The drug company (how did they know? but they should have tested fen-phen), the prescribing doctors (they were unaware of the problems), the FDA (they have no control over such problems), or the Federal government for not giving the FDA a budget to deal with such problems. I vote for the last. Why isn't the FDA given capability to determine use of drugs for purposes other than those originally approved?

Some drugs are bad in one situation, like Thalidomide, which produced terrible birth defects in pregnant women in Europe, but good in another situation. Thalidomide, thanks to an alert FDA staff member never approved for such use in the U.S., is now an experimental treatment for a variety of cancers, including breast, prostate, bone marrow and brain cancer.

The internet for drugs—Is it safe?

Use of the Internet has led to a flourishing electronic drug market, called the "wild west of the web" by *The New York Times* (Chapter 66). Paying by credit card, you can receive an online medical consultation from an online drug company. The company fills out a questionnaire for you. If a company doctor approves the request and the questionnaire, your pills arrive in the mail for a hefty fee. The most common drugs sold online are Viagra, Propecia for baldness, Xenical, a diet drug, and Claritin, an antihistamine.

Ads seek doctors with active licenses who could earn $10,000 a month doing "fully automated online medical reviews." One such cyber-doctor has been put out of business by regulators, and states and Congress are looking for ways to stop or control online medical consultations. Prescriptions from a doctor who has never seen or examined you may be dangerous. The online drug companies maintain doctors oppose online prescriptions because they don't want to lose control of writing prescriptions, but that is not the case. Doctors are interested in protecting your health and safety from schemes that involve selling drugs without seeing you and getting an overview of your health and your other medications. The cyber-doctor has no idea what other drugs you are taking and of possible interactions.

The AMA considers these online prescriptions unethical, pharmacists call them illegal and I think them dangerous. The FDA and state boards have found it difficult to police this problem. Henkel, in the FDA Consumer, recommends that consumers: 1) check with the National Association of Boards of pharmacy at *www.nadp.net* or 847-698-6227 to find if the pharmacist is licensed. 2) Avoid sites that do not require a physical exam or will give you a prescription drug without a prescription or do not give you access to a registered pharmacist to answer questions. 3) Avoid sites without identification or a U.S. address. 4) Beware of sites that advertise "a new cure" for a serious disorder. 5) Beware of sites claiming wonderful results or accusing other parties of attempts to suppress their products. Talk to your doctor about any new medication. Henkel describes a new certification for quality online pharmacies called Verified Internet Pharmacy Practice Sites (VIPPS). Look for their seal. The FDA has published a consumer safety guide for buying prescription medicines online at *www.fda.gov*. Click on buying medicines and medical products online or call 1-888-infofda, 1-888-463-6332.

Do doctors get kickbacks from drug companies?

The answer is not directly but doctors do get benefits from drug companies. The companies spend a lot of money to convince doctors to prescribe their products. Drug companies hire "detail" people who call on doctors in their offices to tell them about new products. Some provide helpful information. Doctors may use this to learn about medications. Of course, the information is biased toward products of the company represented. Detail people leave brochures and samples. Doctors can get a month's supply of a drug to use for themselves, their families or their patients. My office asked "detail" people to leave whatever they wanted, but I would not see them. I did not want to be influenced.

Drug companies sponsor programs, provide food for breakfast and lunch meetings and engage in other promotional activities. In Europe they underwrite or sponsor major meetings. In the U.S., they pay for exhibits at major meetings. Petersen, "a sales representative for Merck says she and her associates were told by superiors they should no longer treat doctors to Broadway plays, weekend trips or other gifts that could be viewed as inappropriate." Drug companies have paid celebrities to recommend their drugs.

On the other hand, drug companies work hard to develop new drugs. Their research and development costs must be built into the cost of the drug. They also show a profit and the big question is: Are their profits excessive? We believe they are.

Many critics believe doctors are too heavily influenced by drug companies. Some have consulting and speaking contracts with drug companies. They give lectures and host conferences about the companies' products, in essence, endorsing the products. Others are financially involved with companies supporting their research. These are conflicts of interest. These doctors use their professional prominence to help sell a product and make a buck. Sponsoring grand rounds (a medical conference) with pens, brochures and refreshments at a V.A. Hospital tripled the use of a drug pushed by the sponsoring company. For hypertension, low cost diuretics and beta blockers are recommended as the first line of therapy. High—priced calcium channel blockers and ACE inhibitors are more heavily advertised, however, and are bigger sellers.

Why do medicines cost so much?

The use of prescription medicines and their prices are soaring, as are costs for health plans covering prescriptions. The Health Care Financing Administration (HCFA) said prescription expenses would rise from 9.4% of personal health spending to 16% by 2010, faster than any other medical category.

Retail pharmacies sold $154.5 billion in prescription drugs in 2001, an increase of 16 per cent. Reasons include: 1) increased use of prescription medicines (42% more); 2) development of new medicines; 3) high cost of brand-name drugs (increased prices of 22%); 4) lack of generic drugs as substitutes for many of the brand-name drugs; 5) direct advertising of prescription drugs to consumers; 6) lengthy patent protection—13 years. Drug companies maintain they need this protection to support research and development of new agents. They do need some protection, but do they need so much? Tanouge writes that new pills may improve quality of life but bust health budgets. The "U.S. developed an expensive drug habit; how to pay for it?" Large employers are worried about this escalation. Myers of the Ford Motor Co. says, "The pharmaceutical industry is being short sighted by not working directly on this problem. I hope they don't assume the pot is limitless, costs can go up forever." Many HMOs for the elderly have cut or abolished drug coverage.

The high prices force difficult decisions on low income people, particularly elderly patients on Social Security. Do they get their medicines or food? Many patients cut corners, decreasing their dose or taking the medicine less often, seeking samples from doctors, paying utility bills late, spending less on food, and cutting back on everything to pay for medicines. Some patients fail to see the doctor to avoid getting prescriptions for expensive medicines. Some patients lose their homes and suffer malnutrition. Middle income people fall through the cracks. Those who can do so go to Mexico or Canada for drugs, where one patient found that a month's supply of Tamoxifen was $15 compared to $95 in the U.S. Talk to your doctor about what you can afford and seek his or her help.

Cohen indicates drug companies' excuse of needing money for research is a bit hollow since research represents less than a third of their costs. Drug companies could reduce costs of marketing, advertising and promotion to doctors without touching research money.

Cohen also points out that the pharmaceutical marketplace has never been free. We are not free to ignore their products. They are milk for cereal. As Angell wrote in the *New England Journal of Medicine* (NEJM), "Just as public utilities are not permitted to charge whatever the traffic will bear, neither should drug companies". "The pharmaceutical industry is extraordinarily privileged. It should be accountable also to society at large."

Fortune magazine ranked the pharmaceutical business the most profitable of all industries. Prescription prices need not be so high. High drug prices have come under attack from Congress. Former Senator Slade Gorton (R) accused drug companies of practicing outrageous discrimination against Americans.

Is there a way to decrease my pill bill?

The *Harvard Health Letter* lists seven ways to cut your medicine bills: 1) tell your doctor you must lower your drug costs; review your drugs with your doctor; 2) use generics if possible; 3) be willing to take medicines two or three times a day using less expensive older drugs; 4) use medications the way they were prescribed; 5) try low-cost brand name drugs; 6) use a pill-splitting device; a large dose in a pill costs the same as a lower dose; 7) shop around, compare prices at chain drug stores, local drug stores, supermarket pharmacies and mass merchant pharmacies, join a drug cooperative, buy pills in bulk from a mail order pharmacy. Some drug companies have introduced discount cards for low-income seniors. They may provide discounts of 25% but it is not clear that they really help.

Will Medicare help with prescription costs? What is the new legislation?

This is a loaded political issue. Everyone knows that Medicare should offer some coverage for prescription costs. The pharmaceutical industry opposes it, saying it will eventually increase costs. What they are really worried about, however, is cost controls. The industry set up and financed its own organization with the Orwellian title of Citizens for Better Medicare, which is, of course, opposed to Medicare drug coverage. In the last political campaign, the drug industry contributed $167 million and Citizens for Better Medicare $4.6 million, mostly to Republicans. Most Democrats support fairly complete coverage of medicines for Medicare patients. The Republicans proposed a partial approach which the Democrats walked out on. Richard Gephardt (D) of Missouri said the GOP prescription plan "is a sham, a hoax, a political fig leaf". My question is: Which party is for the people? Headlines read "Senate kills plan for drug benefits through Medicare".

Now Congress has passed the Medicare Prescription Drug Improvement and Modernization Act of 2003, with a prescription drug plan to start in 2006. The act is complex and difficult to understand. For example, if you have Medicare and choose a prescription drug plan and pay a premium of $35/month, you will pay the first $250 (deductible). Medicare then pays 75% of cost between $250 and $2,250, and you pay 25%. You pay 100% of drug costs from $2,250 to $3,600. Medicare will then pay 95% of costs above $3600. Drug discount cards will be issued in 2004. The NEJM calls this bill a pure Bush power play. The cost is estimated to be over $400 billion, a cost originally concealed by the administration. Democrats, leaders of organized labor and some advocates for the elderly condemn the bill as privatizing Medicare, which may destroy it. It works against Social Security and for drug companies. Will they act to help senior citizens who can't afford their medicines? Don't hold your breath.

Some of the states are also taking action. Maine pledged to cut costs of prescription drugs for uninsured residents. In 2000, eleven states took action on the high cost of drugs. In 2002, thirty-two states offered some type of prescription aid. For information on State Drug Assistance programs go to National Conference of State Legislatures at *www.ncsl.org/programs/health/drugaid.htm*. If your state has a drug-discount program for Medicare beneficiaries, be sure your pharmacy applies it to you.

Why do Americans pay more for medicines than do patients in other countries?

In India, companies pirate the drugs, by copying them, and produce other copies to sell at low prices. Under Indian law, this practice is legal and a big business. The Indians believe if a drug is helpful, it should not be denied to people because of price. A *USA TODAY* survey showed popular drugs cost two to four times as much in the U.S. as in other countries, with much less of a difference for generic drugs (described later). Every industrialized country in the world, except the U.S., has put price controls on prescription drugs.

Cauchon reports U.S. consumers subsidize research and development (R&D) for the entire world. "Our pockets are being picked," Sager says. Drug companies maintain that price controls in the U.S. would severely limit R&D. U.S. drug companies spend huge sums on consumer advertising and the U.S. forbids importing cheaper drugs. The only discounts drug companies give are to the V.A., Defense Dept., Coast Guard, and Public Health Service. Why not to you? U.S. newspapers run ads for ordering cheaper drugs from Canada by a toll-free number. Savings are up to 75%. For example, 100 Premarin tablets 1.25 mg. cost about $86 in the U.S. but only $23.17 in Canada. Glaxo-SmithKline warned Canadian pharmacists it will no longer sell to them if they sell to U.S.citizens. Canada is threatening suit against Glaxo.

Much original research on new drugs is supported by tax payers through research grants from the NIH. Half of the patents for new drugs come from public funds. According to Angell the top ten drug companies spend about 20% of their revenues on R&D and 40% on advertising, but profits are 30% of revenues. This seems vulgar. The drug companies receive the benefit of NIH sponsored research, they can deduct R&D costs and advertising to lower their taxes and they enjoy 13-year patent protection—three bonanzas from the government.

Research and development of new drugs does require large expenditures. If you cut profits, would you slow research? Patents encourage innovation says Surowick, but so does their expiration. The U.S. is responsible each year for development of half of all major new drugs. Sullivan says that of 5000 potential medicines only three get into clinical trials and only one is approved. It costs about $500 million and 15 years to bring a new drug to market. Surowick asks, "Is this the face of evil? Opportunism is more like it." The free enterprise capitalist system is at work.

What are generic drugs?

Generic drugs are the basic constituents of brand-name medicines, produced after expiration of the patents for those medicines and usually sold at lower prices. The savings for generics can be considerable. A drug company bringing a new drug to market gets a patent for 13 years and sells it with a trade-name at an increased cost. For example, the drug Hytrin for hypertension costs $52 a month, the generic version terazosin now costs $23 a month. It earned $500 million a year for Abbott Labs. Prozac 20 mg. pill costs $2.70/pill, whereas the generic fluoxetine costs $0.91. Medicare is promoting generic drugs.

Drug companies try to keep generics off the market. A recent complicated deal between Merck and Schering Plough combined two of their "block buster" cholesterol lowering drugs with patents about to expire, and they got a new patent. The combination may actually be less beneficial for the patient. Drug companies also make a slight change in a drug with a patent about to expire so they can get a new patent. The FTC will study whether makers of brand-name drugs and makers of generics entered into agreements to keep generics off the market. The FTC has filed complaints against seven companies. Consumer groups and states have sued pharmaceutical companies over delaying sales of lower cost generic drugs. Patent protection should allow drug companies sufficient time to recover their research and development expenses only.

There are advertisements in newspapers about drugs that can be obtained only by a prescription from my doctor. Should that be allowed? How does that help me?

It helps the drug company much more than it helps you or your doctor. For years, FDA regulations prevented drug companies from advertising prescription drugs. Pharmaceutical companies began to side-step these regulations. Pilling, in the *London Financial Times,* says the companies tried to create consumer demand through disease awareness campaigns or they advertised a disease without promoting a specific remedy and pushed particular brands without saying what they were for. Advertisements contained a lot of information about diseases, unnamed cures and cures for unnamed diseases.

In August 1997, the FDA relaxed their regulations and drug companies moved into action with Direct Advertising to Consumers (DAC), which has mushroomed into a huge business and may increase the cost of drugs. Many of us are opposed to DAC just as we are to doctors' advertising. DAC promotes drugs, diagnostic studies and high technology screening tests that have not been proven to be effective. Remember, advertising may inform you but it is not medical advice by a professional with your interests at heart. The question is: "Is it education or emotion promotion?" Drug news is often too rosy and overlooks risks and conflicts of interest. The pharmaceutical industry thinks, of course, that DAC strengthens our health care system. The bottom line, as always: Check with your doctor.

In 2001, drug companies allegedly paid $2.7 billion for direct consumer advertising. They believe this informs patients and families but the question is whether it informs or confuses people. In a recent magazine, treatment for diabetes with Rezulin was advertised. The ad said "once-a-day Rezulin may change how your doctor treats Type II diabetes." The suggestion is: Go see your doctor about this. Another is for an anti-allergy drug called Zyrtec which "when allergies are a nightmare, remember Zyrtec for fast relief." Another advertises Procrit a treatment for anemia if you are receiving chemotherapy. These advertised drugs are important medications, approved by the FDA after clinical trials. Are you better off seeing these ads or seeing your doctor? Should you take the ad to your doctor? The chances are your doctor will know about the agent and may order it for you but then again may not. Not all drugs are appropriate for the same purpose in all patients.

Media coverage of drugs is often misleading. Benefits are exaggerated and risks ignored. Ads may create a need for a drug that is not necessary and why not? You can place an ad in a newspaper (i.e., *USA TODAY*) and say whatever you want about medical claims; no verification is needed, no evidence. Just hype! Speaking of hype, an ad in the *St. Louis Post-Dispatch* ran down these topics from *The Big Book of Health Tips*: "When sex can cause temporary blindness, the story's in the book," "Drugs that cause incontinence in the elderly," "The healing power of plants," "Scientific studies prove it," "Why women need chocolate," and "How talking too fast can kill you."

Carey and Mosemak of *USA TODAY* list what consumers should expect in drug ads: 1) risks clearly stated; 2) symptoms to discuss with doctor; 3) information about treatment options and, 4) all necessary information.

For your information, the *PDR Pocket Guide to Prescription Drugs* makes available to laymen some information from the twice-as-big *Physicians' Desk Reference*, used by doctors to check on medications, doses, indications, safety and adverse events. AARP publishes a helpful consumer guide: "How to be Drug Smart." Call AARP at 1-800-424-3410 and refer to stock number D17698.

Section G

About Hospitals; Choosing a hospital—LOS

44. How do I choose a hospital or a clinic? Does it make a difference how often a certain operation is done in the hospital?

W hen I was growing up in the Midwest, it was fashionable, if affordable, to go to a large, proper-named, private clinic either for a check-up or for a serious illness. In the Midwest, this was the Mayo Clinic in Rochester, Minn. The expression was "I think I will go through the Clinic." The patients stayed in an adjoining hotel. Their medical, physical and emotional state was evaluated over the next few days with appropriate diagnostic studies. An interview with a physician provided an overall health evaluation and recommendation. In Boston, such patients would have gone to the Lahey Clinic; in Cleveland to the Cleveland Clinic; in New Orleans to the Ochsner Clinic; in Seattle to the Virginia Mason Clinic and so on.

While prestigious, these organizations were not infallible. My sister-in-law returned from one after a check-up and reported to me that she had a groin hernia. Surgeons do not operate on immediate family members, unless it is a life-saving emergency and no one else is available. I referred her to another surgeon to repair the hernia. A preoperative chest x-ray showed a nodule (a lump, a mass) in the upper part of her lung. I asked her if they did not mention this at the Clinic. She said, "Oh yes, they said it was nothing to worry about." I indicated we would worry about it. A thoracic surgeon performed a right upper lobectomy removing the cancer. Lymph nodes contained tumor cells indicating spread (lymphatic metastases) so she received radiation therapy which controlled the tumor for the next 12 years.

I will use clinic with a capital C to designate a proper-named organization of physicians who practice together. The generic term clinic with a small c describes a place where you may see a doctor. It may be a city clinic for patients with limited means, or offices of a number of doctors. In many cities, physicians join together to provide comprehensive medical care, sometimes representing all specialties. In all clinics, it is important to ask for the qualifications of each doctor you encounter. By and large, they will be capable but do not assume it. Also, you must decide if you are compatible with the physician (chapter 1). Will your health insurance pay for care in such a clinic? Most clinics do not own their own hospitals but are affiliated with or on the staff of a single hospital. Thus, the hospital and clinic go together, and you must accept this arrangement if you require hospitalization.

Hospitals

Hospitals were established in colonial America by most cities (the Philadelphia General Hospital, the Boston City Hospital, the New York Hospital System), by private organizations (the Massachusetts General Hospital, the New York Hospital), or by religious groups to serve their own members or a community. Examples include the Jewish Federation Hospitals and Catholic Hospitals established by men's religious orders like the Alexian Brothers and by religious nursing orders of women, nuns, in many large cities and small towns. The Sisters of Mercy, the Sisters of St. Mary's, and the Daughters of Charity currently represent large national systems. Other religious groups also established hospitals, among them Lutherans, Presbyterians, Congregationalists (the Deaconess system), and Episcopalians. Both the medical and religious needs of a patient could be met by such institutions providing daily Mass, kosher meals, and access to rabbis, priests, or Protestant chaplains.

In the 40's and 50's medical centers grew or started up in urban areas in the U.S. through federal, state and local government support. Every state could point to centers of excellence and often to a number of them. Medical schools, usually part of a university, collaborated with large existing hospitals, acquired such a hospital or built their own, as did many state universities. These so-called teaching centers, teaching hospitals or academic health centers are often associated with schools of nursing, dentistry, public health and allied health professions.

University or medical school hospitals may be owned by the university (Hospital of the University of Pennsylvania; the University of Kentucky Medical Center) or affiliated with the university, as is the Massachusetts General Hospital with Harvard University and the New York Hospital with Cornell University. Other medical schools may maintain only a loose affiliation with a university; the Yale-New Haven Hospital serves as a community hospital as well as an affiliate of Yale University. Hospitals and schools may collaborate with community hospitals that serve as teaching hospitals for medical students and residents.

A teaching hospital offers several potential advantages for patients. The medical staff is usually on the leading edge of what is new and exciting for your care. They have reached a level of capability sufficient to teach students and residents correct, or current, medical practice. Certain operations and treatments may only be available in a teaching hospital, including liver, lung and heart transplantation. Most of the faculty also do research, which keeps them informed.

Another advantage is what I call a fail-safe component. Your doctor knows you, and we assume that he or she is thorough; the specialists should be the same. In a teaching hospital, a medical student and a resident physician interviewing you may uncover new information about you and your health. In their desire to learn, they will question your doctor about your care and alternatives, a beneficial process for you.

A final advantage is that these students and residents often spend the night in the hospital; they sleep there and are available for emergencies. The advantages of teaching hospitals do not mean that non-teaching hospitals are unsafe. They may be excellent institutions with staffs of capable doctors.

Your selection of a hospital depends upon the severity or complexity of your problem. If you live in a small town with a 50-bed hospital, you may receive excellent care for pneumonia, congestive heart failure, appendicitis or other common medical problems. An appendectomy should be a simple, straightforward and relatively uncomplicated operation for a trained surgeon if appropriate anesthesia is available.

For complex problems, you must determine the capability of the staff and the hospital. Are they equipped and trained to do heart surgery on a regular basis? Many doctors believe surgeons should do a particular operation frequently enough to be good at it. How often is enough? For coronary artery by-pass grafts (CABGS), 50-100/year is the minimum number. Fewer than 50 and the surgeon should let someone else do them. For difficult or less frequently done operations or rare medical problems, you should go to a medical center with that capability. Lower operative mortality has been associated with hospitals that do a large number of operations. For complex operations for cancers of the pancreas, esophagus and colon done by surgical teams in hospitals with specialty expertise, the mortality rate is lower. The same is true for heart operations.

Magid, et al, found that patients with an acute myocardial infarction, or heart attack, had a lower incidence of dying if treated within an hour by an angioplasty (dilating the artery) and thrombolysis (dissolving the clot) at a hospital doing these procedures frequently. McGrath et al found Medicare patients who needed a stent, or tube, inserted into a narrowed coronary artery did better when it was done by doctors that did it frequently. Allison et al showed that elderly patients with heart attacks had a better chance of survival at a teaching hospital. Be sure the hospital and doctors you select have frequent experiences with your problem.

The title Medical Center or Health Center is self-designated. Anyone and any institution can use such a name. No regulations or requirements apply. Some academic medical centers, part of a medical center complex, now call themselves Health Sciences Centers to indicate that they are more than a medical school and hospital. However, it would be difficult to imagine a Health Sciences Center without a medical school, a hospital and patients. I like the German word for hospital: *Krankenhaus*, or sick house. The place you go for care when you are sick. The designation health center is not quite correct since most of us go there only when we are sick, although we hope to leave healthier than when we came.

The evolution of hospital and specialty care

Many operations, procedures, diagnostic tests and complex therapy were developed in academic medical centers. That is one of their major purposes: research and advancement of your care. The other is education of the next generation of health care professionals. When new procedures become established therapy, the young specialists in training in academic centers learn them. They then establish the therapy in community hospitals, where it becomes available to more patients. This is the evolution of specialty care in the community. At one time heart surgery was only done in medical school hospitals or at several large clinics in the United States. Now it is done well in many good community hospitals.

Other hospital systems are available for certain patients. The Veterans Administration (VA) oversees an extensive network of hospitals available for veterans of military service who cannot afford care elsewhere. VA Hospitals are usually affiliated with medical schools, which helps assure good care. Some evidence indicates that the VA is trying to get out of running hospitals and wants to privatize the care of veterans. The U.S. military uses a network of hospitals for active duty and retired military personnel. Public health hospitals are available in various locations primarily close to Native American reservations to provide care for our first citizens.

Collaboration by medical schools and large city hospitals once helped assure good care. Most of these hospitals have been phased out or closed. The buildings were often old, in need of replacement, and expensive to run; many hospital patients depended on Medicaid, Medicare or other health insurance. Many cities provide programs for the poor and needy in private hospitals. This solution is still being implemented in some cities and may not be totally satisfactory where you live.

45. There are things I would like to know about hospitals and don't know where to ask. What are for-profit hospitals? How far should I have to travel to a hospital? Do hospitals compete? What does LOS in a hospital mean?

Not-for-profit or tax-exempt hospitals may not make much money but they must at least break even. The head of a large religious hospital system once said, "no margin—no mission." To cover expenses, not-for-profit hospitals depend almost totally on payments from patients, insurance companies, HMOs or government. To pay for special purposes, like new buildings, comforts for patients, or care for patients with no resources, they turn to fund raising campaigns—charitable events, dances, parties, golf tournaments, celebrity events, and the like.

Both not-for-profit and for-profit hospitals take care of some patients with no money or insurance, in hospital jargon self-pay patients. Hospitals may try to limit the number of their self-pay patients. However, the law requires a hospital emergency facility to admit any patients needing care, sending them to another hospital only if the patient's HMO has a contract with that other hospital. In some states, part of the hospital budget must be devoted to "charity" or "indigent patient" care to maintain tax-exempt status. Charity care may help meet an IRS test for that status.

For-profit hospitals

Until the late 1960s, all hospitals were not-for-profit institutions. Since then, corporations have been buying hospitals and operating them for a profit. Publicly traded companies built networks of hospitals that were expected to make a return on stockholders' investments. Humana, Tenet, and Hospital Corporation of America have developed large systems across the country. Some university hospitals were acquired by corporations, including Louisville General Hospital, Creighton University Hospital, Tulane University Hospital and, in 1998, Saint Louis University Hospital, where I was Professor of Surgery. Calling it a serious ethical issue, Catholic leaders protested the sale of this teaching hospital to a for-profit, but to no avail.

The impact of for-profit health care is uncertain. It definitely has increased competition among hospitals. Despite an initial belief that increased competition would decrease the cost of care, however, no evidence has come forward to support that claim. For-profit health care puts it in the market place as a business. Caring for the sick was once thought to be a sacred task. Now a patient is a consumer. I may be a doctor, but I am called a health care provider.

Now, for-profit companies have shed some of their hospitals, which went back to being public or private institutions. The for-profit movement is not better than the not-for profit tradition; maybe it is not worse, but it certainly is different. Could such institutions become more interested in profits than caring for patients? Souba wrote that we may be curing without caring. Reinhardt wrote, "patients can be viewed as biological structures yielding future cash flows . . . . cost cuts at Tenet leave workers and patients unsatisfied."

How far should I have to travel to see a doctor, go to an emergency facility, be hospitalized, see a specialist or be hospitalized for specialty care?

Years ago the U.S. wrestled with the popular concept that health care, doctors and hospitals should be available in all communities. The result was the Hill-Burton Act of 1946, a Federal program providing for hospitals of 50 beds or so in any community without a hospital. Health care facilities spread into smaller communities but doctors did not always follow. Many small towns tried and failed to get doctors. The government solution was to create more medical schools, which did not solve the problem. Doctors practice not only where communities need them, but also where their families wish to live and where they can use their skills and not feel isolated professionally. Many small towns will never have a doctor. The best recourse for a small town is a nurse practitioner capable of treating minor problems and referring major ones. A group of small towns could have a doctor with a group of nurse practitioners, which could provide excellent health care for rural areas. If you decide to retire or live on a beautiful but remote Caribbean island without health care facilities, you are taking your chances. You can't have it both ways: beautiful, quiet, isolation and full service health care.

The movement in health care is no longer centrifugal, spread out and made available everywhere. It is now centripetal, centralized for better care, but you may have to travel to get it. Is it unreasonable to drive 15 minutes or 30 minutes or even an hour to a good, well-equipped and staffed hospital? How often do you need it? How far do you drive to go to a shopping mall? How far do you travel to go to Wal-Mart or B-J's or a rock concert? Are you willing to travel as far or a little farther for excellent health care?

In England after World War II, the government developed the National Health Service (NHS) providing free health care for all citizens. For patients in remote areas, buses went out every day brought them to clinics and hospitals and took them home at the end of the day. The English, by and large, like this system. The U.S. has not been willing to provide such services for its citizens. As a young surgeon, I worked for the NHS. I found patients liked it and felt it was doing a good job.

Competition among hospitals

Because of a decrease in length of stay (LOS) for many operations, illnesses and deliveries, the census of hospitals, the number of patients/day, has decreased. Hospitals maintain empty beds at considerable cost because of the number of people needed for care: physicians, nurses, orderlies, nurses' aides and maintenance workers. Equipment and supplies are expensive. Many hospitals have closed beds—rooms, wards or nursing units. Many communities or regions are "overbedded, with too many hospital rooms or beds. In fact, we now have too many hospitals and tertiary care institutions.

This has brought about fierce competitions for you, the patient. Advertising has increased. Hospitals all have "marketing" departments. What was once a charitable, benevolent and caring institution has become a business, albeit one that may still take care of you in a professional and caring way.

A hospital may keep beds full and make the budget by developing loyalty in the medical staff so that they will admit all their patients to that hospital. To this end the hospital provides special services to the staff, such as free reserved parking, an attractive staff lounge to hang out in, delicious lunches, occasional cocktail or dinner parties and other amenities. A hospital, however, cannot pay a doctor for admitting you to that hospital. The Fraud and Abuse Act of Medicare does not allow it. Hospitals can however, buy the practice of a doctor or they can buy an entire multi-specialty clinic or group of doctors. The doctors are employees of the hospital and, hopefully, will use only that facility. Frequently, offices are provided adjoining the hospital, which is convenient for the doctor and also for you. If you are a patient in that hospital, your doctor is close by.

Call-a-nurse is a marketing device to promote a hospital and medical staff—call if you wish to go to that hospital and see a doctor on their staff, otherwise look elsewhere. These programs do not provide expert opinions but rather a list of the medical staff and specialist to refer you to.

You might ask why more hospitals don't close given the surplus. The neighborhood around a hospital may feel a great loyalty to the institution or the medical staff may wish to continue there. A tradition or pride of a religious group or a Board of Trustees may enjoy the prestige or community involvement. A hospital closed recently because it was not needed and not being used. The community around the hospital organized itself and developed a campaign which reopened the hospital. They insisted on having a hospital close by even though other hospitals were within 10-15 minutes. Why doesn't a hospital decrease its bed capacity? Human foibles enter in.

A full service hospital with all specialties represented requires a minimum number of beds, perhaps 300 to 500. In order to maintain full capability, a number of operations, such as heart operations, should be done every month. Hospitals may join in a system with a core tertiary care hospital and "feeder hospitals." Institutional pride plays a big role in the issue of capability. When I was Chief of Surgery at the Yale-New Haven Hospital, I was invited to meet with the Trustees of a neighboring community hospital. They asked if I would help develop a cardiac surgical program at their hospital. I suggested we could take care of all their heart patients in our cardiac surgical program at Yale. We had extra capacity, and our hospital was only 30 minutes away. The Chairman of the Board said I misunderstood: They wanted a heart surgery program in their hospital. Asked why this was so important, they said the other hospital in their community had a heart surgery program and they wanted one too. It was a matter of institutional pride.

A large tertiary care hospital in a major urban area realized they did not need so many beds. Instead of closing some, they joined forces with an adjoining hospital, which they then closed so all patients came to the larger institution. The small hospital was destroyed to save the bigger hospital. Members of the religious community that founded the smaller hospital were distraught and withdrew support.

Some state hospital and health care commissions control expansion of hospitals and duplication of services. They review requests for capital expenses above a certain amount for new buildings, facilities, beds, operating rooms etc. They can limit expansion but cannot mandate decreases or close hospitals. If lack of need for your hospital made it a candidate for closure, how would you react? Shift loyalty, or fight for it? In the midst of abundance, we have more health care available than we are told we can afford. This over-abundance has led to fraudulent activities: payment of kickbacks to doctors to raise the number of patients eligible for Medicare and Medicaid, inflated hospital costs and charges to the government. HCA, a for-profit company paid almost one billion dollars to the government for fraud. Recently, Tenet has been fined large sums for fraudulent practices.

What does length of stay (LOS) in a hospital mean?

Gradually over the years the LOS has decreased. We know now that patients can safely leave the hospital soon after a major operation. If your postoperative pain is controlled with medicine taken by mouth, you may enjoy being at home more than in a hospital. Now minimal operations are common. Removal of the gallbladder can be done by laparoscopy with only three or four very small incisions. You may be able to go home the next day. Other operations in the abdomen can be done that way. Some operations in the chest can be done by thoracoscopy. Certain heart operations can be done by minimal surgical techniques.

Other factors influence LOS. In the past, hospitals were reimbursed for the days you were in the hospital: for your care, medicine and dressings and other supplies. Patients were billed for expenses plus extras to allow hospitals a small surplus to cover expenses of patients who could not pay. Now hospitals can no longer do this.

Medicare adopted a policy of paying a set amount of money for a particular health problem, or diagnosis-related groups (DRG's). Thus, they would like to get you out of the hospital as soon as possible although I hope no hospital will send you home if your condition is unstable or it is not safe for you. DRGs further reduce LOS, which has become very short.

In the past, a woman might have stayed in a hospital for five to seven days after having a baby. Now some insurance companies require a woman to go home the day after, sending in a nurse to indicate in her chart that tomorrow she must be discharged. That may or may not be in her best interest. She may not feel able to go home, particularly if she has had an episiotomy, an incision in the mouth of the vagina. Her doctor may have to protest to the insurance company. Some states require insurance carriers to let her stay in the hospital for two days. Your doctor is your best protection against premature discharge from a hospital.

Your nurses, doctors and the hospital do not want complications to develop because you left too soon. They keep track of patients readmitted because of complications and try to avoid them in the future by making sure it is safe for you to go. Taheri, et al, reviewed the costs of hospitalization related to LOS and found costs attributable to the last day of stay are insignificant. Reducing hospital stay by a day decreases total cost by only three percent. They urge a de-emphasis on LOS and attention to better use of capacity and care during early days after admission.

If you live alone and are concerned about getting along by yourself, ask your nurses to arrange a meeting for you with the hospital social worker, for "discharge planning." If you can get along at home but need help to bathe or prepare meals, a home health service can help. If your hospital does not have such a service, they can arrange for it. If you are limited in what you can do for yourself, a convalescent home may be appropriate for a few weeks before you return home.

ICUs

46. What are intensive care units (ICUs) like? Why do they scare some people? What is nosocomial infection?

If you or a member of your family has been a patient in an ICU, you may feel that ICUs are cold, impersonal, mechanical and noisy places. You may remember the beeping of monitors, the whooshing or gurgling of ventilators, and the ringing of alarms, but ICUs are now becoming quieter, less intimidating places. Newer respirators and monitors, except for alarms, run quietly.

Years ago, the visiting hours were restricted to a few minutes every few hours later in the day. Mornings were reserved for treatment of patients. Now family members are not considered visitors and can visit when they wish, although when procedures are being done or doctors are examining you (making rounds), your family may be asked to wait outside momentarily. The size of the room limits the number of visitors at one time; for large families, the number visiting at one time may have to be limited. Otherwise, immediate family—spouse, parents and grown children—should have complete access to see and be with you.

Florence Nightingale wrote, in 1852, "It was valuable to have one place in a hospital where postoperative and other patients needing close attention could be watched." Ninety years later her advice was followed. The first post-anesthesia recovery room was set up in Rochester, Minnesota, in 1942.

Forerunners of ICUs include rooms for iron lungs used during the polio epidemic in the 50s. A patient lies inside an iron lung with head and neck protruding; the production of negative pressure within the tank expands the chest and pulls air into the lungs. No longer manufactured, iron lungs are used by only about 50 patients in this country today.

A special hospital unit to care for patients requiring artificial ventilation or ventilator support with the first Angstrom ventilators was set up in Scandinavia in 1952. Doctors there developed the apparatus and methods for artificial ventilation or ventilatory support. A four-bed respiratory care unit was established at the Massachusetts General Hospital by Dr. Pontopidan in 1960, and one of the first patients admitted to that unit was a patient of mine whose chest had been crushed in an auto accident.

The first general ICU was established in the Baltimore City Hospital in the early 60's. Coronary care units followed. Now all hospitals provide intensive care—a small general unit for all patients in smaller hospitals, medical and surgical units in larger hospitals, and ICUs for every specialty in large teaching hospitals: coronary care, pulmonary care, neurology and neurosurgery, general medicine, general surgery, cardiothoracic surgery and so on.

The purpose of an ICU is to help you recover from a major operation or a life threatening illness by supporting and monitoring organ function. If your lungs fail, an endotracheal tube is inserted into your windpipe and attached to a ventilator which will breathe for you. Your heart rate, ECG and blood pressure are displayed on a monitor. Drugs and fluids are given through intravenous catheters to support blood pressure, heart and kidney function. A catheter, or tube, inserted into your bladder collects urine and measures each hour how much your kidneys are making to help determine kidney function and fluid balance. A small catheter may be placed in your back, an epidural catheter, to control pain with the injection of narcotics. Other measurements and monitoring devices may be used.

Alarms sound with marked changes in the ventilator, your heart or blood pressure. A nurse is always close by. If your heart stops beating (a cardiac arrest) an alarm will sound and a team will rush to resuscitate you. They will begin by thumping on your chest and then rapidly depressing your chest wall and breast bone with their hands in an external cardiac massage. The massage may cause the heart to beat; if not, the masage will be continued to circulate blood throughout the body. Drugs will be given to stir the heart into activity. The name for a cardiac arrest is a Code. If you hear over the public address system "Code Red—emergency ward" you are hearing a call to a team to resuscitate someone in the emergency ward whose heart has stopped. If the patient left an order not to be resuscitated (do not resuscitate order—DNR) the patient will be allowed to die quietly if a cardiac arrest occurs.

ICUs are frightening for some patients even though they are necessary and often life-saving. The major stressors in ICUs are pain, inability to sleep and the discomfort of tubes in the nose, mouth or elsewhere. Your nurses are taking measurements on you, moving you, bathing you, feeding you etc. Newer ICU rooms include windows, but if you are in a room without one, you may not know whether it is night or day. You may not sleep well or at all.

Psychiatric problems are common in ICU patients, caused by the severe illness that brought you there. These problems include depression, anxiety, fear of death and disorientation. Pain, fear, anxiety, lack of sleep, tenseness, inability to speak/communicate, lack of control, nightmares and loneliness can be bothersome. Ask for or try to get help.

ICUs should not be frightening. Your nurses can keep you comfortable and your room quiet. Your pain can be controlled and you can be sedated to rest. Ask for pain medication if you need it or sedation if you would like it. Your nurses call button must be at your fingertips. If you cannot talk because of a tube in your throat to help you breathe, you may write out requests or use sign language. Your arms may be secured so that in your sleep you cannot accidentally pull out any of the tubes or separate yourself from the ventilator. When your nurse or family is in your room, your arms and hands may be free so you can move them. The first consideration is your safety followed by your comfort.

Problems arise if you are so sick you are not fully alert or able to call for help. Your nurses should either be at your bedside or close by. Your immediate family can help. It is common for very sick patients to become confused and lose track of time, the day and even of where they are. Don't worry if that happens to you. Recovery from your illness will bring you back to reality.

If your illness is very serious and one from which you may not recover, hopefully you have provided an advance directive, a living will and your thoughts about resuscitation, should a need for it arise. (Chapters 49, 50) Your family must be closely involved. Your clergyman or religious peson can be of great help to you. (Chapter 13) The training of doctors to help a family understand, deal with and accept death is important.

ICUs strive to maintain quality care by assessment programs to reduce errors and nosocomial problems, or complications in the ICU, and improve quality of life and functional status. Changes are taking place to make ICUs more comfortable and humane for patients and more supportive of their families. Efforts are underway to control night time light and noise levels although for safety reasons these annoyances can't be completely eliminated. Volunteers are assigned to waiting rooms; nurses are assigned to communicate with families about the condition of the patients. Physicians and nurses recognize that patients' families may suffer more than the patients, experiencing anxiety or depression. Some hospitals provide sleeping rooms for families adjacent to waiting areas.

What is nosocomial infection?

It is an infection occurring in the hospital or ICU. In an intensive care unit, you are exposed to bacteria brought into the unit by other patients. In spite of scrupulous attempts at cleanliness, with nurses and personnel washing their hands before they come into your cubicle, bacteria may be brought in. They could get into your lungs or the tube that helps you breathe and cause nosocomial pneumonia. This is a hazard of all ICUs and one from which the personnel try to protect you. These bacteria may be resistant to antibiotics. If such a problem is recognized you will be treated vigorously.

Other infections should not be a problem in a clean, well-run ICU. Personnel should wash their hands before they come in see you. They should wear sterile gowns, masks and gloves when they do procedures such as insert catheters or change dressings. Tell your doctor if they don't.

MISTAKES

47. How big a problem are mistakes in hospitals and in health care? What should be done about it?

You may have read about a surgeon amputating the wrong leg of a patient. Another surgeon, operating on a patient with a groin hernia on one side, ended up making the repair on the other side. In two cases surgeons operated on the wrong side of the brain. Growing up with medical lore, my son refused to be put to sleep for a vein operation on one leg until the surgeon entered the operating room. "It's my right leg," he told the surgeon.

Error in medicine is not common, but, like all human error, it happens. Errors can occur in diagnosis and treatment, with medication the most common source. In the hospital a doctor writes an order for medicine in the order book at the nursing station. A clerk transmits it to the pharmacy. The pharmacist prepares the medicine and sends to the nursing station where a nurse or aide gives it to you. Errors can occur all along the way. The doctor's writing may not be clear, the transmission through the computer to the pharmacy may be faulty, the pharmacy may fill the order incorrectly or the nurse may give the medicine without checking the order, or too fast or by the wrong route. Many procedures in hospitals guard against such errors; the main protection is to check, double check and check again. The nursing profession has stressed to nurses to do so before giving a medicine. Some authorities have said that if nurses do not know the medicine they should not give it. Under a new proposal, hospitals and pharmacies would use medicines with barcodes from pharmaceutical companies. Accurate communication is the big need.

An article in the *Institute of Medicine* (IOM) estimated medical errors kill between 44,000 and 98,000 people a year in U.S. Hospitals. This seems to overstate the problem. Upon close examination, many of these deaths turned out to have occurred in very sick people who would have soon died anyway or would have been dead within three months after leaving the hospital. The estimates used no control subjects. What were death rates in similar sick patients with no errors? Thus, a patient may die with an error occurring but not die from the error—a big difference. Only 22% of the deaths appear to have been potentially preventable and only 6% definitely preventable.

The IOM report served as the basis for media descriptions of medical errors as the eighth top killer in this country, costing up to $8.8 billion a year. The majority of these incidents reflect classic systems failure, however, and not true human error. The IOM called for a national effort to report errors without punishment, as is done in the airline industry through the confidential Aviation Safety Reporting System run by NASA. Hospitals are drawing upon standards of the aviation reporting system to reduce or eliminate systematic, ICU and medication errors.

A major problem in the reporting of errors is the potential for malpractice law suits against nurses, doctors or hospitals. Brennan said the IOM report could do harm without liability reform. I believe medical errors are a problem that should be addressed by all in medicine but are not as big a problem as stated by the IOM. Their figures are based on estimates, not facts.

In an article titled "Why some doctors may be hazardous to your health," one of a spate of articles and editorials about good and bad doctors after publication of the IOM estimates, Bernard Gavzer wrote that one can separate doctors into two groups: good and bad doctors. It would be nice if it were that simple. The truth is that doctors are real people, and people make mistakes. The fact that even good doctors on occasion make mistakes should not astound patients. Good doctors' mistakes may be evident only after the fact or in retrospect. For example, if I recommend an appendectomy to a young woman with abdominal pain on the basis of my preoperative diagnosis but I find at operation a ruptured ovarian cyst, I am in error. It is an acceptable error, however; it did not harm the patient.

Errors have occurred with prescriptions written by doctors and filled in drug stores. Doctors' handwriting has been blamed but the use of abbreviations account for some of the confusion. For example, q.d. means "every day" but if pharmacists read the period after the q as i the abbreviation becomes q.i.d., quadrupling the dose to four times a day. A pharmacist not sure about a prescription should call the doctor. This has happened with prescriptions I have written, and I appreciated the calls.

A major campaign is underway by hospitals, doctors, nurses, pharmacies, and nursing homes to develop ways to eliminate errors. Errors are investigated so that they are not repeated. Hospitals better monitor and report adverse reactions to improve drug safety. The FDA has increased staff for the Division of Pharmacovigilance and Epidemiology, now the Office of Post-marketing Drug Risk Assessment, to better monitor adverse drug and device reactions. The Institute for Health Care Improvement (IHCI) held a National Congress on reducing adverse drug events and other topics. (135 Francis Street, Boston, MA 02215. Telephone 617-754-4800)

For years, surgeons have attended weekly or monthly meetings in which all patient care is reviewed. Why did complications happen? Why did diagnostic problems occur? All deaths are reviewed in detail to determine whether anything else could or should have been done or whether the patient died of a disease that could not be treated further, such as metastatic cancer.

Residency programs are increasing supervision of young doctors to cut down on errors and, citing fatigue among physicians, have decreased working hours for residents. The IOM Report calls for a national center for patient safety, which Congress has so far not created.

You also can help to eliminate errors in your care. Be sure everyone knows where your problem is, which side it is on, etc. Ask about your medicines. Ask about what is being done to you. Report any adverse reactions to medicines or treatment promptly. Most errors may produce inconvenience but are not particularly harmful. Rarely is an error life-threatening.

Be familiar with reactions such as drug toxicities, allergic reactions, drug interactions, interactions with foods and possible medication errors. If in doubt, ask your doctor or pharmacist. Take only drugs you need. Keep a record of all of them. Read and understand your prescriptions. Check before you leave the pharmacy and understand the medicines, their purposes and the need for any special precautions. Alternative medicines (herbs, etc.) can cause reactions. Ask questions about your care. Insist on answers. The *Harvard Health Letter* gives the following advice by Gordon.

Staying Safe in and out of the Hospital

You need to know:

- the name and purpose of each medication
- how much to take, how often, and for how long
- what side effects are and how to deal with them
- special instructions for use, such as taking the drug with food or avoiding sunlight

Keep an updated record of your medications, especially if you have a chronic condition:

- include nonprescription drugs
- note adverse reactions to individual medicines
- consider purchasing a drug reference book

Use one pharmacy:

- make sure the pharmacist's computer has a list of all your current medications, including over-the-counter drugs you take regularly
- alert the pharmacy to any allergies or chronic conditions
- ask for written information about each prescription and review it with the pharmacist

If admitted to a hospital:

- bring your medication record
- bring medicines in their original containers
- ask the doctor the name and dose of prescribed drugs and write them down
- before taking a medication, ask what it is and make sure its effects correspond with what you were told to expect
- examine medicines before you take them so you learn the way they look and can spot an unfamiliar one
- never remove your identification bracelet and make sure a nurse checks it before giving you a drug
- let staff know of adverse reactions you have had to medications or dyes used in diagnostic tests such as angiography
- indicate in the operating room or mark with ink which side is to be operated upon
- ask what procedure is to be done and why.

Four useful books describe the need to use more open reporting systems and to fail-safe all aspects of hospital care. *Protect Yourself in the Hospital,* by Thomas Sharon, a registered nurse (Contemporary Books); *Health Smart of a Hospital Handbook,* by Dr. Joseph Sacco, a medical director (Alpha Books); *Dr. David Sherer's Hospital Survival Guide,* by David Scherer, an anesthesiologist, and Maryann Karnich (Claren Books); *The Truth behind America's Terrifying Epidemic of Medical Mistakes,* by Drs. Robert Wachter and Kaveh Shojania (Rugged Lard).

Privacy

48. Is there no privacy or modesty in a hospital? Those hospital gowns are terrible.

I agree the gowns can be a problem, those open in the back with ties at the neck and waist leaving your rear exposed. They do provide you with some cover, however, while giving your doctor unrestricted access to the areas of the body that need to be examined.

Another interference with privacy comes with the assignment of two or more patients to a room to save on hospital building costs and on nursing care, since two patients can be checked in one visit. It was also thought patients would like company. The charge is greater for a single room so most insurance companies and HMOs will only pay for a double room. In actual fact the cost to a hospital of a single room is really not much more than that of a double room. Today the arguments for double rooms are no longer persuasive. When I am sick, I don't want company. How about you? Some hospitals are converting to all private rooms. As occupancy in many hospitals decreases, why not move toward that?

Doctors, nurses, and aides should preserve your privacy and modesty. I always knocked on the door of a patient's room before entering. I never checked on a patient in a bathroom. If the curtains were drawn around a bed, something private was being done—a bedpan or dressing change—my rule was to stay out. When I examined a bed patient I asked them to use the bed sheet and gown to expose only the part to be examined—the abdomen, the chest, the wound etc.—and to keep everything else covered. After an operation or during convalescence you may certainly use your own nightgown or pajamas rather than the hospital gown. The secret to comfortable use of the gowns: Wear two of them, one tied in back and one tied in front. Then you are covered. If a nurse or therapist helps you walk in the corridor, your fanny won't be hanging out.

If you prefer to see no visitors or only family, a note to this effect can be displayed prominently on your door. The privacy act does not allow the hospital to tell a caller you are in the hospital or to give out your room number. The hospital cannot tell your clergy person that you have been hospitalized. The worst assault on patient privacy came recently when the Justice Department under John Ashcroft issued subpoenas demanding that at least six hospitals in New York City turn over hundreds of patient records for certain abortions. The Attorney General has absolutely no need for this information. He has no business second-guessing sensitive medical decisions.

Section H

End of Life Decisions

"It is not death that people fear as much as dying."

Peter Downs

"It's not that I am afraid to die. I just don't want to be there when it happens."

Woody Allen

"Everyone knows they're going to die but nobody believes it. If we did we would do things differently."

WNET—NY On our own terms.

CALLING IT QUITS.

49. Can I call it quits if I wish? What is—Do Not Resuscitate— DNR? What is meant by "pulling the plug"? What is euthanasia? Is physician-assisted suicide ethical?

Can I call it quits if I wish?

You may be called upon to make end-of-life decisions for yourself or for loved ones. You may have to decide whether to consider such options as a Do Not Resuscitate order (DNR); terminal sedation; pain control; voluntarily cessation of eating and drinking; withdrawal of life support; physician-assisted suicide; and voluntary active euthanasia.

The first and most important question is: Have you reached the end of life? Do you have an illness from which you absolutely cannot recover or one from which you could recover and enjoy life again? Your doctor can help you with information about the nature of your illness. Perhaps you have been sick for a long time and do not want to continue living but do not wish to commit suicide. You can choose not to continue.

As a nursing home patient in his late 80's, my grandfather could not get up and around, slept most of the time and clearly was not enjoying life. One day he stopped eating and drinking; he refused everything. The nurses and aides wanted to start intravenous (I.V.) feedings and/or transfer him to a hospital. His doctor and I, with the agreement of his daughter, my mother, said no to that. We believed he had decided it was time to go. A few days later he died peacefully in his sleep.

Some nursing homes may insist on giving a patient I.V. fluids or feedings by a tube inserted through the nose into the stomach. Patients with severe loss of mental faculties, confusion, disorientation or stupor (dementia) may have difficulty in swallowing and eating and consequently may not want to eat and drink. Yet some doctors and nursing home personnel have insisted on force feeding such patients. This is cruel.

Elderly patients with clear minds and severe medical problems but no trouble in swallowing also may not wish to go on, and they too should have the right to refuse food and drink. It is *not* a bad or cruel way to die. I believe calling it quits is different from suicide. Suicide is a deliberate act to end life: an act of commission. Calling it quits means "enough is enough." It is an act of omission.

What is a "do not resuscitate" order—DNR?

If a patient suffers a cardiac arrest or stops breathing, under a DNR order the patient will not be resuscitated and will be allowed to die. The order is appropriate in the event of a health problem from which patients cannot recover, like end-stage or metastatic cancer; irreversible, uncontrollable heart or lung disease; or strokes that left them unresponsive. Patients, if they are able, and/or their families should make the decision to ask for DNR orders, in consultation with their doctors; they may ask in advance for DNR orders under terminal circumstances, in living wills. Clergy can be a great help in these decisions. Upon agreement by all concerned, an order would be written in the hospital chart. Some patients wear hospital wrist bracelets that say DNR.

At the age of 90 my father-in-law was failing with congestive heart failure and wanted to die at home. Sons who had not seen him for some time insisted he be sent to a hospital and his wife was afraid of his dying at home with her alone. He was admitted to a hospital where acute problems developed and aggressive interns and residents put him on life support in the ICU. After a few days, he recovered sufficiently to leave the ICU and life support. My wife who knew her father's wishes because he told her, "please don't let that happen again," went to the hospital and had it clearly stated in his chart and made known to all doctors and nurses he did not wish further resuscitation. He died several nights later in his hospital bed, alone.

No one wants their life prolonged unnecessarily, particularly if suffering or comatose. What is unnecessary suffering: uncontrollable pain or an irreversible coma? Many attempts have been to define futility in the care of a patient— almost futile attempts! Few signs other than brain death indicate absolutely that a patient on life support will die, but if the electroencephalogram (EEG) is flat, and the patient has no reflexes, the patient is dead, no matter what the heart is doing. What if my doctor and my family and I disagree about the patient's chances? What do we do then? (Chapter 60 on Ethics, and Hospital Ethics Committees? and Chapter 52.)

Most ethical doctors separate permissible acts of omission—we do not order a treatment, or we omit therapy such as a ventilator—from impermissible acts of commission. We believe it wrong to take direct action to end a patient's life.

What is meant by "pulling the plug"?

The practice of withholding or withdrawing life-sustaining treatment is generally well accepted. Life support systems are generally plugged into electrical outlets, and discontinuance of their use is referred to in the slang expression "pulling the plug," a crude way to put it in the opinion of some people.

Withholding life support is the right of patients who do not want it and make their wishes known before a crisis occurs. The family can make the decision if the patient is not capable. Doctors, however, will not make such a decision without agreement by the patient and/or the patient's family. We always err on the side of sustaining life even if the outlook is dismal and always institute life support for a patient unless we have a clear directive not to do so.

Withdrawing life support is another patient/family/physician/cleric decision. It is made after careful determination of the hopelessness of the patient's case: a terminal illness; untreatable malignancy; stroke; little brain function; brain death; multiple organ failure (the need for a ventilator, kidney dialysis, liver failure, circulatory failure) or end-stage AIDS with deterioration foreshadowing a fatal outcome in an old or tired patient. Frequently, such a patient will be unresponsive and unable to participate in the decision. If the decision is up to the family, it is not made suddenly but reviewed over some days.

Some family members may accept the inevitable, believing the patient has suffered enough. Other family members, however, may not be able to give the patient up. Such feelings may be based more on guilt than on love: A child who has not seen or supported a parent for many years may step in at the end to "protect" the parent. I have seen a number of such interventions. They can be difficult.

If a family agrees on the need to withdraw life support, but the doctor does not, I suggest you get another doctor.

The criteria I use for stopping life support are: (1) brain death, (2) metastatic end-stage malignancy, (3) a severe stroke in an adult who is unconscious and requires ventilatory support with no improvement over at least a week's time, (4) severe failure of many organs—lungs, liver, kidneys, heart, or brain (multiple organ failure) (5) Alzheimer's disease with limitations before life support, (6) elderly patients with limited capability before the beginning of life support or (7) other end-stage diseases. Strong determinants of withdrawal of ventilation are: physician's perception that the patient preferred not to use life support, low likelihood of survival, use of inotropes or vasopressors and high likelihood of poor cognitive function.

Some people argue it is too expensive to keep someone alive unnecessarily and a lot of health care dollars are spent (wasted?) on patients in their last month or weeks of life. But who should decide whether someone is being kept alive unnecessarily? Certainly not an economist. How do you know it is the last month or weeks of your life? That determination is made in retrospect after you die.

When the time comes and all agree to stop life support, the ventilator is disconnected first. If the patient struggles, sedation is given. If the patient gets along without the ventilator, other support is continued. More frequently, however, the patient becomes less responsive, stops breathing and dies quietly with the family at the bedside.

Doctors are now learning and trying to help. I recommend a four-part PBS series from 2000: "On our terms: Moyers on dying" by Bill and Judith Moyers, available on tape from PBS on *www.pbs.org/on* our terms/ or from—On Our Own Terms Discussion Guide, Thirteen/WNET New York, PO Box 245, Little Falls, NJ 07424-9766. The discussion guide provides an excellent list of outreach programs, including Americans for Better Care of the Dying, (phone 202-530-9864), (*www.abcd-caring.org);* Hospice Association of America (phone 202-546-4759 or *www.hospicefoundation.org).* The SCCM ran a special supplement to the *Journal of Critical Care Medicine* titled "Compassionate end of life care in the ICU," with 11 articles on blending science and compassion. Another source of information for members is the AARP, 601 E. St. NW, Washington, DC, 20049, with booklets *Understanding the Grief Process, Caregiver Survival Resources,* and *Supportive Care of the Dying.*

What is euthanasia?

The word "euthanasia" comes from the Greek "eu," meaning well, and "thanos," meaning death. It is a well or good death, an easy, painless death, putting a patient to death painlessly. Is euthanasia synonymous with physician-assisted suicide? Big differences exist between these practices. If a patient with a terminal illness is suffering with severe pain or discomfort, and a doctor gives pain medication in sufficient quantity and frequency to control the suffering, it may lead to earlier death of the patient. Many pain medications depress breathing. A doctor may give a patient a prescription for such medications and, if the patient takes too much, it could lead to death. The doctor's intention in this circumstance is to give the patient relief. Many of us find this acceptable. The doctor's intention was not to kill the patient. The patient suffered from a necessary complication of the relief of suffering. Technically, the result could be called euthanasia.

A major problem, I believe, is for patients with widespread or terminal malignancy and severe pain. These patients should receive sufficient pain medication for pain relief, with no concern about addiction. If the pain medication shortens their life by a few days or weeks, at least they will die pain free. Hospices will help (Chapter 52).

Is physician-assisted suicide ethical?

Physician-assisted suicide, on the other hand, is a deliberate act to end a patient's life. It follows from the intent to kill. The patient may or may not be suffering and may or may not have a terminal illness. Maybe the patient is depressed or does not want to live but cannot summon up the will to commit suicide himself so wants a doctor to commit what many of us call murder.

In our judicial system, first-degree murder is the charge for killing someone deliberately and intentionally, with premeditation or with reckless disregard for human life. I believe that taking a direct action to kill a patient, with the intent to do so, even though the patient wants to die, is first-degree murder. Former Surgeon General C. Everett Koop, said, "Doctors are healers, not killers. The power to heal should be kept separate from the power to kill. People won't trust their doctors if assisted suicide becomes legal." Many physicians feel this way. I can omit some aspect of treatment but I will not purposely kill a patient. Some physicians, however, believe that physician-assisted suicide is acceptable. Dr. Jack Kevorkian is the best known advocate and has led the way, helping over 120 patients die. He is serving a 10-25 year sentence for second degree murder.

The courts have tried to equate competent, terminally ill patients who require life support with those who do not. Forgoing life support is not the same as physician-assisted suicide. The Supreme Court ruled a patient does not have a constitutionally protected right to have a physician assist them in committing suicide. Laws in 38 states define assisted suicide as a crime. In seven other states it is illegal under common law. State codes are silent on this issue in North Carolina, Ohio, Utah and Wyoming. Oregon allows physician-assisted suicide but it is carried out infrequently.

Dr. Charles McKhann, a good friend, colleague, and Professor of Surgery at Yale, argues in favor of the practice in *A Time to Die: The Place for Physician Assistance in Support of Physician-Assisted Suicide*. Another proponent is Marcia Angell, Deputy Editor of *The New England Journal of Medicine*. In an editorial titled "The Supreme Court and Physician-Assisted Suicide—The Ultimate Right," she writes: "by permitting the cessation or stopping of life-sustaining treatment, we stepped originally on a slippery slope". Physician-assisted suicide puts us farther down a slippery slope. So how do we answer the question: Is physician-assisted suicide ethical? I say it is not ethical. Drs. Angell and McKhann say it is. We have no final answer. and the argument will continue. Table 1 lists groups supporting or opposing physician-assisted suicide.

Physician-assisted suicide in the Netherlands has been reviewed and described in detail and used as an argument both for and against physician-assisted suicide in the United States. Van der Maas summarizes this in the *New England Journal of the Medicine*:

> "Physician-assisted suicide and euthanasia are illegal in the Netherlands and punishable by fine or imprisonment. However, physicians carry these out and report their cases which are investigated but not prosecuted. So long as they observe guidelines set up by the Royal Dutch Medical Association, they are not prosecuted.
>
> These guidelines are:
>
> (1) The request must be voluntary.
> (2) It must be well considered.
> (3) The desire to die must be enduring.
> (4) The suffering of the patient must be unbearable with no alternatives.
> (5) The physician involved must consult a colleague.
> (6) There must be a fully documented written record."

Van der Maas estimates about half of the physicians in the Netherlands have carried out physician-assisted suicide. They receive about 25,000 requests for information and formal applications for assistance from about 9,000 patients a year, but provide it for only about 3,000 patients. Only about 2% of annual deaths in the Netherlands are due to physician-assisted suicide. Despite opposition, the Netherlands Parliament has approved a bill which legalizes physician-assisted suicide. The Vatican has called the law "a sad record for Holland" . . . which "violates human dignity". The Hemlock Society, of course, welcomed the action. Switzerland, Colombia and Belgium tolerate euthanasia. Van der Maas believes the Dutch system cannot be transplanted to the United States because of so many differences in our societies.

These arguments have produced some good fallout. Physicians have now begun to study and emphasize the need for better care of dying patients. Cohen cites a report by the IOM titled "Approaching Death: Improving Care at the End of Life." Azevedo, in a balanced review of physician-assisted suicide, recounts the experience of an 84-year-old man with excruciating pain from cancer whose doctor would give him nothing more than Tylenol. The patient went down to the basement and shot himself. This tragedy is the fault of the doctor. The man wanted pain relief not physician-assisted suicide so he did it himself. Doctors must recognize adequate pain management is important. Elderly and minority patients in nursing homes may have inadequate treatment of cancer pain.

The AMA described "eight elements of quality care for terminally-ill patients" (cited by Downs): (1) the opportunity to discuss and plan for end-of-life care; (2) trustworthy assurances that physical and mental suffering will be carefully attended to and comfort measures secured; (3) assurance that preferences for withholding life-sustaining intervention will be honored; (4) assurance there will be no abandonment by the physician; (5) assurance that dignity will be a priority; (6) assurance that burden to family and others will be minimized; (7) attention to the personal goals of the dying person; (8) assurance that care providers will assist the bereaved through early stages of mourning and adjustment.

Patients terminally ill with cancer may be depressed, have a feeling of hopelessness and the desire for a hastened death. It is important to recognize and provide treatment for them, as part of adequate palliative care. More information and help can be obtained from the Compassion in Dying Federation which supports patient empowerment and expansion of end-of-life choices at 6312 SW Capital Highway, Portland, OR 97201. A guide to end-of-life financial decisions is available for $5 from Legal Council for the Elderly, Inc., PO Box 96474, Washington, DC 20090-6474 (make check out to LCE Inc.) For a Medicare guide call 1-800-633-4227. To find your state agency for Aging Call U.S. Dept. of HHS 1-800-677-1116 or *www.aoa.dhhs.gov*

Elizabeth Barrett-Connor and Stuenke wrote: "Everyone dies too early or too late." How do you define dying at the right time? I provide selective references to writings on end of life decisions and care. The reference list is not exhaustive because if it were it would take up the rest of this book.

Table I

Groups which Support or Oppose Physician-Assisted Suicide

FOR	AGAINST
The Hemlock Society	Center to Improve Care of the Dying at
American Civil Liberties Union	George Washington University, Washington, D.C.
A Compassion in Dying Group	Americans for Better Care of the Dying
	The American Medical Association
	The California Medical Society
	The American Foundation for Suicide Prevention
	120 Wall Street
	New York, NY 10005

Table II

Request for help in dying requires:

1. Evaluation for depression and other psychiatric conditions
2. Evaluation of the patient's decision-making competence
3. If the patient is competent, discuss the patient's goals for care.
4. Evaluate the patient's "total suffering," physical, mental, social, spiritual, and the patient's response to it.
5. Provide full information and deliberation, hospice care, professionals, etc.
6. Consult professional colleagues.
7. Be sure that care plans are followed.
8. Decline physician-assisted suicide "because it is not justified by the principle of non-intrusion or by the obligation to relieve suffering." Also, it is against the law in all states but Oregon.

LIVING WILLS

50. Should I have an advance directive? What is the difference between a durable power of attorney for healthcare and a general durable power of attorney? Should I be an organ donor?

Here is a good definition of the two types of advance directive, from a brochure given to patients on admission to the St. Louis University Hospital (SLU):

A Durable Power of Attorney for Healthcare allows you to designate another person (known as a proxy or agent) who is at least 18 years of age to make medical decisions for you in the event you are unable to do so. These decisions may include, but not limited to withholding or withdrawal of life-prolonging procedures.

A Living Will or Healthcare Directive allows you to state in advance your wishes regarding the use of certain medical procedures and treatments and becomes effective when you are unable to make your own decisions and can no longer communicate such decisions. It serves as a guide to your family or the person you name as your agent.

All states now have laws on advance directives, first proposed over two decades ago. The statutes provide ways for people to decide what treatments they do not want and to name proxies to decide for them if they become incompetent. You may obtain forms for advance directives from libraries, hospitals, and state bar associations. Your doctor or lawyer may provide you with forms as well, although you do not need to hire a lawyer to fill them out. You must sign both your living will and durable power of attorney for healthcare in the presence of two qualified witnesses and in most states a notary public. Your doctor and his/her staff, among others, cannot serve as witnesses. Keep copies at your doctor's office and at the hospital where you go for health care.

The 1991 Federal Patient Self-Determination Act (PSDA) requires hospitals to inform adult patients on admission of their rights to participate in decisions about their care. The PSDA was also intended to help reduce high costs of caring for people in the last few weeks or months of life. As Sister Louise Lears has pointed out, advance directives initially were received with enthusiasm partly because "They had the potential to . . . help resolve some fears about ineffective or overly burdensome life sustaining treatment."

"Patients fear losing their lives in the medical system," said Henry Perkins. "They dread being trapped in insensitive medical institutions, tethered to inhumane machines, robbed of personal privacy and subjected to accompanying indignities."

Some people believe that the scope of living wills is too broad. The goal should not be to extend autonomy further than reason allows anymore than it is to extend life regardless of its quality. Tonnelli writes there may come a time when we will be unable to direct our own lives. That is true but we can record our wishes and hopes.

Review your living will with your doctor. You may find older doctors to be uncomfortable with the discussion, however. They are more concerned about keeping you well and alive. Younger doctors, having studied medical ethics, will be more receptive. Ask your doctor if he/she is comfortable with your wishes and will support you if and when you become incompetent. If your doctor has problems with that, ask why. As a last resort, get a new, better doctor.

Many of my friends and family members have completed living wills to avoid prolonged life support in an ICU, linking this directive to the occurrence of "terminal illness," "end-stage malignancy with continuous pain," "incurable illness," "severe incapacitating illness," and the like. It is important to mention such compelling circumstances. For, after prolonged life support in the ICU, many patients fully recover, and the next thing you know they are back on the tennis courts. Some 50% or so of patients who stay in an ICU for longer than two weeks are enjoying life at home a year later.

It can be appropriate for you to state, that given any of the above incurable conditions:

- I do not wish to be placed on life support (ventilators etc.) or to be kept on life support if this has happened to me as an emergency procedure. But make it clear that this applies only in the event of terminal illness or other compelling circumstances. Do not say: I don't ever want to be on a ventilator; a few days on a ventilator may get you over an acute problem like pneumonia and help return you to health again.

- I do not wish to be fed intravenously or through a tube in my stomach. Again, do not say that in general you do not want to be fed intravenously (IVs); a short course of IVs may get you through an acute illness and help speed you to a full recovery.
- I do not wish to receive antibiotics or other medications which may prolong my life.
- I wish to be kept comfortable and free from pain by whatever medication is necessary, even though such medication may shorten my life.

All of the incurable conditions require assessment. Your family can participate in that process but ultimately it is your doctor who will make the prognosis that will help your family come to a decision. Your doctor must approve the decision; under federal law, hospitals and nursing facilities can provide only the care ordered by patients' doctors. Some aggressive doctors believe only death is the terminal event for an incurable condition; patients are to them soldiers in the battle against cancer. This approach may be wrong for you.

Gearon, writing in the AARP publication *The States*, gives these tips for making your wishes known:

1. Discuss your wishes with family members, doctors and caregivers.
2. Avoid generic advance directive forms; complete and update documents with your doctors.
3. Pick a health care agent or proxy who will act aggressively on your behalf; the person closest to you may not always be the best choice.
4. Sign each directive, date it and have it witnessed according to the laws in your state.
5. Put copies of your advance directives in your medical records and make them widely available to family and care providers.
6. Choose a new doctor if yours is not willing to abide by your wishes.

You can revoke your living will simply by telling your doctor you want to do so, as did my late sister-in-law. She developed recurrent lung cancer which could not be treated by operation. I hoped a short course of x-ray therapy would relieve her pain and allow her to go home for however long she would live. While the radiation therapist was trying to understand what I had in mind, the patient developed lung failure, was intubated with a tube in her throat and put on a ventilator. It was obvious that she could not survive without the ventilator. To keep her as comfortable as possible, we requested a tracheotomy so that we could put the tube to help her breathe into her throat, or trachea or wind pipe, through a small incision in her neck rather than through her mouth. A semipermanent epidural catheter was placed along her spinal cord for injections of pain medications to control her severe pain.

Now she was comfortable and breathing easily with the ventilator but it was apparent she could not recover and would always require use of the ventilator. She could live in this condition for weeks to months. Her living will stated that she did not wish to be kept alive on a ventilator. Her mind was clear; she was competent. Her family told her she could not live without the ventilator. Did she wish it removed? She clearly shook her head no. No one knew whether she knew she had terminal cancer.

She continued to enjoy visits with family and was even moved, ventilator and all, to a waiting room with a piano which she played for her grandchildren. This went on for some weeks. Eventually, however, when she became somnolent and unresponsive, the family unanimously decided to stop the ventilator. Her children and sister were with her when the ventilator was stopped. She died about eight hours later. Was this protracted struggle worthwhile? The patient apparently thought so, and her family had more time to adjust to the fact that their wife, mother, grandmother and sister would die.

What is the difference between a durable power of attorney for healthcare and a general durable power of attorney?

A durable power of attorney for healthcare applies only to health matters, providing for the appointment of an agent or proxy to make decisions about your medical care if you are unable to make them. In a general durable power of attorney, you grant your agent specific powers to make decisions for you in financial matters if you are no longer competent. Generally, a durable power of attorney is given only to a spouse or, in the absence of a living spouse, to a child.

You can designate a spouse, a child, another relative or a trusted friend to make health-care decisions for you when you are no longer competent. I recommend that you pick someone who loves you so much that they do not want you to suffer unnecessarily or to be on life support only to prolong your life. Remember, this person is not you and may not think like you. If the person you ask says "I can't bear to think of you dying," select another proxy. Review your living will with your proxy and ask whether they agree with you and will support your wishes when the time comes. Give your proxy several copies of the will.

Sometimes, however, physicians do not listen to designated proxies or family members or disagree with them. Doctors differ on what is considered futile care. They may not be aware of your wishes or may choose to ignore them. That is a major reason why you need an agent or proxy to support you. In the end, however, proxies may be unable to select or stop treatment consistent with your wishes.

H. J. Silverman and P. N. Lanken have asked if advance directives are fulfilling their purpose. They note low completion rates, with only 15% or so of patients hospitalized in certain circumstances have or fill out a living will. Many patients don't understand the need for one or expect family members to make decisions. Some suspect a living will takes away their rights. Hospitals may fulfill the letter of the law, but do not really give patients much information or ask for their participation. Completed advanced directives may not be available in the nursing home or hospital. Your physician may be reluctant to initiate discussions about advance directives.

Some advance directives fail to meet specific criteria under state law. In North Carolina, for instance, a living will must contain two specific statements to be valid. It must say that you do not want your doctor to use extraordinary means or artificial nutrition to keep you alive if your condition is terminal and incurable or if you are in a persistent vegetative state. It must also say that you are aware that the will authorizes your doctor to withhold or discontinue extraordinary means or artificial nutrition or hydration. In making a living will, be certain to check the statutory requirements of your state.

Also, when does the advance directive take effect? The determination of when you become incompetent can be difficult. Who is to say: your family— your physician? If a state of incompetence occurs suddenly, as with a stroke, determination is easy. If it develops slowly as with senility or Alzheimer's disease, it may be difficult. Legal battles have been fought over this question. Your proxy and your doctor should protect you and make every effort to keep it out of the courts. Courts deal with law, not your wishes.

To sum up: Think about your hopes for the future, your health care in the future and how you would like to be treated if you have an illness which will result in death. Some of you may want everything possible to be done. You may decide to travel to other medical centers, seek other opinions and alternative medical treatment (Chapter 42). This is your option. Others may want to be kept comfortable, to be at home surrounded by family if possible. Some call this a "good death" or a "death with dignity". Many are not afraid of death but are afraid of dying and particularly of dying alone. Remember, your family may be physically incapable of caring for you in your home, even with a hospital bed and visiting nurse care. A hospice may be the answer. (Chapter 52)

For further reading or information please see:

- Choice In Dying, 200 Varick St., New York City, 10014-4810, (800) 989-will, a national not-for-profit organization, has a website devoted to end-of-life decision-making issues, "http://www.caregiver.on.ca/choice_in_dying.html".
- Supportive care of the dying. 503-215-5053. care of dying.org
- National Federation of Interfaith Volunteer Caregivers 816-931-5442. nfivc.org
- The Well-Spouse Foundation. 800-838-0897. www.wellspouse.org

- The AARP, 601 E St., N.W., Washington, D.C. 20049, (202) 434-2277, lists on its home page a section with information on advanced directives, *http://www.aarp.org/programs/advdir/adirhow.html* or *www.aarp.org/ontheissuesadvdir.html* For 10 dollars a year you can become an AARP member—aarp.org/lsn; 800-424-3413.
- Partnership for Caring provides information and forms for advance directives for each state for a small fee. www.partnershipforcaring.org; 800-989-9455; 24 hour hot line.
- The AMA's booklet on advanced directives, produced in association with the AARP and the American Bar Association, is available at the End of Life Resources home page, "http://www.changesurfer.com/BD/Death.html". The title is "Shape your health care with health care advance directives—download this booklet from *www.abanet.org/ftp/pub/elderly/ad-ftp.wpd*

Should I be an organ donor?

The decision about donation of any of your organs must be made by your family or surrogate since you will not be competent at that time. It is helpful to indicate your preferences beforehand. In many states you can do so on your driver's license and in an advance directive.

The shortage of organs is a major problem. Many patients die while waiting for a transplant. Kidneys are more available because two are removed with each donation, hearts, livers, or lungs less so. Some family members have sidestepped shortages, when tissues match satisfactorily, by donating single kidneys and also parts of livers and lungs to other family members.

If you can see your way clear to become an organ donor, you should do it. You should approve organ donation on behalf of a family member if the decision is up to you. Transplant centers maintain a high ethical code and will give you and a loved one every consideration. Organs are removed only after brain death or cessation of circulation.

AUTOPSIES

51. When are autopsies done? Should I sign for one for a family member who died? Does anyone really learn from them? Is it true the family must pay for one? Do life insurance companies require an autopsy before they pay benefits?

An autopsy is an examination of a body after death. It requires incisions in the abdomen, chest and back of the head, which are afterwards repaired. Done with care and respect, an autopsy is a serious medical activity. If an autopsy is required, it must be done before the embalming of the body. If you wish to have a wake and viewing of the body, an autopsy will not interfere. The person may still look quite natural.

The purpose of an autopsy is to determine the patient's cause of death and any other diseases or problems. An autopsy may uncover problems that could not be identified prior to death. The problem for which the patient was receiving treatment may not be the cause of death. A cancer patient, for instance, may actually have died from a heart attack or blood clot to the lungs. Autopsies help doctors learn more about diseases, their causes and manifestations. For patients who die in an ICU, an unsuspected infection is a frequent cause of death but one diagnosed only at autopsy. Articles in the medical literature recently emphasize the need for autopsies and the importance of the information gleaned from them like diagnoses not suspected clinically. An autopsy may help you and members of your family learn about problems that tend to run in families, like arteriosclerosis, cancers and various organ diseases.

If the cause of death is uncertain or death is sudden and unexpected, I recommend an autopsy. If the patient had widespread cancer which had been diagnosed, or if an elderly patient gradually fails and dies, not much would be learned from an autopsy. The relative responsible for the body of the patient must agree in writing to have an autopsy. If a patient requests one before dying, the living relative does not have to agree. An autopsy can be limited to the chest, abdomen or head. If the patient had a recent operation you can limit the autopsy to that area.

In my experience with deaths in my family, relatives objecting most to autopsies had maintained little recent contact with the patient. After death, they were going to make up for that by doing something for the relative. If a patient has undergone a number of operations or procedures in an ICU, a relative may say the patient has gone through enough. Some may even say the patient has suffered enough but an autopsy does not make a person suffer.

In most circumstances, the cost of an autopsy is borne by the insurance carrier or hospital. I have heard of rare circumstances where a family was asked to pay. Ask about that before you agree to the procedure.

Life insurance companies do not require an autopsy. They require a certified death certificate provided to you by the funeral director and the doctor. If the death is sudden, unexpected, mysterious or a possible homicide, a medical examiner may order and perform the autopsy. They do not need your permission. A suicide does not require an autopsy unless the cause of death is unclear. If you have any doubt about what happened to your relative, request an autopsy.

Section I

Nursing Homes, Hospices and Home Health Care

HOSPICE—NURSING HOMES—CARE AT HOME

52. What is the difference between a nursing home and a hospice?

For many years, institutions have cared for the elderly, the seriously handicapped or retarded people—those without family or who could not be cared for at home. Many institutions were developed and supported by religious organizations: Altenheim, or an Old Folks Home, by the Lutheran Church; Emmaus Homes by the Evangelical and Reformed Church; the Roman Catholic Carmelite Homes and the Jewish Centers for the Aged (JCA). Religious institutions originally cared for severely retarded or handicapped persons. State and local government provided facilities for the mentally ill and destitute, with Poor Farms. The prevailing practice, however, was to care for our family members, our loved ones at home as long as we could. Many elderly and sick individuals prefer to die at home. Handicapped, retarded children or with Down's syndrome grew up with their siblings at home. Many families consider such children as a gift, not a burden.

Changes in society, with both parents working and with people living longer and moving about more, increased the need for alternatives to home care. Nursing homes and skilled nursing facilities (SNF) helped fill this need. Nursing homes care for the elderly. SNF help recently discharged hospital patients with recovery and rehabilitation from illnesses and operations, like stroke and hip replacement; patients leaving SNF return to their homes and an independent life. Many nursing homes and SNF are no longer religious-based but are instead associated with hospitals, community organizations or private groups.

Some patients come to SNF from step-down facilities, founded to meet the needs of patients after early discharge from expensive hospitals and ICUs. Step-downs include special facilities for patients who require a ventilator to breathe—ventilatory support. They also offer ambulatory kidney dialysis; treat head injury, respiratory and spinal cord injury; and serve as rehabilitation centers. Some such patients recover sufficiently to go to a SNF or home. Others die in the facility.

Now we have retirement communities. An older individual or a couple can rent or buy an apartment or a condominium in the facility and live independently. Residents who need take-out meals can obtain them from the central facility. With further aging or disability, residents may move to a room in a facility with nursing care available for the rest of the individual's life. With this kind of "Graded Care in a Retirement Center," residents can meet all of their medical needs without going elsewhere.

What are hospices?

Many patients with terminal cancer require such frequent pain medication that they cannot be cared for adequately at home. No patient near the end of life should be required to suffer. At that point no one should be concerned about drug addiction or the likelihood that drugs to keep them pain free contribute to the shortening of their life. Modern hospices were developed to provide pain medication and other care for the terminally ill and support for their families. They provide a wonderful service. Support the hospice in your community.

The word "hospice" comes from the Latin words for "hospitality" and "guest" and originally referred to medieval refuges established by Christian monastic orders for the weary and sick on crusades. In the nineteenth century the Irish Sisters of Charity founded the forerunners of modern SNFs, small, quiet and home-like shelters for patients not in need of an acute-care hospital. Others were established in England and France. At St. Christopher's Hospice in Syndenham, England, Dr. Cicely Saunders promoted the concept of seeking "quality of life" for patients rather than prolonging it almost beyond endurance. In 1961 Dr. Saunders came to Yale University to give a lecture on hospice care at the invitation of Florence Wald, Dean of the Yale School of Nursing. After a visit to St. Christopher's in 1969, Wald returned to New Haven to study terminally ill patients, with the help of Dr. Ira Goldenberg, a Yale surgeon, and brought hospice care to the U.S. in creating the Connecticut Hospice in 1971. Today the National Hospice and Palliative Care Organization of Alexandria, VA represents over 2000 hospices throughout the United States. They are at 1700 Diagonal Road, Suite 625, Alexandria, VA 22314. 800/646-6460.

Some commentators have said that hospices just mark a return to old values. In the past most cancer patients died at home, their families with them. Then health care shifted to hospitals and intensive care units. Hospice programs provide assistance for terminally ill patients to stay at home for as long as possible. After that, the patient moves to a home-like environment in the hospice with families always an important consideration. Hospices emphasize comfort, relief of symptoms, total welfare of the patient and family, and "dying with dignity," as described by Elisabeth Kubler-Ross. Acceptance of death by you, if you are terminally ill, may be difficult if you also have hope. Are these incompatible? Can you hope for the best and still accept the inevitable? Can any of us in such a situation believe death is best? If we have in ourselves or a loved one a failing body, weight loss, weakness, and need for large doses of pain medication, death may be welcome. In many older people that is the case.

In the past some hospital patients with terminal illnesses were given overenthusiastic treatment by some doctors and were isolated and neglected by others. Families and medical personnel alike did not inform patients of their terminal situation, leading to denial in many patients. This is where the hospice movement and hospice institutions can be helpful, in showing patients and their families how to deal with the realistic possibilities ahead of them.

In 1979, Joseph A. Califano, Jr., then Secretary of Health, Education and Welfare (now Health and Human Services) visited the hospice in New Haven, CT. He said he went with the idea a hospice was about dying. "I came away realizing that hospice is something far more. It is about living, a way of living more fully and completely, embraced by human support, up to and through the end of life." Dr. Kenneth Liegner who visited St. Christopher's in 1974 said that he expected a terminal care or death house environment, with lonely and depressed patients. Instead he found patients in colorful wards (no private rooms), part of an active community of staff, families and children.

Kathleen Breeding, Director of Social Services for the Beacon of Hope Hospice in St. Louis, set forth these criteria a patient must meet to be eligible for a hospice: (1) A patient must have a terminal illness where life expectancy is less than six months if the illness runs its expected course; (2) The patient must express a desire to enter hospice care and understand the care is palliative— providing symptom relief, pain control, comfort and support—rather than curative; (3) For a diagnosis to meet specific Medicare criteria, the hospice will complete an assessment visit to determine if appropriate criteria are present. If so the patient is admitted to hospice care. If the patient improves significantly and no longer meets required criteria, the patient may be discharged from the service with the right to change his/her mind about hospice and the possibility for hospice care in the future. The hospice team encourages the patient and family to do as much as the patient may tolerate for the highest possible quality of life. Many hospice patients stay at home and continue to garden, cook, manage personal affairs, and so on. Only when they are no longer able to carry on do they go to live at the hospice center. Family members report a better experience for dying loved ones who received care at home with hospice services.

Medicare, Medicaid in most states, and many private insurers entitle a patient to hospice benefits. A federal law gives patients access to a list from which they may choose a hospice program. Currently, however, health policy discourages use of a hospice for dying patients from nursing homes. Policy changes and reimbursement incentives are needed to improve access for these needy people. Palliative and hospice care is also needed for children with life-threatening conditions. Problems of understaffing of both nursing homes and hospices have been reported.

Hospice is described as the comfort team by the AARP publication *Modern Maturity*, with a succinct description of what can be done in an article titled

"Start the Conversation". Information about Hospices can be found at All about Hospices: A Consumer's Guide, 202-546-4759 or *www.hospice-america.org*.

Publications about facing the end of life for patients and for families include *The Rights of the Dying: A Companion for Life's Final Moments*, by David Kessler, Harper Perennial, 1998; *The Good Death*, by Marilyn Webb, Bantam, 1997; *Death and Dying in America, In Hospice: A Photographic Inquiry*, by Marilyn Webb, Little Brown, 1996.

Following are children's books recommended by the Hospice's Child and Family Support Program. Stacey Orloff, Crossroads of Life, 3:18-19, 1998.

Books for Children

> *Everett Anderson's Good-Bye*, Lucille Clifton
> *Geranium Morning*, Sandy Powell.
> *Badger's Parting Gifts*, Susan Varley.
> *The Tenth Good Thing About Barney*, Judith Viorst.
> *It Must Have Hurt A Lot*, Doris Sanford.
> *The Lighthouse*, Dyan Blacklock.
> *The Fall of Freddy the Leaf*, Leo Buscaglia.
> *Charlotte's Web*, E.B. White.
> *William and the Good Old Days*, Eloise Greenfield.

How Can I Get Health Care at Home?

House calls by physicians carrying a little black bag of medicines, once common, are now a rarity. Nowadays a doctor can do little for you in your home. Modern medicine requires a laboratory, an x-ray facility and a pharmacy. Although it might be comforting to you for your doctor to come to your home, from the doctor's point of view it is time consuming, inefficient, poorly reimbursed and not cost effective. More patients live far apart in urban and rural areas and no longer in small communities where a doctor could see many patients in a short time.

Nurses moved in to fill the gap. They can do many things in your home that allow you to stay there and not go to a nursing home. This home health care was originally provided by Visiting Nurse Associations (VNAs). Now many hospitals and other groups provide nursing services. Nurses can change dressings; check incisions and your temperature, blood pressure, pulse; and help with bathing and other personal activities during convalescence after an illness or operation until you can care for yourself. Periodically, insurance carriers, HMOs and Medicare decide to not support home health care adequately, causing nurses to drop out because they are not adequately reimbursed. Whether home health care will allow you to stay in your home with infirmities is an unanswered question. If you are alone you may enjoy life in a nursing facility with company for meals, bingo, card games, musical programs, exercise classes and other sociable activities. If you seek help at home, call your nearest hospital and ask if they have that service. Check on visiting nurses alliances or associations.

Recently there is renewed interest in house calls by physicians. The Deaconess Family Medicine Program at the Forest Park Hospital in St. Louis includes house calls as part of its residency program for family doctors. Dr. John Glick, a resident there said, "The patients just love it and it helps me establish rapport with them." Dr. Richard Schamp, the Director of Geriatric Training in this program, believes house calls will come back again. The major problem is financing. Many doctors believe house calls are effective in patient care to assess patient function and safety in the home setting. Simple structural modifications in a home may make it easier for the elderly to get around safely. Some doctors also make home visits to pregnant women and during the first two years of the child's life, to help prevent child mistreatment, domestic violence, emergencies and the need for hospitalization.

Section J

Our Health Care System

RIGHT TO HEALTH CARE—HMOs, MEDICARE

"Every criminal has a right to a lawyer, but we don't feel every sick person has a right to a doctor"

Jocelyn Elders, Former U.S. Surgeon General

53. Do I have the right to be given health care? What are managed care and health maintenance organizations (HMOs)? Why can't I sue an HMO for denial of health care I need? Can you help me understand Medicare and Medicaid? What about medical insurance? What do I do if I have no health insurance and am ineligible for Medicaid?

Do I have a right to be given health care?

It should be a right but currently in the U.S. it is more of a privilege. If you are employed, your employer may provide you with health insurance. If you are unemployed or in a job that pays a minimum wage, you may be eligible for Medicaid, a welfare program for the needy that helps pay for doctor bills, medicines and hospitalization. Administered by the states with some financial support provided by the Federal Government, Medicaid differs from state to state. Inquire at your local office about eligibility. As for Medicare, you are eligible when you reach 65 years of age.

Periodic attempts are made to set up a single payer system so that the Federal Government would provide everyone with health care insurance as it does for the elderly with Medicare. President Bill Clinton pushed for this early in his first term but Republicans in Congress have been unwilling to consider such a program. Most western countries—Canada, England, France, Germany, and the Scandinavian countries—provide health care for all. The U.S. is the only industrialized nation that does not. In some of these countries, particularly England, the costs of public health care led to rationing in the form of long waits for operations and other care. Canada limited the health care available, particularly for elective operations. In general, conservative politicians oppose universal health insurance and liberal politicians support it.

It is estimated that 44 million Americans lack health coverage even though many of that number have jobs. The hardest-hit are working families and children. The number of uninsured rises yearly. U.S. health care is not the best in the world—far from it. A study of health in 13 countries ranked the U.S. 12th, with higher rates of newborn and infant mortality and generally lower rates of life expectancy. The uninsured are slow to seek medical care, forgo necessary care for serious symptoms, and run an increased risk of death due to lack of treatment for chronic illnesses such as diabetes. A relationship between lack of health insurance and decline in overall health in late middle age has been reported. The best U. S. health care is excellent but many people can't get it.

What are managed care and HMOs?

During World War II, a wage stabilization board prevented inflation with wages fixed at the level at the beginning of the war. Industry, to do something for their hardworking workers, offered health benefits, which didn't cost much then. Thus began health care as a benefit of employment.

Since then, traditional fee-for-service care from doctors and hospitals has become increasingly expensive. More care and procedures could be provided and were perhaps required or requested. This escalation led American business, the principal payer for health insurance through work, to consider ways to control rising health care costs. Some people blame doctors for the rapid rise in health care costs even though doctors control only 35 per cent of health care costs, exerting little control over 65% of costs. Some people blame consumers, with patients seeking more care and more diagnostic studies. The truth is that excellent health care is expensive.

The upshot has been the emergence of managed care delivery systems that have taken control of both delivery and cost of care, replacing control by doctors, hospitals and patients. Policies from traditional private medical insurance companies like Blue Cross/Blue Shield and Mutual of Omaha are still available and afford considerably more freedom in choice of doctors, hospitals and health care. They are more expensive, however, unless you join a group policy for a corporation, a university or some other organization.

Managed care is also known as "prepaid health care," with a prepaid and/or capitated (so much paid per person per month or year) payment structure to reduce use of health services and expenses. The major principle is control by financial incentives, penalties, and administrative oversight to provide "a comprehensive approach to provision of health care combining clinical services and administration in an integrated, coordinated system for timely access to primary care and other necessary services in a cost effective manner." The Health Maintenance Organization (HMO) is the major structure, a prepaid health plan providing comprehensive health care for members at a fixed cost with periodic prepayments. Up to 80 million Americans use HMOs for their health care, about 85% of the work force with insurance.

According to the HMO Act of 1973 (US Public Law 93222), an HMO comprises: (1) an organized system in a geographic area which ensures delivery of health care; (2) agreed on set of basic and supplemental health maintenance and treatment services; (3) a voluntarily enrolled group of people; and (4) reimbursement by a predetermined fixed periodic prepayment for each person without regard to services provided. An early example is the Kaiser-Permanente system on the West Coast, a prepaid group practice that owns its own hospitals and employs doctors as well. The largest not-for-profit HMO in the country, it began in WWII as a plan for all the workers in the Kaiser ship-building company.

While HMOs take many forms, a leading example is the staff model, which hires mostly primary care doctors and contracts with hospitals and specialists for emergency and specialty care. As a member of a staff model HMO, you must go to their primary care doctors and the specialists, emergency department and hospitals on their list. If you seek care elsewhere, they will not pay for it.

Many plans involve a co-pay; you pay so much for visits to your primary care doctor, so much for prescriptions, so much for emergency room visits, as well as deductibles for the hospital, specialists and tests. Hopefully, your HMO offers quality assurance programs, preventive care and health promotion programs, but in my experience, HMOs do not live up to the name of Health Maintenance Organizations. Many HMOs have not stressed health maintenance and control of risk factors with programs to stop smoking, lose weight, exercise, and improve health. They simply deal with sickness as it occurs.

Prudential Health Care Plan, Inc., advertises a Disease Management and Preventive Care Program that covers advice for expectant mothers, asthma education, influenza and pneumonia immunization, complex case management, diabetes self management and bike helmet safety. No real health maintenance programs were listed. The fine print reads "may be subject to deductibles, co-pays or coinsurances." The reason for deductibles, co-pays and co-insurance is to decrease use and save money. If you must pay for part of the diagnosis and treatment, you may think twice about whether you want to proceed.

HMOs have lessened the rate of increase, or escalation, in health care costs but have led to other problems. Your HMO may give you no choice of doctors. Your family doctor may not be part of the plan. Especially troubling is the role of HMO primary care doctors as gatekeepers who reduce costs by reducing patient referrals and, in so doing, may receive a financial incentive for controlling costs. You cannot see a specialist or go to a hospital or an emergency facility without their approval. Patients object if a doctor is forced to act as a gatekeeper. In a survey almost 13, 000 California patients said doctors acting as gatekeepers would undermine their trust and confidence in their medical care. Primary care physicians now called PCPs should be coordinators of your care, not gatekeepers.

Your HMO may disallow certain services, tests or medicines. If you had a health problem in the past, it may not be covered for some time—maybe years. Some HMOs try to exclude very sick or elderly patients. Recently one-hundred HMOs dropped 450,000 patients. Many HMOs dropped out of providing care for a million or more Medicare patients saying reimbursement is too low. Extra money provided to them by Congress may not go to patient care; Medicare officials now insist on reviewing Medicare mailings by HMOs.

Dr. David Himmelstein et al. compared the quality of care in 248 investor-owned, for—profit HMOs to that of 81 not-for-profit HMOs. Using data from the National Committee for Quality Assurance (NCQA), an independent organization that monitors the quality of care in HMOs, the authors concluded that investor-owned HMOs deliver lower quality of care than not-for-profit plans. The dilemma in health care is how to provide all the health care your doctor wants you to have and still control costs.

In "utilization review," HMOs, Blue Cross/Blue Shield, and Medicare all use their definition of medical necessity to decrease utilization of hospital services for health care. As cited by Wells, the AMA defines medical necessity as: ". . . health care services or products a prudent physician would provide to a patient for the purpose of preventing, diagnosing or treating an illness, injury, disease or its symptoms in a manner: (1) in accordance with generally accepted standards of medical practice; (2) clinically appropriate in terms of type, frequency, extent, site and duration; and (3) not primarily for the convenience of the patient, physician or other health care provider." So far we cannot be confident that the HMOs use a sensible definition of medical necessity.

Most plans use utilization reviews to make sure you leave the hospital as soon as possible. If you plan to enroll in an HMO, check the details, although many of you may have no choice of the plans available to you because they were selected by your employer. Read the fine print. Determine if doctors are restricted in services they can provide for you. Try to determine what the HMO will cover or will not cover. The problem is you may not know what you will require in the future.

If you are enrolled in an HMO, you may be happy with the care you receive. Many people are not so happy. Be sure you know what you will receive and where you must go for care. My advice to you is to be persistent in seeking and obtaining quality care.

Many doctors object to HMOs because they are told what they can and cannot do for you. Worse yet, these decisions are made by non-physicians. As stated by Samuel Wells of the American College of Surgeons (ACS): "Physicians and surgeons have been deeply frustrated by the fact that non-physicians have substantial powers to restrict the medical doctors' ability to manage patient care." He goes on: "This may represent the practice of medicine by those who are neither educated nor licensed to do so."

Some doctors call managed care "unmanageable care." As described by Dr. Jerome Kassirer, "Frustrations in their attempts to deliver ideal care, restrictions on their personal time, financial incentives that strain their professional principles, and loss of control over clinical decisions are a few of the major issues. Physicians' time is increasingly consumed by paperwork they view as intrusive and valueless, by meetings devoted to expanding clinical reporting requirements, by the need to seek permission to use resources, by telephone calls to patients as formularies change, and by the complex business activities forced on them by the fragmented health care system. To maintain their incomes, many not only work longer hours, but also fit many more patients into their already crowded schedules. These activities often leave little time for their families, for the maintenance of physical fitness, for personal reflection, or for keeping up with the medical literature."

Managed care and HMOs create a number of ethical problems. As described by Kassirer, physicians are asked to adopt a "distributive" ethic in which the principle is population or group based to provide the greatest good for the greatest number of patients within the allotted budget. The AMA maintains no matter what their plan structure, doctors must remain dedicated to the care of their individual patients (an individual ethic). Kassirer states, "When physicians are forced to choose between their personal finances and the welfare of their patients, they should reject a distributive ethical construct."

Doctors are rebelling against insurers. Many won't take HMO patients. Many are retiring early. Some are giving discounts to patients that pay cash and avoid insurers. Managed care can undermine the physician-patient relationship. Some HMOs' physicians, by contract, cannot tell patients about treatments that are not approved. (Chapter 32)

The Federal Government and states have considered legislation to protect you from arbitrary decisions of managed care companies. The Labor Department requires a health insurer to answer in 15 days if a treatment or procedure is not covered; for urgent claims it is 72 hours. Prior authorization may be required. If a claim is denied, the insurer must tell you why. You have the right to a speedy appeal if your HMO denies you care that you seek. You may have to be persistent. If you are turned down by an HMO, you can go to your state insurance commissioner's office at www.naic.org/consumer/state/usamap.htm (the National Association of Insurance Commissioners).

Why can't I sue an HMO for denial of health care I need?

You should have the right to sue an HMO but this has been a very divisive issue (Chapter 62). The Supreme Court of the U.S has ruled you can't sue in federal court but you may do so in a state court. A class action suit has been filed against the Humana Company on matters of coverage. The American Association of Health Plans (AAHP), a national organization of HMOs, mounted an expensive TV campaign to try to stop passage of a bill allowing patients to sue HMOs for denying care. They claimed premiums would go up if they could be sued. An editorial in *USA TODAY* describes their campaign as spooking patients and distorting facts.

Congress and the Health Care Financing Administration (HCFA), the federal agency that administers Medicare and the federal government's role in the Medicaid program, want to use risk adjustments so that HMOs with younger people get paid less. The HMOs, of course, use risk avoidance to decrease costs. As Kassirer and Angell write, "It makes no sense to have a health care system in which the name of the game is to avoid caring for sick people." Dr. C.Everett Koop, former U.S. Surgeon General, wrote, ". . . managed care hampers patients by emphasizing the bottom line."

Higher prices, lower payments to doctors and abandonment of unprofitable Medicaid and Medicare patients are "paying off in higher profits," the Associated Press reports. In *Parade Magazine*, the caption for a cartoon showing HMO executives read, "Of course we want to make a profit. Do you think we are in this for our health?"

Defenders of managed care and HMOs, such as Ubell, maintain you can get quality care from an HMO if you carefully evaluate the plan, study coverage limitations and find the right doctor, look for special features, get references and be ready to go at them if they won't pay for certain treatments. Young says managed care provides a foundation for a quality health system by continuous improvement. Lipina, a nurse, believes HMOs can offer benefits in spite of the heavy criticism. Moore even believes that managed care can benefit academic health centers. Not many doctors or administrators agree with this.

Kevin O'Rourke writes, "Lest I seem to be a lobbyist for managed care, let me add two factors:

1) To date, managed care has not found a way to care for the uninsured. There are almost forty million people (now more) in our country who do not have adequate access to health care. This is a much more serious issue than controlling health care costs;

2) No system of providing health care will be perfect. There must always be checks and balances to develop a fair and effective system. Every worthwhile health care system will emphasize the motivation of health care professionals must be to patient benefit rather than profit for providers."

The Kennedy Institute of Ethics at Georgetown University runs a course and programs on Ethical Challenges in Managed Care. For more information about managed care and HMOs call NCQA at 1-888-275-7585 or visit *www.naqa.org* on the web. If you have a problem with your HMO, physicians assigned to it, reimbursement and other matters, contact your local county medical society. This association of doctors works hard to provide excellent care for you and their organization will look into problems with HMOs, hospitals and other physicians.

Can you help me understand Medicare?

The 1965 Amendment to the Social Security Act established a two-part program of health insurance for the elderly called Medicare providing a health safety net for older people: Part B covers doctors and some diagnostic tests and Part A covers hospitalizations. Both have deductibles and yearly maximums. People can participate in Part A, the hospital insurance program, if they are 65 years of age or older, receive retirement benefits under Title II of the Social Security Act or Railroad Retirement Act or qualify under the special transitional program. People who are not qualified as above and are 65 years or older may participate by paying premiums themselves. Anyone 65 years of age or older who is a U.S. citizen or a permanent resident alien for five years may decide electively to enroll in Part B, a program of supplemental medical insurance. Part A is a program of hospital insurance benefits financed by contributions from employers, employees, and the self-employed. Care is covered for a number of days in hospitals and extended care facilities for each benefit plus post-hospital home care. Entitlement to this benefit is automatic but claims must be presented for reimbursement.

Part B is supplemental medical insurance covering a substantial part of physician and other practitioner services, medical supplies, x-rays and laboratory tests incident to physician services as well as some services not covered under Part A such as ambulances, prostheses, etc. Enrollment in Part B is voluntary and is funded from equal contributions by those electing to enroll and the Federal Government. All benefits are subject to a deductible and a 20% co-insurance amount. Originally, Medicare did not cover medicines but now offers coverage under the drug bill that recently went into effect. (Chapter 43).

Dire predictions have been made about Medicare going bankrupt. Congress recently could have shored up benefits for everyone but decided on a tax cut instead. Present support for Medicare will continue at least through the year 2005. In 1999, Medicare trustees estimated that the Hospital Insurance Trust Fund (Medicare Part A) will remain solvent until the year 2015. They expressed concern, however, about the Supplementary Medical Insurance Trust Fund (Medicare Part B) and the recent rapid cost increases. They urge Congress to control these costs.

For elderly persons with only social security income these extra expenses may preclude the care and medicines they need. Many older individuals should, if financially able, buy private insurance as a Medicare supplement. Blue Cross-Blue Shield, the AARP, Mutual of Omaha and other organizations provide such supplements. Compare and select carefully. Look for a balance between appropriate care and cost control, which sometimes gets out of balance.

Although Medicare is a federal program with pre-determined benefits, the programs are administered by regional companies that determine the eligibility of doctor visits, hospitalization and other items. They then pay only a percentage of what you are charged. If your doctor is a participant as a Medicare provider, he/she cannot bill you for anything more than what Medicare pays. If not signed up as a Medicare provider, he/she can bill you an additional amount.

For help with Medicare and health insurance counseling call Medicare at 1-800-633-4227 or *www.medicare.gov*.

What about medical or health insurance?

Private companies sell health insurance of many different kinds and levels of coverage. Some provide excellent coverage, others do not. If you have coverage, check and ask what is provided. Almost all plans now have deductibles and co-pays. The cost of health insurance has become out of reach for many people, and many employers have dropped or decreased health insurance benefits. HMOs usually have the least expensive and broadest coverage but also the most restrictions on what they cover. In spite of increased costs to you or your employer for coverage, HMOs report healthy profits and their executives pull down huge salaries as they cut costs at the expense of care. If the federal government took this over, profits and high salaries would not be necessary. Many of us believe this is the only satisfactory long-term solution. In the meantime some states, Missouri for example, provide low cost insurance for children.

What do I do if I have no health care insurance and am ineligible for Medicaid?

Call your city or county health department and ask what you can do. Many communities operate public clinics where you can see a doctor, get immunizations and prescriptions. Most public hospitals have now closed but many cities have made arrangements for you to get care at private hospitals. Again, call the Health Department of your community and ask for their help. If you have an urgent or emergency problem, go to the closest emergency ward. By the Emergency Medical Treatment and Labor Act (EMTALA) of 1985, they cannot turn you away. All Medicare participating hospitals must provide a medical screening exam, and an emergency health care problem must be stabilized. Hospitals must have a physician call schedule for all specialties. Not-for-profit hospitals will take care of some indigent or needy patients but they can't take care of everyone on that basis. If you've been on welfare, then get a job and go off welfare, remember you may lose your Medicaid coverage.

For further information:

The AARP has published an excellent summary of "Your Medicare Rights" available from them at 601 E. Street, NW, Washington, DC 20049, www.aarp, org. They also publish a helpful booklet titled "Nine ways to get the most from your managed health care plan." AARP membership is open to anyone over the age of 50 for $10 per year, even though you are not a "retired person." As a member for many years, I have found membership valuable and recommend it.

For more information on managed care: 1) *Consumer's Guide to Health Plans,* Center for the Study of Services, Washington, DC. Call 1-800-213-7283. $12.00; 2) *Guide to Top Doctors,* Center for the Study of Services, Washington, DC. Call 1-800-213-7283. 3) *Choosing and Using a Health Plan,* U.S. Agency for Health Care Policy and Research and Health Insurance Association of America. Call 1-800-358-9295. Contact AARP Fulfillment at 601 E. Street, NW, Washington, DC 20049 to request:

> Making Medicare Choices   (stock #D 16747)
> Checkpoints for Managed Care   (stock #D 16342)

Websites include:

www.aarp.org—AARP
www.medicare.gov-www.hcfa.gov/quality/8b.htm. and homepage *www.hcfa.gov.*
HCFA, oversees Medicare
www.ncqa.org—NCQA, evaluates health plans

www.jcaho.org—JCAHCO, evaluates health plans

www.aahp.org—American Association of Health plans, national trade association for health plans.

www.consumer.gov/qualityhealth—Quality Interagency Coordination Task Force represents all federal agencies to improve the quality of health care in a coordinated way.

Medicare and Home Health Care—A book by Health Care Financing Administration Publication No HCFA 10969. 7500 Security Boulevard, Baltimore, Maryland 21244-1850.

Medicaid is a joint state and federal program to provide care to low income people who would otherwise be uninsured. Each state runs its own program with their regulations and rules under broad federal guidelines. People on welfare are usually eligible for Medicaid, as are pregnant women and children eligible for Aid to Families with Dependent Children (AFDC) and the disabled. Managed care programs may be required. Every state is different. Check with the Agency for Healthcare Policy and Research (AHCPR) *www.AHCPR.gov/consumer* or toll free 1-800-358-9295 and your state office.

THE AMA—ORGANIZED MEDICINE

54. What is organized medicine? Is the AMA a doctor's union? What do I do if I have a complaint against a doctor? Does the medical profession police itself?

Usually, organized medicine is thought of as the American Association of Medical Colleges (AAMC), the American Medical Association (AMA), state and county medical societies, the American Board of Medical Specialties (ABMS) that oversees the 24 specialty boards providing special education and examination, and the many specialty societies such as the American College of Surgeons (ACS).

What can I do if I have a complaint or a grievance about a doctor?

Report it to your county medical society, or, if your county doesn't have one, to your state medical society. A committee will investigate such matters, take action and report back to you. If the investigation reveals a significant problem with a doctor, the medical society may revoke the doctor's membership and report the revocation to the state licensure board for review. If the wrongdoing is serious enough, the state board will revoke the license of the doctor to practice. It is illegal to practice medicine in a state without a valid license.

What are the various colleges or societies of each specialty?

A board or governing group determines the educational or training requirements to become a specialist in each discipline. They prepare and give examinations. Doctors who meet the educational requirements and pass the examinations become diplomats of the boards, qualified to practice the specialties.

Each specialty also has its own college or society. To qualify for membership, physicians must be caring and responsible practitioners in their specialties. The ACS, for example, is dedicated to raising the standards of surgical practice and improving the care of surgical patients. To that end, in recent years it has worked with legislators, consumer groups, hospitals, accrediting organizations and others to support national patient safety legislation, a goal still unrealized as of 2004. The specialty societies also provide continuing medical educational (CME) programs for their members, residents and medical students to keep them up-to-date for excellent patient care.

If you have a complaint against a specialist, write to his or her specialty society and make your complaint. If a patient makes a complaint to the ACS against a surgeon, it is investigated thoroughly and a report given to the patient. Action is taken if necessary; but a society or college can only eliminate the individual from membership. They have no legal standing to do anything further on their own but they will report their findings to the state licensing board, which can take action about the surgeon's license.

These boards and societies are all voluntary and private, started and supported for your protection by doctors and not by the federal government. They were developed to be sure anyone who claims to be a surgeon, for example, received proper training in surgery and can draw upon extensive knowledge in that specialty.

A license to practice medicine in a state requires only one year of internship after four years of medical school and passage of a general medical examination. Federal, state and local governments set no further direct limits on what a doctor can do. Broadly speaking, as far as the government is concerned, any doctor could perform brain surgery without any training in neurosurgery. However, the government will not provide funds for Medicare or other programs to a hospital not approved by the American Accreditation Healthcare Commission (AAHC), a nationally recognized non-government group. The AAHC will not approve hospitals that do not meet its generally accepted standards, and these include allowing only qualified individuals or board-certified doctors to practice specialties.

What else protects us from doctors doing more than they are trained to do? Here are other safeguards:

1. Aberrant doctors will incur lawsuits and may lose insurance coverage.
2. Residency review committees from the Accreditation Council for Graduate Medical Education (ACGME), comprising representatives from all specialty societies, boards and the AMA, visit hospitals to be sure they meet ACGME standards for residency training in each specialty. This is a voluntary effort by doctors to be sure you get good health care from properly trained doctors.
3. The AAMC supervises medical schools to be sure students receive a good education before becoming doctors.

Some people feel the boards and specialty societies exist to restrict the numbers in a specialty and decrease competition. This is not true. They are dedicated to be sure those who practice the specialty have the capability and education to provide good care for you. These groups police themselves and wait to hear from you about problems with any specialty doctor.

The specialty boards have developed programs for re-certification. If a doctor is certified as a surgeon in 1995, the question is: How do we know that surgeon has kept up in the year 2005? Most certificates now last for only 10 years. Specialists must renew them by passing recertification courses and examinations—another effort to protect you and provide better care.

Is the American Medical Association (AMA) a doctors union?

Sometimes, in its history of more than 150 years, this voluntary organization of doctors of all specialties has acted like a doctors' union. The old AMA seemed more interested in preserving the status quo, the world that doctors knew and liked. Previously they fought for fee-for-service payment of medical costs, which, among many other things, contributed to escalation of health care costs. In the past, the AMA opposed all government funding of medicine as socialized medicine. Although the AMA has always been interested in good care for you and good medical education, they are now more actively championing your rights as patients. It is my observation that the AMA speaks for a consortium of doctors, who are most interested in good quality care for you.

One Clear and Determined Voice for Quality Patient Care—Your 1999 Guide to the AMA, states two principles:

1. "The integrity of the patient-physician bond is preserved and renewed through the power of physicians working together.

2. As we look toward the next millennium, we reaffirm our commitment as stewards of medicine and caring advocates for our patients and our profession."

The AMA enforces a Code of Medical Ethics; helps with medical education; endorses patients' choice in a patients' bill of rights; supports medical research, particularly breast cancer research, mounts opposition to binge drinking, tobacco use and substance abuse and addresses other public heath problems. They have worked to rid television of the promos for boozy, dangerous student spring breaks and of liquor ads for adults and children.

The AMA has said that physicians hope to prevent managed care from making profits more important than patient care. The association takes a strong stand that you should have free choice of physicians-a nice principle but under managed care how do you have free choice? They further oppose the limitations of managed care in favoring the return of medical decisions to physicians and their patients and an increase in patients' choice and responsibility. They want to insure the availability of quality medical care to all, by providing among other things individual ownership of health plans and innovative progressive solutions to your health and care.

The AMA has gone to court to support an individual's constitutional right to refuse medical or life-prolonging treatment and contest other issues. They support rational medical judgment as the standard in protecting rights of patients with communicable diseases. Under the American Disabilities Act, they supported protection from discrimination against patients infected with HIV. In many other ways they support what is best for your health and for your doctors' ability to take care of you safely and adequately.

The AMA includes sections on medical schools, medical students who participate in deliberations, resident physicians, young physicians, and international medical graduates who provide excellent medical care in this country. They offer programs on minority affairs, women physicians and senior physician services. Practice and personal services for members include insurance coverage and information on streamlining practice management and other business and office aspects of medicine.

The AMA has shown itself to be rigorous in its background checks of applicants for membership, as notably shown in the case of the infamous Dr. Michael Swango. Evidently, a license to practice medicine is only a starting point. No matter how impressive the applicant's resume, how illustrious the medical school, how outstanding the academic record, the Swango case shows that the AMA goes out of the way to protect the public by looking for signs of trouble others might have missed.

Perhaps the AMA reaches its highest public profile in its outstanding *Journal of the American Medical Association* (JAMA), often cited in the media for medical news. JAMA provides research and clinical updates for your doctor. It also contains information for you in its patient's page, available from your doctor. JAMA carries monthly reports from the Center for Disease Control and Prevention and the Federal Drug Administration.

Some efforts are underway in the United States to develop unions for doctors. In Los Angeles, the Service Employees Union is forming a new branch called National Doctors Alliance and hope to represent doctors in bargaining with HMO's and managed care organizations. According to the Rev. Kevin O'Rourke, another group is eyeing the St. Louis region as a favorable area for union recruitment. In a review of the ethics and morality of doctors' unions, O'Rourke suggests a guild equivalent would be a better way to organize physicians so that they can continue to take good care of you in the face of changes representing hazards to the practice of good medicine. The medical and specialty societies should be able to provide that assurance. Although the AMA has suggested the need for doctors to form an affiliated national labor organization, they have not pursued it. Many of us are opposed.

AMA publications are available at 515 North State Street, Chicago, Illinois 60610, (800) AMA-3211 or at www.ama-assn.org. They provide information about health care and activities of the AMA.

Does the medical profession police itself?

It is sincere and diligent about disciplining or getting rid of bad doctors. The medical profession is becoming less tolerant of physician misconduct for it reflects badly on all of us. However, the authorities must know about the problems in order to deal with them, and hospitals don't always report problems with doctors on their staffs. Perhaps a doctor brings a lot of his patients to a hospital and, wanting this to continue, the hospital turns a blind eye. This kind of conniving represents a serious conflict of interest. Incompetent, corrupt, dishonest or unethical conduct by doctors must be made known and dealt with. If you know about any such conduct, you must report it.

The case of the serial killer Dr. Michael Swango represents an especially egregious breakdown of the hospital peer review system. Between 1983 and 1997, it is estimated that this handsome and charming psychopath murdered from 35 to 60 hospital patients, while going from one university hospital to another, three in all.

Before offering Swango a place in its psychiatric residency program in 1993, the Stony Brook Medical School of the State University of New York should have looked him up in the National Practitioner Data Bank (NPDB) as required by federal law. In the NPDB they should have found an entry for Swango, noting his dismissal as a resident from the University of South Dakota at Sioux Falls upon the discovery of his conviction of assault in Illinois for poisoning co-workers.

It was Swango's application for membership in the AMA, incidentally, that had brought the poisoning to light. Taking his word for nothing, the AMA did their own background check and upon finding that his assault conviction was not for inadvertently getting caught up in a barroom brawl, as he had claimed in job interviews, they notified the university.

Although federal law requires hospitals to report information on disciplinary actions and malpractice claims against health-care providers to the NPDB, perhaps 75% of hospitals, fearing liability, never file such reports. The law should impose penalties for failure to report dangerous doctors, and doctors should be on notice to report aberrant colleagues. Limiting liability for reports to the NPDB would help.

THE FDA—GOVERNMENT HELP

55. What does the Food and Drug Administration (FDA) do? How are new drugs tested? What other help does the Federal Government provide for health care? Where can I get information about trials of new drugs for cancer and other diseases?

The FDA is the U.S. government agency that is supposed to protect you from unsafe drugs, foods, cosmetics and medical devices, as well as from untrue claims for products. The agency comprehensively explains their mission in a pamphlet, as follows:

"What does FDA do?" FDA ensures that our *food* is safe and wholesome, our *cosmetics* are not harmful, and *medicines, medical devices,* and *radiation-emitting products* such as microwave ovens are safe and effective. FDA also monitors *feed and drugs for pets and farm animals.* Authorized by congress to enforce the Federal Food, Drug, and Cosmetic Act and several other public health laws, the agency monitors manufacture, import, transport, storage, and sale of $1 trillion worth of goods annually, about a quarter of the US economy, at a cost to taxpayers of about $3 a person.

"How big is the FDA?" FDA employs over 9,000 employees, in 157 U.S. cities with 2,100 scientists, including 900 chemists and 300 microbiologists, in 40 laboratories across the country. About 1,100 FDA investigators and inspectors visit 15,000 facilities a year as part of their oversight of the 95,000 U.S. businesses regulated by the FDA.

"What does the FDA do with defective products?" About 3,000 products a year are found unfit for consumers and are withdrawn from the marketplace, either by voluntary recall or court-ordered seizure. These products usually are destroyed, or in some cases, are reconditioned to be in compliance with FDA regulations.

"What should I do if I have a food or drug product that has been recalled?"
Take it back to the place of purchase and ask for a refund. Stores generally have a return and refund policy when a company announces a recall of its products.

"Whom can I call with questions about food safety?" Call the FDA Consumer hotline at (800) 532-4440, for general food safety questions; the FDA Seafood hotline at (800) FDA-4010, for a question about seafood; the US Department of Agriculture (USDA) hotline at (800) 535-4555, for questions about meat or poultry products. If the situation is critical, phone the FDA emergency number, (301) 443-1240, staffed 24 hours a day. For more on food safety, go to FDA's Center for Food Safety and Nutrition home page.

"Does the FDA control pesticides in foods?" The Environment Protection Agency regulates sale and use of pesticides. The FDA regularly tests foods to determine if pesticides are present in unacceptable amounts. If so, the agency takes corrective action.

"Does the FDA regulate illegal drugs?" The federal Drug Enforcement Administration (DEA) controls the illegal use of "street" drugs such as heroin, cocaine and marijuana. However, if a street drug is to be studied for legitimate medical uses, the FDA would regulate it as an investigational drug. FDA-regulated prescription drugs such as barbiturates and amphetamines are sometimes abused and wind up as street drugs. They then fall under DEA jurisdiction.

"What should I do if I've had an adverse reaction to an over-the-counter or prescription medicine?" Contact your doctor right away and urge him to report the problem to the FDA MedWatch hotline, 1-(800) FDA-1088 or fax 1-800-FDA-0178 or modem 1-800-FDA-7737. Your doctor, however, is not required to report to the FDA. Consumers can report problems directly. For more information, visit the *MedWatch* Web site www.fda.gov/fdac/special/newdrug/medwatch.html.

"How can I participate in the FDA's process for making its rules?" Any citizen can submit comments on rules the FDA proposes. The agency announces rules in the Federal Register and accepts comments for 60 days. The Federal Register is available in many libraries or at *www.acces.gpo.gov/su_docs/*. The FDA urges consumers to participate in the rule-making process. For more information about submitting comments, call the FDA Dockets Management Branch at (301) 443-7542. The FDA includes patient representatives on its review committees. They meet in Washington, D.C. and the FDA will fly you in and put you up at a hotel at government expense if you participate. If you wish to volunteer go to *www.fda.gov/oashi/patrep/patbroc.html* for information.

"How can I make a Freedom of Information Act (FOIA) request to the FDA?" They are best made by sending a letter specifying exactly what material you seek from the FDA, Freedom of Information Staff (HFI-35), 5600 Fishers Lane, Rockville, MD 20857. For more on FOIA requests, call (301) 443-6310 or a look at the *Handbook for Requesting Information and Records from the FDA* on the Web site.

"How can a regulated industry complain to the FDA about an agency action?"
Contact the FDA Office of the Chief Mediator and Ombudsman, (301) 827-3390. If the complaint concerns human drugs, call Jim Morrison at (301) 594-5443; for biologics, call Joy Cavagnaro at (301) 827-0379; for veterinary drugs, call Dr. Marcia Larkins at (301) 827-0137."

How are new drugs tested?

Development of new drugs requires trials. First, the drug is evaluated in animals for safety and side effects. Some people object to the use of animals to find safe, new medicines but the use of animals is a critical first step (Chapter 86). In animals with a disease similar to the target of treatment by the drug, the drug can also be tested for effectiveness. If the drug is safe in animals, studies begin in humans.

A Phase I trial is done in normal volunteers who are willing to take the medicine, often for a fee. This trial is to evaluate again safety and side effects. If the drug is safe, then a Phase II trial gives the agent to patients with the disease to see if they respond favorably. A Phase II observational trial surveys the outcome in many patients who have taken a drug over time compared with patients who have not taken it. Such results are suggestive but may be only associations—the drug effect and outcome may occur together but not as cause and effect.

If patients respond sufficiently during Phase II, a Phase III trial is undertaken. To prove an effect, a Phase III randomized, controlled, double-blind trial is necessary. Patients that agree to enter the trial are randomized by a secret computer system of allocation to a group receiving the active agent or the other group receiving a placebo, a harmless inactive substance that looks the same as the active agent. The patients and investigators do not know who is in which group. When the study is complete—weeks, months or years later, depending on the disease—and each group evaluated to determine results, the code is broken. If a lot of adverse events have occurred, the code could be broken early to see if the agent is causing the trouble, and if so the trial is stopped. Expensive to carry out but necessary, these trials contribute to the high cost of developing new medications. Many trials are negative, indicating that the medicine is not worthwhile for that particular purpose. If the Phase III trial is positive, the drug will be approved by the FDA.

After products are approved and marketed, the FDA is supposed to continue to review the products for new problems that may come up. Reports from health professionals and manufacturers have been a critical part of this process. The FDA has required labeling changes, warnings on the drug package, product recalls and withdrawals, medical alerts, safety alerts for medical devices and warnings through the *FDA Medical Bulletin*, the press and letters to doctors. If products are not made and labeled correctly, the FDA can force a company to stop selling them.

The FDA had been criticized for the long time it took to approve new drugs, formerly up to three years. The delay reflected a shortage of drug reviewers; the agency did not have enough money to pay for adequate staffing. Since 1992, however, an agreement between the drug industry and the FDA has speeded up the process, providing the agency with millions of dollars from the industry in the form of users' fees for FDA studies of new drugs. (For information—*www.fda.gov/fdac/special/newdrugs/benefits.html* or *newdrugs/ testing.html*. Critics, however, charge that this emphasis on the approval of new drugs has reduced necessary oversight of drugs already approved and in widespread use. They point to the agency's delay in uncovering the detrimental effects of the popular, widely-advertised painkiller Vioxx, a Cox-2 inhibitor drug for arthritis, as an inevitable result of this shift in emphasis. The *New York Times* has described this pharmaceutical/FDA relationship as industry distortion of the FDA.

In 2004, four years after FDA approval of the blockbuster Vioxx, Merck voluntarily withdrew the drug in light of a four-year follow-up study arranged by Dr. David Graham, a director in the agency's office for drug safety. The study found that patients taking Vioxx doubled their risk of heart attacks. Dr. Graham estimated that use of Vioxx has led to the deaths of some 55,000 Americans.

"I would argue the FDA as currently configured is incapable of protecting America against another Vioxx," Dr. Graham said in Senate hearings on the debacle. "We are virtually defenseless."

In shifting resources to tests of new drugs and cutting costs elsewhere, the FDA has ended collaboration with independent drug safety experts and academic groups capable of monitoring drugs already on the market, as reported in the *New York Times* for December 6, 2004. More money for testing of new drugs has meant less money for finding problems in drugs that might turn up only after use by millions of people. With adequate funding, it is said, the Vioxx study could have been done in two years rather than four, thereby reducing exposure of the public to the dangerous drug that much sooner. Millions of people also took another arthritis drug Bextra before the agency asked its manufacturer, Pfizer Inc., to pull it in April 2005, citing heightened cardiovascular risks associated with the drug. Now another arthritis drug, Celebrex, carries a warning about those possible risks.

Dr. Jerry Avorn, a professor at Harvard Medical School, noted that the agency needs courage more than money. When doubts arise about the safety of a medicine, he said the FDA should insist that drug makers pay for independent tests. If companies refuse, then the agency should call a press conference to inform doctors and the public of problems with the medicine and of unsuccessful efforts to get the drug makers to do clinical trials. "The FDA has moral authority and extraordinary public relations power if they choose to use them," said Dr. Avorn.

The FDA has also been criticized for not getting on top of the flu shot problem. In October 2004 the British government shut down a Chiron facility in the UK after identifying bacterial contamination in vaccine manufactured there. Although the facility was to have provided half of our supply of flu shots, the FDA did not determine that it could not assure sterility of the Chiron lots until two weeks later. It appears that the FDA finds it difficult to provide adequate inspection of plants abroad.

Meanwhile, however, the FDA has enjoyed its share of successes. Perhaps its greatest triumph came in the 1960s, in keeping thalidomide off the US market and saving American children from the birth defects that were to afflict thousands of European children, causing them to be born without arms or legs. Frances Kelsey, now 86 and still working at the FDA in an advisory capacity, had just joined the agency in 1960 when she received as her first assignment review of thalidomide, a pill for morning sickness. Drawing upon laboratory studies she had done on pregnant rabbits, she came to believe that thalidomide might be unsafe for pregnant women and fetuses, and she steadily refused to approve it, despite increasing pressure by the manufacturer who went over her head to complain to her superiors. Her eventual vindication led to new legislation strengthening the FDA. In 1962 she received the President's Award for Distinguished Federal Civil Service from President Kennedy.

The FDA, working with the Centers for Disease Control (CDCP) and Canadian Public Health officials, tracked down parsley grown in Mexico as the source for the bacteria, shigella, causing outbreaks of food poisoning in California and Minnesota. Importation of the parsley was stopped.

The FDA has published concern about taking too much acetaminophen (Tylenol) or taking it with alcohol, in which case it can damage the liver. Another drug, Lotronex, was great for some patients with irritable colons but resulted in the death of others. The FDA ordered a warning for the label but the manufacturer withdrew the drug from the general market. Because it is so effective for patients with irritable bowel disease, Lotronex is now available on a limited basis with ample warnings. Acutane, a powerful agent for acne, can produce birth defects and psychiatric problems. In spite of this, women on the drug do get pregnant. The warnings on the label have not done the job.

The FDA issued the following public health advisory on phenylpropanolamine (PPA), commonly used as a decongestant and as an appetite suppressant: "PPA is unsafe for continued use." The advisory came on the heels of a study associating its use with an increased risk of hemorrhagic stroke, or bleeding in the brain.

Consumer Healthcare Products Association, which helped pay for the study, later had some doubts about it, however, thinking the evidence tenuous. In the meanwhile, stores pulled the products from their shelves and manufacturers reformulated their PPA products to eliminate the drug.

Up until recently, drug trials had been confined to adults, and drugs were given to children without any information about their safety or effectiveness for children in particular. Now the FDA is issuing new rules for carefully monitored and controlled trials in children, although an ethical concern is children may not be able to give informed consent. A randomized trial will be done of the stimulant Ritalin, given to many kids with attention deficit hyperactivity disorder. A childhood vaccine for pneumococcal meningitis has been approved for children under the age of two years.

The FDA has tightened up on the review and approval process for medical devices, recalling over 1000 devices each year after reports of problems. FDA scientists test hip implants, for hip replacements, in fatigue testing machines to see how soon they might wear out. Wheelchairs are checked for safety.

Illicit use of prescription drugs, especially pain killers, poses a big problem. The Office of National Drug Control Policy has called for a crackdown. The most commonly abused drugs are OxyContin and Vicodin, possibly coming from foreign countries. Many are obtained illegally by students, using stolen prescription pads and making calls to pharmacists under assumed names. Nurses can call for themselves. This illicit use of prescription drugs creates shortages making it more difficult for those that need those drugs to get them.

Counterfeit drugs brought in from abroad or produced by fraudulent companies represent another big problem. These drugs, which include fake Lipitor, Procrit, Neupogen, Botox and Viagra, may contain few or no active ingredients. If you have a problem with a drug, report it. The government hopes to solve this problem by strengthening licensing requirements for wholesale distributors and requiring an electronic product code on every bottle of drugs to be sold in the U.S.

FDA Consumer is a bi-monthly magazine published by the FDA with information on how to get health and safety information and how to get healthy and stay healthy. It covers topics on diet, nutrition, new medicines, cholesterol, osteoporosis, vaccinations, cell phones and brain cancer (no relationship), and health claims for food. A subscription is $12 per year, available from the Superintendent of Documents, PO Box 371954, Pittsburgh, PA 15250-7954 or at 1-302-512-1800 or fax 1-202-512-2250.

The FDA makes information available to you by phone at (301) 827-6630, *www.fda.GOV*, www.fda.gov/opacom/faqs.html or by mail to The PHS, FDA, HF-2, Rockville, MD 20857. MedWatch is the FDA Medical Products reporting program for adverse events and product problems and relying on professionals and you to report problems or reactions to drugs, medical devices and other products. (1-800-FDA-7737) Remember, errors can occur in prescriptions and in hospital pharmacies. Always check out any problems with your doctor and pharmacist.

What other help does the federal government provide for health care?

A great deal of information and help is available from many agencies of the government. The addresses, phone numbers and web sites are listed in Chapters 56 and 66. Your state also has a Department of Health and many cities have health departments. They will be happy to direct you to health care facilities or provide other information.

The U.S. DHHS offers many programs to help you. One is Healthy People 2010—Understanding and Improving Health, obtained for $10 from the U.S. Government Printing Office, Superintendent of Documents, Washington, DC 20402-9382, stock number 017-001-001-00-550-9, visit the webside *www.health.gov/ healthypeople/* or call 1-800-367-4725. Their focus areas are listed in Table I based upon 467 objectives to improve health. An extensive bibliography for all these areas is found in their publication Healthy People 2010. Their leading health indicators are listed in Table II.

A government guide of health information sponsored by America Online is available at *www.governmentguide.com*. The PHS, the Surgeon General and the NIH work to eliminate global health disparity, improve minority health and racial, socioeconomic and ethnic differences in health care.

The NIH in Bethesda, Maryland, operates large research institutes and programs supported by the government that help monitor and approve research grants to private universities and research institutes. This is one of the largest and most effective research efforts in the world. Americans can be proud of it.

The Public Health Service (PHS) of the U.S. celebrated its 200th anniversary in 1998. It has eight operating divisions: NIH, FDA, CDCP, Agency for Toxic Substances and Disease Registry, Indian Health Service, Health Resources and Services Administration, Substance Abuse and Mental Health Services Administration, and the AHCPR. The PHS provides periodic reviews and reports on health and prevention in Prevention Report. Information about subscribing to this publication can be obtained at *http://odphp.osophs.dhhs.gov*. If you want e-mail advisories send your e-mail address to U.S. DHHS, Hubert H. Humphrey Building Room 738G, 200 Independence Avenue SW, Washington, DC 20201.

Table I

Healthy People 2010 Focus Areas

1. Access to quality health services
2. Arthritis, osteoporosis, and chronic back conditions
3. Cancer
4. Chronic kidney disease
5. Diabetes
6. Disability and secondary conditions
7. Educational and community-based programs
8. Environmental health
9. Family planning
10. Food Safety
11. Health communication
12. Heart disease and stroke
13. HIV
14. Immunization and infectious diseases
15. Injury and violence prevention
16. Maternal, infant, and child health
17. Medical product safety
18. Mental health and mental disorders
19. Nutrition and overweight
20. Occupational safety and health
21. Oral health
22. Physical activity and fitness
23. Public health infrastructure
24. Respiratory diseases
25. Sexually transmitted diseases
26. Substance abuse
27. Tobacco use
28. Vision and hearing

Table II

Leading Health Indicators

- Physical activity
- Overweight and obesity
- Tobacco use
- Substance abuse
- Responsible sexual behavior
- Mental health
- Injury and violence
- Environmental quality
- Immunization
- Access to health care

Where can I get information about trials of new drugs for cancer and other diseases?

Patients and their families often seek information about new treatments or clinical trials particularly for cancer. Information about clinical trials can be obtained from—*http://clinicaltrials.gov/* developed by the National Library of Medicine (NLM). The FDA has an Office of Special Health Issues (OSHI) to help you (1-888-INFO-FDA—voice mail—2-3-3 or 301-827-4460 or email at OSHI @ oc.fda.gov). Now the NLM has opened a simpler site for trial information at ClinicalTrials.gov. For cancer trials the site is cancertrials.nci.nih.gov. For new drugs there is *www.centerwatch.com* and for mental disorders *www.nimh.nih.gov*. Actis.org gives information about AIDS; also call 1-800-874-2572. Information and studies of arthritis therapy can be obtained from the Arthritis Foundation at *www.arthritis.org*. If you agree to participate in a study be sure to ask what you can expect—benefits, complications, risks, how often will you be seen, why is this research being done, etc.?

Should I enroll in a clinical trial?

The Harvard Health Letter describes volunteering for a study as a great public service, but remember it is an experiment. Those that volunteer do so to help find a cure to a disease or to advance science. You may get a free physical exam and be paid. They provide five tips: 1) Take the informed consent form home and read it carefully. 2) Understand the type of trial. 3) Remember, you're allowed to quit. 4) Know who is paying for the study. 5) Ask yourself if you really have the time.

56. Medical information about health—Where to find it?

What is the best source of medical or health care information? What is the Physicians Committee for Responsible Medicine? What is hype in medical reporting? What are magic bullets? Can I trust the internet for health information and prescriptions? Should drug companies be allowed to advertise medications direct to consumers that require a doctor's prescription?

What is the best source of medical or health care information?

Health care information is everywhere: the morning and evening news on television, newspapers, brochures, pharmaceutical advertisements, websites, and federal government publications. Many medical schools publish excellent health care magazines. Be wary, however, of the many commercial books and magazines about your health. These books must make big money for so many of them to exist. They promise to reveal secrets to health or home health remedies recommended by doctors, but can they deliver on these promises?

Some commercial publications do not list the doctors who made the recommendations. Others cite authorities with dubious credentials like one William Castelli, M.D., promoted as "a respected physician" and a lecturer of preventive medicine at Harvard Medical School. I am a graduate of the Harvard Medical School and, checking with the alumni office, I found that Dr. Castelli is not and never has been on the Harvard faculty.

Dr. Castelli says he has no financial interest in the book. That may be a dodge, however: the question is how much was he paid directly for the endorsement? What does he know about all the other diseases he writes about? The 22-page advertisement for the book shows people in white coats with stethoscopes around their necks. Are they real doctors or actors, playing doctors on TV, so to speak? What are their names? What are their credentials? What is the evidence of effectiveness for their 2,005 proven ways to block the onset of illness and pain? Look for references to clinical trials that clearly show their recommendations to be better than taking a placebo.

Health Secrets, published by Bottom Line/Health, describes "27 healing breakthroughs that can save your life—and 10 blunders that can kill you." All you need to do is order their book: *The World's Greatest Treasury of Health Secrets* for $29.95, which lists a group of legitimate doctors but does not say whether they contributed to the book. Some of the recommendations in the book may work but be careful.

Prevention promotes a book by Dr. Shapiro called *Picture Perfect Weight Loss*, which tells you how to walk off 10, 20, even 100 pounds, for just three installments of $9.99 each plus postage and handling. Shapiro says, "It's sweeping the nation".

Recently, I went to a bookstore to get new copies of books I had given to friends with terminal illnesses. While there, I looked at the shelves of health-care books, reassured to see that some of them were very worthwhile: the *AMA Encyclopedia of Medicine* and its *Family Medical Guide*; the *Johns Hopkins Family Health Book*; the *Mayo Clinic Guide to Self Care*; the *Merck Manual for Patients*; and the *Harvard Medical School Family Health Guide*. Less reassuring, however, was *Family Health for Dummies*.

In all, the store contained 80 long shelves of books on holistic and alternative medicine; 80 shelves of books on illness; 10 shelves of books on women's health; and 15 shelves of medical references, including medical dictionaries and encyclopedias. Thus, many books on every subject related to health and medicine are available to you. One purpose of this book is to allow you to learn what you wish to know without buying so many books.

If a report appears in a respectable medical journal like the NEJM, the JAMA, *Archives of Surgery* or *Internal Medicine*, you can be sure it has been thoroughly reviewed by doctors. *Reader's Digest* and *Parade* often carry articles by medical authorities that can provide useful information. Your questions about an article should be: Who wrote it? What are their credentials? Is it nothing more than a commercial? Several years ago in *Parade* Dr. Isadore Rosenfield gave what I believe continues to be sound advice about insomnia: "If you and your doctor decide you need a sleeping pill, use one that is short acting, doesn't leave you with a hangover, works quickly and doesn't accumulate in the body. Don't take it for more than three weeks, and never 'borrow' a pill from a friend." He says evidence is lacking for the claim that melatonin is helpful for insomnia.

Although tarnished in selling the now-withdrawn drug Vioxx, the Merck pharmaceutical company to its credit publishes a superb, nonprofit book of reliable medical information: The *Merck Manual, Home Edition* for $29.95 at bookstores. It is up-to-date and accurate.

Many doctors rely on reliable, nonprofit publications like the *Harvard Health Letter*, the *Johns Hopkins Medical Letter*, the *Tufts University Diet and Nutrition Letter* and the U. of California, Berkeley *Wellness Letter* to keep up in the field

The helpful *Physicians Desk Reference* (PDR) books include the *PDR Medical Dictionary*, the *PDR for Nonprescription Drugs and Dietary Supplements* and the *Basic PDR* obtained from PDR, PO Box 10689, Des Moines, IA 50380-0689. Recommendations from Surgeon Generals of the U.S. also can be very useful. You can rely on a simple test. If the article is by an identified doctor and provides documented information and not hype, it is probably accurate.

The most extensive book about health and human biology is the *Encyclopedia of Human Biology (2nd edition)*, Academic Press, Orlando, FL) in seven volumes. Hopefully you can find it in your public library. http://www.apnet.com/human. (800) 321-5068. Another good source for health and safety information is *Staywell* at San Bruno, CA. www.staywell.com (800) 333-3032. The DHHS developed a magazine called *FDA Consumer* (Chapter 55).

What is the physicians' Committee for Responsible Medicine (PCRM)?

It is a source of good information about nutrition and health. This voluntary, not-for-profit group comprises over 5,000 physicians and 100,000 lay people, "doctors and lay persons working together for compassionate and effective medical practice, research and health promotion." They offer active programs in preventive medicine for cancer and other diseases and in promotion of healthful eating, research advocacy, and broader access to medical services for everyone. Membership is open to the public through

PCRM, 5100 Wisconsin Avenue NW, Suite 404, Washington, DC, 20016. http://PCRM@PCRM.ORG. (202) 686-2210.

I have reviewed several of their publications, including "Vegetarian foods—powerful for health," "A better health pyramid: The new four food groups," "Cancer pain," "Racial bias" and "Federal nutrition policy," "The medical costs attributed to meat consumption" "A vegetarian start kit," and "Good nutrition for kids" by Dr. Spock. They are all quite sensible and worthwhile. I intend to join the group.

PCRM recommends a low-fat vegetarian diet and provides evidence in support of their recommendations. Such diets decrease the risk of arteriosclerosis, cancer, hypertension, diabetes, gallstones, kidney disease and food-borne illnesses. PCRM takes off the top of the U.S.D.A. Pyramid of Foods, removing (1) fats, oils and sweets, (2) milk, yogurt and cheese, and (3) meat, poultry, fish, dried beans, eggs and nuts group, and leaving a "better health trapezoid of" (1) dark green, dark yellow, and orange vegetables, (2) whole grains—bread, rice, pasta, cereal, corn, millet, barley, bulgur, buckwheat, grits, tortillas, (3) fruit, (4) legumes—beans, peas, lentils, etc.

What is hype in medical reporting? What are magic bullets?

Many careful reporters are accurate and realistic in reporting. Some, however, blow a new medicine or procedure out of proportion by calling it a medical breakthrough even though it has not been tested in patients. This kind of reporting gives people false hope and ends in great disappointment for them. Patients with end-stage diseases facing death cling to every bit of new information. It is cruel to suggest to them a cure may be available soon when it is years away, if ever. Moynihan, et al. report "news media stories about medications may include inadequate or incomplete information about benefits, risks and costs of drugs as well as financial ties between study groups or experts and pharmaceutical manufacturers.

Some examples come to mind of hype, short for "hyperbole" or extravagant exaggeration. In 1998, Joseph Palca stirred up a lot of political and ethical discussions by reporting on NPR that a physicist, Richard Seed, was seeking support to set up a clinic to clone people. This was a publicity stunt. People should have recognized that Seed was a physicist, not a biologist, with no background in cloning and no idea whether it would be possible to clone people. On the front page of the *New York Times,* Gina Kolata reported that a breakthrough in the cure for cancer was on the horizon, a story heard and reprinted around the world. Nobel Laureate James Watson added to the hype by saying it looked like a great breakthrough and so did Richard Klausner, the NCI Director. The basis for the story was the work on mice, not humans, of a distinguished investigator, Dr. Judah Folkman.

Dr. Folkman has worked all his life on the angiogenesis factor, which produces blood vessels for both tumors and normal tissues. Using inhibitors of the angiogenesis factor, or angiostatin, in mice, he found that tumors were inhibited. In *Scientific American* he said, "In animals, angiostatin can stop nearly all blood vessel growth in a large tumor or metastases." Evidently, Kolata overlooked the important qualifier "in animals."

In *Science* Marshall wrote about the power of the front page of the *New York Times*. He said U.S. cancer clinics were swamped with phone calls from desperate patients seeking the two new drugs they heard about through the news media. Marshall pointed out as did others that neither of these drugs had been tested in humans. Many agents produce good results in animals, but never help patients. Asked to comment on all of this, Dr. Folkman said, "If you have a mouse with cancer, we may be able to cure it but that's all."

Advances, as with beauty, are in the eye of the beholder. When does a scientific advance occur? Is it when a new technique is discovered but is yet to be tested? Is it when animal experiments produce exciting results? They may not apply to man. Is it after the first few clinical trials? They may not last. Is it when we have clinically established something as being useful for patients? Yes, that seems to be an advance. But only time will tell if it is a temporary or permanent advance.

Be wary of news about medical breakthroughs. Ask: Has it been tested in man? Has it been subjected to a rigorous clinical randomized trial in which some patients receive a placebo? Only then will we know if it will be clinically useful. Some people say a cure for some cancers may be developed but a cure for "hype" never will be.

What are magic bullets?

These are agents or drugs thought to be breakthroughs for therapy, as was penicillin. Many, however, never get FDA approval because they don't help with a variety of diseases. Some when used for a specific purpose help a lot, as does the agent anti-TNF antibody which helped patients with rheumatoid arthritis but did not help all patients with infections. Many good new agents treat specific ailments. None so far has been good for all of a variety of problems.

Can I trust the internet for health information?

Yes and no. An estimated 19,000 web sites are devoted to health care, with more appearing all the time. Many legitimate private, not-for-profit, and government agencies provide useful, factual and true information about pharmaceuticals, health care and disease prevention. Other organizations sell products or give information to sell their services or products, some of which may be legitimate. Some for-profit companies may give truthful information and sound advice about their products. The reader must be careful, however. Look out for grandiose claims and hype. Beware of sales pitches. Look out for undocumented claims. Buying prescription drugs on the Internet can be dangerous. The internet doctor does not know you, your illness or condition, your allergies, or other drugs you are taking. You face some real hazards in buying drugs over the internet (Chapter 43).

In a study of the reliability of health advice on web sites, investigators at the University of Michigan Health System found some good sites but others that led to confusion and misunderstanding. Half the information had not been verified by medical authorities. A small percentage had major inaccuracies. Thus, be careful about such advice.

Commercialization is another problem. The former U.S. Surgeon General Dr. C. Everett Koop took in $40,000 from each health care institution listed as one of the best on his website www.drkoop.com He has allegedly now cleaned up his act.

Jeremy Buhle suggests that in the future, just as some people have a personal shopper, they may have a personal health agent who keeps them informed about health information, related financial matters and other things. Carrns gave examples of information leading people to worry so much about diseases that they become cyberchondriacs.

Reliable Organizations:

Physicians Committee for Responsible Medicine
 5100 Wisconsin Avenue NW, Suite 404, Washington, D.C. 20016
 URL—*http://www.PCRM.org/*

Nutrition Action Health Letter
 Center for Science in the Public Interest
 1875 Connecticut Avenue NW, Suite 300, Washington, D.C. 20009-5788
 URL—*http://www.cspinet.org*

Institute for Health Care Improvement
 135 Francis Street, Boston, MA 02215
 fax—(617) 754-4865, email-dberwick@ihi.org, URL—*http://www.IHI.org*

The Institute for Health Care Improvement is an independent nonprofit organization working to "improve health care quality in the U.S., Canada and Europe by fostering collaboration rather than competition among health care organizations." Its goals include improving public health, achieving better clinical outcomes, reducing costs without compromising quality, providing greater access to care, creating an easier to use health care system and improving satisfaction among individuals and communities. They publish a news magazine called *Eye on Improvement* from PO Box 2730, Chino Valley, AZ 86323 with "11 Worthy Aims for Clinical Leadership of Health System Reform" by Donald W. Berwick, M.D., "Continuous Improvement as an Ideal in Health Care," by Dr. Berwick, "Physicians as Leaders in Improving Health Care: A New Series" in Annals of Internal Medicine by Berwick and Nolan, "Understanding Medical Systems" by Nolan, "Building Measurement and Data Collection into Medical Practice" by Nelson, et al., "Developing and Testing Changes in Delivery of Health Care" by Berwick, "Physicians as Leaders in the Improvement of Health Care System" by Reinertsen, and "Cooperation: The Foundation of Improvement" by Clemmer, et al. Programs on reducing costs and improving outcomes guides are Reducing Delays and Waiting Times, Reducing Cesarean Section Rates, Improving Asthma Care, Reducing Adverse Drug Events and Reducing Costs and Improving Outcomes in Adult Intensive Care. A program in telemedicine has been developed.

American Council on Science and Health
1995 Broadway, Second Floor, New York, NY 10023-5860
tel—(212) 362-7044, fax—(212) 362-4919
URL—http://www.acsh.org, email—*acsh@acsh.org*

Government agencies: The federal government's health portal link to quality on-line health information: http://www.healthfinder.gov.

FDA links: Please see Chapter 55
National Institute for Occupational Safety and Health (part of CDC) email—
pubstaft@cdc.gov, tel—1-800-356-4 674, http://www.cdc.gov/niosh/homepage.html
National Center for Chronic Diseases Prevention and Health Promotion (CDC)
CDCP, 1600 Clifton Rd., Atlanta, GA 30333. Public Inquiries: tel—(404) 639-3311, (404) 639-3534, (800) 311-3435 URL—http://www.cdc.gov/
U.S. DHHS—URL—http://www.hhs.gov/
U.S. EPA—email—public-access@epamail.epa.gov URL—http://www.epa.gov/

Office of DPHP
U.S. DHHS, Hubert H. Humphrey Building, Room 738G 200 Independence Avenue SW, Washington, D.C. 20201 URL—http://odphp.osophs.dhhs.gov
The Healthy People 2000 and 2010 Program http://web.health.gov/healthypeople/

Substance Abuse and Mental Health Services Administration Helping children and young adults avoid substance abuse. tel—(800) 729-6686, URL—http://www.health.org.

Council of Public Representatives of the NIH URL—http://www.nih.gov/welcome/publicliaison

Women's Health:

AHCPR—Consumer information and clinical practice guidelines; topics of concern to women include mammograms and smoking cessation. email—info@ahcpr.gov URL—http://www.ahcpr.gov/consumer/

NHLBI—Publications on women and heart disease. email—(NHLBIinfo@rover.nhlbi.nih.gov). URL—*http://www.nhlbi.nih.gov/nhlbi/edumat/pub_list.htm*

National Center for Complementary and Alternative Medicine www.nccam.nih.gov

NIA—Publications related to women's health, including menopause. Public Information Office, NIA, Building 31, Room 5C27, 31 Center Drive, MSC 2292, Bethesda, MD 20892-2292 email—niainfo@lkacc.com, tel—(800) 222-2225, (800) 222-4225 URL—http://www.nih.gov/nia/health/health.htm

Office of Research on Women's Health, NIH—Directory of academic and community aspects of women's health so they can network with each other. Building 1, Room 201, Bethesda, MD 20892, URL—http://http://www4.od.nih.gov/orwh/

Women's Health Interactive At www.womens-health.com, women can communicate directly with health care professionals, join a discussion group, or assess their situation through the use of health profiles. tel—(970) 282-9437, fax—(970) 282-0023, email—whi@womens-health.com

National Women's Health Information Center—URL—http://www4.woman.org

Other:

AHCPR—Your Guide to Choosing Quality Health Care—available at: URL—*http://www.ahcpr.gov/consumer/qntool.htm*

National Library of Medicine—*http://www.nim.nih.gov/medlineplus http://clinicaltrials.gov*—information on more then 4000 clinical trials

NIH—*www.nih.gov*—provides free access to Medline—nine million references and abstracts

Partnership for Prevention—Initiative to eliminate racial and ethnic disparities in health. URL—*http://www.prevent.org*

AHA—AHA, National Center, 7272 Greenville Avenue, Dallas, Texas 75231, email—URL http://www.amhrt.org/resources.html

CancerTrials
Information on studies of cancer treatment., URL—http://cancer
trials.nci.nih.gov

MedMark: *Medical Bookmarks* Links to medical sites for clinical preventive
services. Examples: MedExplorer, Medlinks, MedWeb, Yale Medical
Library, Medinet, WebDoctor, MedNexus, Medical Reference Library
URL—http://www.medmark.org/main.html

Medscape: An online resource for better patient care. Institute for Health
Services, Research and Policy Studies, 339 East Chicago Avenue, Room
712 Chicago, IL 60611, phone 312-503-0420, fax 312-503-2936,
www.medscape.com

Heart Disease and Stroke: The NHLBI Information on ways people with heart
disease can lower their cholesterol. URL—*http://www.nhlbi.nih.gov/chd/*

**The Health and Human Services Panel on Interactive Communication and
Health** *http://www.scipich.org*—Ask for a copy of the report on information
in cyberspace.

PHS operation divisions of the U.S. PHS are following: NIH, FDA, CDCP,
Agency for Toxic Substances and Disease Registry, Indian Health Service,
Health Resources and Services Administration, Substance Abuse and Mental
Health Services Administration, AHCPR—all reached through the U.S. PHS:
330 C Street S.W., Room 2132, Washington, D.C. 20201.

Web sites with information for specific diseases—Healthcommunities.com,
a physician—developed and monitored program provides information on
more specific problems such as:

> *www.hiv.channel.com, www.urologychannel.com, www.oncologychannel.com,
> www.radiologychannel.net, www.neurologychannel.com, www.resident
> channel.com, www.residentchannel.com, www.podiatrychannel.com,
> www.cardiologychannel.com, www.sleepdisorderchannel.com, www.pulmonology
> channel.com, www.dermatologychannel.net, www.womenshealthchannel.com,
> www.alternativemedicinechannel.com.*

Web sites for Hepatitis C include: **American Liver Foundation**, CDCP, tel—
(800) 465-4837, Hepatitis Hotline—(888) 443-7232.

Harvard Health Publications web site—*www.med.harvard.edu/publications/
health_publications.*

For cancer risk—your cancer risk.Harvard.edu—Distance learning @ Harvard. Edu
Academic Medical Centers—*www.aamc.org/better_health*
CBS Health watch for patients—*www.cbshealthwatch.com*

Dr. Steven Barrett founded *www.quackwatch.com* to expose cases of health fraud.
The online medical dictionary—*www.graylab.ac.uk/omd*
Family doctor—familydoctor.org
Information on most licensed physicians—*www.ama-assn.org/aps/amahg.htm*
AMA information about health—Medem.com
AARP web site: explore health—*www.aarp.org/*
Rating web sites—health scout at www.healthscout.com

The Arthritis Foundation provides information on treatment of arthritis at *www.arthritis.org*, the American Cancer Society on treatment of cancer at *www.cancer.org*, and the American Heart Association on treatment of heart disease at *www.americanheart.org*.

Information about cognitive impairment or memory problems can be obtained from the NIH www.nih.gov. The Alzheimer's Association web site is www.alz.org.

Dr. Koop provides a web page (www.drkoop.com) rating 1500 web sites for credibility, content and opportunity for feedback and medication information—www.healthfinder.gov or www.fda.gov.

The Aetna Insurance Co. provides information on health and virtually every drug in the pharmacy both for primary care physicians and for patients at *www.intelihealth.com*. Find better sites through *www.healthscout.com*.

Helpful books include the *Oxford Medical Companion*, Oxford U. Press, England, 1999; *Getting the best from your doctor—an insider's guide to the health care you deserve*, by Schwartz, et al., Harper Paperbacks; the *Big Book of Health Tips*, by Frank Cawood and Associates; *Take Off*, on losing weight, the FCNA Publishing Company in Georgia; *The Internet 2nd edition*, by Smith and Edwards, published by Springer; *Wellness Made Easy—365 Tips for Better Health*, by the U. of Ca., Berkley Wellness Letter; and Gerteis, et al, *Through the patient's eyes—understanding and promoting patient-centered care*, by Jossey-Bass Publishers, San Francisco, Ca.

The British Medical Journal in London, England, has published online *Clinical evidence—international source for the best available evidence for effective health care* at *www.clinicalevidence.org*. Payer's *Medicine and Culture* reports the variety of treatment in the United States and Europe. From Henry and Company, New York, Napier, et al, and the American Council on Science and Health comes *Cigarettes—what the warning label doesn't tell you—The first comprehensive guide to the health consequences of smoking*. The American Council on Science and Health has a website at *http://www.asch.org*. *Healthwise Handbook* by Kemper, et al, Healthwise, Inc., Boise, Idaho is in its 12th edition. The Consumers Union, New York, publishes *Consumer Reports—The best of health—275 questions you have always wanted to ask your doctor*, by Marvin M. Littman, M.D.

PRIMARY CARE

57. What are primary, secondary, tertiary and now quaternary care? Do I need a primary care physicians?

P rimary care doctors may be family doctors, internists, or doctors trained in both internal medicine and pediatrics. Obstetricians and gynecologists could also be primary doctors but would not treat a case of the flu. Furthermore, if you belong to an HMO, it is necessary to see your primary care physician first, for referral to an ob/gyn doctor. Thus, primary care is what you receive for all of your general health problems.

Secondary care is provided by surgeons for gallbladder disease, for example, or by a cardiologist for chest pain or by a dermatologist for a persistent skin rash. Any specialist seeing you for a common problem provides secondary care.

Tertiary care includes unusual treatment such as cardiac surgery or a coronary artery angioplasty. Specialists in teaching hospitals provide tertiary care. The boundaries and definitions are inexact, blurred and unimportant. The important thing is that you have a good family physician you trust who can refer you to qualified specialists when needed.

Super-specialists perform operations and diagnostic procedures that most of you will never require, such as heart, lung, liver or pancreas transplants, positron emission tomography (PET Scanning) to determine spread of cancer, neurosurgical operations for Parkinson's disease, or lung volume-reducing operations for emphysema. I call such super-specialized procedures quaternary care. Such care is beyond the capability of most hospitals and requires specialists and medical centers with special equipment. Many approaches border on experimentation.

There is a general belief that we have too many specialists and not enough primary care physicians. An excess of specialists may contribute to the high cost of health care. More primary care physicians could strengthen community health centers for the needy and provide medical care for small towns and rural areas.

Government and some medical organizations are seeking the education of more primary care doctors and fewer specialists. The interest in primary care physicians has led medical schools to emphasize the selection of students for their humanitarian rather than for just their scientific capabilities, students who want to care for patients rather than to star as high-powered surgeons, cardiologists or scientists. Incentives for more primary care residencies may come from limiting Medicare reimbursement to hospitals for training residents in the specialties. Whether this move will improve your health is not known.

I believe that excellent health care in the U.S. requires the availability of a sizable number of specialists. Do you stay with a family doctor or go to a cardiologist if you have severe coronary artery disease? Perhaps you need both. Excellent and high-powered surgeons, orthopedists, cardiologists and other specialists can be wonderful, caring people, and many of them are. Other excellent and celebrated cardiac surgeons operate well but never talk to patients or their families before, during or after operations. Take your pick. Do you want an excellent surgeon who will see you only in the operating room or an excellent and also caring surgeon who regards communication with you as part of your care? You can have either.

If you and your family are healthy, you may not have a doctor of your own. You may go only to specialists as needed: obstetricians for childbirth, pediatricians for your children, orthopedic surgeons for broken bones. I know families who have a family plastic surgeon for cuts and injuries. You may feel you do not need general doctors. As you and your family get older, you may need advice about your health or which specialist to see or what to do about maintaining your health. If you know a doctor or a friend who is a doctor, you may be able to get advice about other things that bother you. If not, you should have your own doctor. I recommend developing a relationship with a doctor before you need one. (Chapter 1)

PROBLEMS IN HEALTH CARE AND THE SYSTEM.

58. What are the problems with health care on the national level?

The primary problems are its increasing costs and its lack of availability for many people. Total health care costs in the U.S. now top $1 trillion a year, or 14% of gross national product, with a doubling to $2 trillion predicted for 2007. John Rother, of the AARP, said the health system of the future is a mixed bag: The upside is the possibility of living longer, healthier lives with the downside that it is likely to cost a lot more.

In the U.S., everyone is unhappy with health care. Patients complain about the lack of care at bargain prices or without charge. Doctors complain about fights with insurance carriers and bureaucrats and the burdens of paperwork. Hospitals complain about their compulsory role in solving society's problems by taking care of the indigent. Insurance companies complain about patients who don't want to pay, or can't pay, for their care. Employers tell insurance carriers to hold the line on costs and, when the carriers do, everyone else accuses them of unfairness or cruelty.

Meanwhile, responsibility for payment has shifted from patients to insurers and the government. In 1960, 55% of health care was paid out of pocket by patients, 23% by private insurance and 22% by government; in 1997 this was 19%, 36% and 45% respectively. Sixty percent is now paid by the government.

Why do the costs go up so much?

Health care costs go up more rapidly than the rate of inflation due to increased demand for services and care and improvement in medical capability, with more effective instruments, diagnostic procedures, operations and other advances. We all want expensive high-tech medicine. In addition, we probably have more doctors and hospitals than we need. Hospitals have empty beds, with occupancy estimated at only 60%. Some people believe a lot of end-of-life care is futile, marginal, or unnecessary but who is to define this? It is true that we spend a lot on end-of-life care but how do you know when it is the end of life?

Paul Ginsburg, head of the Center for Studying Health System Change, describes "a medical arms race" in which doctors, hospitals and insurers all compete to provide the latest technology, in "Health Costs Going out of Control." Not mentioned are for-profit hospitals, insurers and HMOs, the high cost of drugs and the unwillingness of the American public to accept rationing. We want care now, and we don't want to be put on a waiting list, standard procedure for patients in England. Bone marrow therapy for cancer of the breast is helpful and expensive. Should it be limited? Not if you are a woman with breast cancer.

> The burgeoning of surgicenters in the community provides greater access to surgeons and procedures. Do we have too many and are they doing too much? Many diagnostic centers offer x-rays, CT scans, MRIs and nuclear studies. An advertisement once offered 25% off for a full body scan for diagnosis of almost anything. This is a waste of resources.

The Institute of Medicine (IOM) made these recommendations in "Report: Health System Broken," as cited by Karen Davis and Julie Appleby: High quality medical care for all Americans must be "reinvented;" computer technology must be adopted; communication between doctors, nurses and other professionals must be improved and team concepts developed; care must be made available when patients need it 24 hours a day by internet, phone or face to face; patients should be given more control of treatments and medical reports; and quality should be rewarded with financial incentives. Shouldn't you be able to e-mail your doctor? The major obstacles to such changes are cost and resistance to change.

Many hospitalizations can be avoided by preventive programs and earlier treatment. Healthy lifestyles, exercise, weight control, control of tobacco, prenatal care for all pregnant women, vaccination for all children, and disease prevention will help. Some people say we can't afford all the health care we want. Richard Lamm, former Governor of Colorado, says: "Modern medicine must recognize resources are limited and choices are inevitable." He quotes Victor Fuchs: "The divergence between what is beneficial for the individual and beneficial to society as a whole is the key element in the current health care debate. The best medicine for an individual is not always the best health policy for society."

What about lack of availability of health care coverage for many?

It is estimated that 43 million Americans lack health-care coverage. The IOM reports over 18,000 deaths in the U.S. yearly due to lack of health insurance, which does not include costs of human suffering. The uninsured may be poor and unemployed, or if employed without health-care coverage, unable to afford it on their own. Workers with health plans often pay more and end up with plans that are flawed. Unlicensed insurers prey on people desperate for lower rates. Medicare does not pay doctors well, and as a result some doctors will not take Medicare patients. Health care and insurance premiums increase 13% or more a year while hospital administrators often make more than a million dollars a year.

Sad tales tell of people selling their homes to pay for health care or, if unable to pay, of declaring bankruptcy. They can't afford health insurance, or if insured, can't afford the increasingly higher co-pays, and do not see a doctor when they should. Some patients receive care at public clinics or hospital emergency wards but often not until it is too late and possibly at higher costs for hospitals. If a young pregnant girl does not get good prenatal care and delivers her baby prematurely, the premature baby may cost hundreds of thousands of dollars in an ICU.

Some children go without vaccination, at great cost to their health. A white American boy born in St. Louis in 1990 can expect to live to age 75, whereas, lacking good health care, the average African-American boy born there in the same year will die before the age of 60.

Widows and middle-aged people from 45-65 years of age can be hard hit. A patient with internal bleeding who spent 34 days in the hospital incurred a bill of $5.2 million. A man scraped together $145,000 from friends to buy a kidney. Uwe Reinhardt of Princeton writes, "What this country is doing is gradually driving the lower third of the wage and income distribution out of health care."

In "Red Flag Signals Major Jump in Health Care Insurance Premiums," Julie Appleby cited as causes demand for prescription drugs, an aging population, legislative requirements that insurers offer certain services, a growing ability of doctors and hospitals to demand pay increases and loosening of some of the tight controls of the early HMO era. What she did not cite is more and better treatment for many diseases, particularly cancer.

A coalition of the AFL-CIO, AMA, U.S. Chamber of Commerce and other consumer advocates is forming to support national measures to cope with the problems of health-care coverage.

Shouldn't everyone have some basic health care coverage or care?

Certainly, but who will pay for it? The federal government is trying to cut costs, particularly Medicare, through measures such as the balanced budget act. The Administration and Congress are again producing budget deficits. A proposal for a single-payer system in which government pays for basic health care for everyone has not met with success. Opponents ask: Who wants the government running everything? Look at the problems with the Post Office, which led to the offering of alternatives like FEDEX and UPS.

Dr. Quentin Young, national coordinator for Physicians for a National Health Plan, is working to get a single-payer system. Daniel Callahan, the cofounder of the Hastings Center for biomedical ethics, asks, "Why are we so terrific on the technological side and so regressive on the social side?" His answer is that Americans stress individualism and profit and do not share. The solution will not be quick or easy. Ultimately, however, every American must have basic health care coverage, and many Americans now agree. (Chapter 43, 53)

European countries provide health care coverage for everyone. Isn't that a better way?

Universal health care sounds great but has its problems. Canada cut back on services because of costs, primarily in specialty care. Patients may have to wait. To avoid that, patients who can afford it come to the U.S. The Aetna Insurance Co. sells supplemental health-care policies to many Canadians for care in the U.S.

The National Health Service in England provides health care for everyone but its many problems include long waits for care as well as fiscal concerns. In England and France, health—care costs represent 30 percent of the national budget, and they continue to rise. No system or solution is perfect. As for the U.S., national health insurance will arrive only with a major change in social climate to a more liberal approach to social welfare.

Recently, in the *St. Louis Post-Dispatch*, John Carlton described four ways you can talk about health care. With his permission and that of the *Post-Dispatch*, I have reproduced this table.

Table I

Four ways you can talk about health care

What's the problem?	Perspective #1 The health care "system" is fragmented, irrational and confusing. No one	Perspective #2 People want the best possible care, but they're unwilling or unable to pay for it.	Perspective #3 Hospitals, HMOs, insurers and the government do a bad job of allocating	Perspective #4 Market incentives are driving the problem. Health care is a commodity and can't
	The system has grown up haphazardly, leaving too many players and programs to ever work together coherently. Services are wastefully duplicated. Patients are left unable to figure out how to get the care they need. Patients who need expensive care are treated like hot potatoes, because no hospital or insurer can afford to be stuck for their bills. The uninsured, poor and unlucky fall through the very large cracks.	People balk at the high cost of health care, but demand access to treatments costing hundreds of thousands of dollars. They can't have it both ways.	Institutions and insurers are spending more than they need to on overhead and taking millions in profits out of the system. We're also spending too much on specialists instead of family practitioners, and too much on expensive hospital care rather than preventive medicine.	Companies are motivated by profit and prestige, not altruism. This has led hospitals to move out to the suburbs in search of well-insured patients, leaving poor people without access to care; insurers to cherrypick among clients; and HMOs to pay out earnings in dividends and salaries, rather than reinvest in plant, equipment and personnel.
What should be done?	Either create a single-payer system to end the need for cost shifting and to reduce overhead so more money can be devoted	Either accept the need to pay more for health care than we already are paying.	Spend more on preventive medicine, and gradually cut back oon expensive hospital care.	Either let government run the health care system.
	Or give state government a stronger hand in approving new health care spending on facilities to reduce duplication of services.	Or make the difficult cost-versus-benefit choices of how to ration care, whether to accept second-best drugs and technology,	Trim management and administrative staff, and hire more health-care professionals.	Or recognize health care as a public utility, subject to strict government regulation.
			Make sure health care is delivered by the least expensive appropriate personnel (e.g. physicians' assistants rather than doctors, etc).	And rethink government repayment plans to better align market incentives with what we actually want health care companies to do.

Why this course of action?	Only by centralizing our current system can we hope to fix it.	If we don't decide, the ever-rising cost of health care will bankrupt us all. We can't make informed decisions about how to reform the system until we decide what our priorities are. Oregon has done it, so can we.	There's no need to wait for big changes or better coordination in the health care system. Increasing efficiency is just good business, and preventive care will reduce the number of people who need expensive hospital services.	The government already provides health care to millions of poor and elderly Americans, spending far less on administration than private insurers do. In Europe and Canada, where doctors are well paid but not rich, every citizen has health insurance and basic health care. If we took the drive to maximize profits out of our system, we'd have enough money to provide much better care.
What do critics say?	Some inefficiency is the price we pay for choice. Centralizing control of the system might well force people to accept second-class care and create "socialized medicine"	We're already spending enough to provide everyone with equal access to health care; the problem is we're not spending the money wisely. If we reduce overhead and emphasize preventive medicine, we can continue receiving world's best care.	We spend nearly twice as much per capita on health care as the Canadians do. While individual hospitals, doctors and insurers could certainly spend their money more wisely, we can't find that kind of savings here. And as to preventive medicine, just try to get Americans to exercise more.	Get real. Do we really think the government would do a better job at a complicated task like this? Greater government control will stifle creativity of health care companies and reduce the quality of service.

Section K

Ethical Issues in Health Care

59. Why so many ethical issues in health care now?

Ethical issues in health care and research are mind-boggling, with advances in scientific research creating scenarios not yet accepted on ethical grounds. The possibility of human cloning is a prime example. Transplantation of organs is another, forcing the issue of how to make sure that someone is an eligible donor, that is to say, that available tests are accurate in determining death. Organ transplantation involves yet another ethical issue. While selling organs or body parts is illegal, fees are charged for processing the parts. Some for-profit companies associated with transplant and research programs at hospitals or medical schools charge large fees that are returned to the hospital programs. Some of these fees are excessive and thus unethical.

The list of issues continues with genetics studies and the human genome, liberty and privacy, feminist concerns and managed health care. Is boxing ethical? Is it really ethical for doctors to advertise? Is every person in the U.S. entitled to health care? Is it a right or a privilege? If it is a right, who will provide it and who will pay for it? (Chapter 53)

Denial of legitimate treatment to the sick is an ethical problem, as is lack of continuity of care. These problems arise now that many providers of health care are for-profit companies who seek to limit the amount of health care you can get. Perhaps we can't afford to pay or will not pay for all the health care we would like to have.

Patient autonomy, advance directives, determination of incompetence and end-of-life care raise issues with ethical implications. Some concern centers on the use of scarce or expensive medical resources in the last few weeks or days of a patient's life. The problem is who knows it is the last few weeks of life? Attempts to define futile care or futility are also cause for concern. How do we know when care is futile? Who defines it as such? It is certain that a patient with a cancer spread throughout the body with no response to any known therapy, deterioration and pain, needs care: sedation, pain control and comfort. It is also certain that a patient with permanent coma is brain dead. Many doctors believe that permanently comatose patients should not be kept alive by artificial means such as a ventilator.

Father Kevin O'Rourke indicates a surrogate decision-maker, a family member or friend, does not have to force physicians to keep such patients alive. He says "from an ethical perspective, the surrogate is the person promoting the dignity of the patient and ensures respect for the patient even when the patient cannot speak for himself."

A National Bioethics Advisory Commission (NBAC) reviews and makes recommendations about ethical issues in medicine, particularly research with humans as subjects. NBAC comprises lawyers, Ph.D.s and M.D.s who are bioethicists. They hold meetings every month and post reports at *www.bioethics.gov/pubs.html.*

Great crimes against individuals have been committed by using them as subjects of research without their understanding of what was being done to them. In Nazi Germany during World War II, gruesome experiments were carried out on captives in concentration camps. In 1932 the US Public Health Service began the infamous 40-year-long Tuskeegee studies of poor African-American patients with syphilis who were not treated but simply watched to see what happened to them. No proven cure for the disease existed at the start of the study, but even after penicillin became the standard cure in 1947, the researchers withheld it. (Chapter 61.) More recently, we have learned about government employees working with radioactive substances who were not told of possible risks. Many of them later developed serious health problems or died. Now laws protect us from such tragedies. In succeeding chapters you will learn about such protection and the importance of ethics for you.

Further information on ethical issues in medicine can be obtained from the sources indicated below and from *Health Care Ethics*, published by the Center for Healthcare Ethics, Saint Louis University, 221 North Grand Boulevard, Room 20, St. Louis, Missouri, 63013.

1. The Center for the Study of Bioethics at the Medical College of Wisconsin at *www.mew.edu/bioethics*.
2. Center for Bioethics at the University of Pennsylvania at *www.med. upenn.edu/bioethics/index.shtml*.
3. Western Institutional Review Board at *www.wirb.com*.
4. University of Virginia Center for Biomedical Ethics at *www.med.virginia. edu/medicine/inter-diss/bio-ethics/home.html*.
5. The *Journal of Clinical Ethics* at *www.cliniclethics.com*

Sometimes a company choosing a sound ethical approach finds it is not good business. The Smith & Wesson Co. entered into an agreement with the federal government to put locks on all of its hand guns, implement "smart gun" technology and tighten procedures for selling weapons. According to Jeffrey L. Seglin, the company was vilified by its customers, retailers and the NRA and forced to cut back. The company president said, "Would I put locks on our guns if it would save one child?" His answer was yes. No other gun maker has taken such a stand.

In other chapters, I respond to your questions about the right of health care (Chapter 53), end-of-life issues (Chapter 49, 50), physician-assisted suicide (Chapter 49), and related ethical problems. Ethical issues also arise with the use of tissues from human embryos in stem-cell research, genetic testing and counseling and gene therapy (Chapters 63, 64).

PROFESSIONAL ETHICS

60. Professional ethics-how does it affect me? What is bioethics? What do hospital ethics committees do?

Professional ethics require your doctors and nurses to put your well-being and care first and foremost in their relationship with you. Your rights, concerns and care take precedence over any of their relationships with third parties that might also involve you. Be sure your doctor feels that way. Be sure your doctor doesn't have contracts with an insurance company or HMO that conflict with your doctor/patient relationship.

The word "profession" comes from the root "profess" which means to avow before, to swear a sacred oath. Students graduating from medical school swear to devote themselves to the care of the sick and to the service of humanity by invoking the Oath of Hippocrates, Maimonides Prayer, or the Declaration of Geneva 1948. The Harvard Medical School Class of 1997 showed their dedication to upholding the ethics of the medical profession by writing their own oath (Chapter 41). By 1994, every medical school in the U.S. offered a program in medical ethics in its curriculum. Many medical specialties now teach ethics in their residencies.

Members of professional groups take pledges to place the welfare and rights of their patients above all else. The American College of Surgeons (ACS) uses a central judiciary committee to maintain professional conduct of its fellows. Sanctions for misconduct include admonition, censure, probation, suspension and finally expulsion. The important role of the ACS in promoting ethical behavior has been reviewed by Dr. C. Rollins Hanlon.

The AMA observes a code of ethics and has established an ethics institute. In the Journal of the American Medical Association (JAMA), Dr. C. Bruce Baker et al. wrote they "deplore the current corporate mentality and excess interest in efficiency and profits that threaten to preempt the personal comfort of professionals and more fundamentally still, the moral dimension of the patient-physician relationship—the main challenge facing medicine today is insuring free market medicine remains moral medicine."

Managed care and HMOs cause ethical problems for many physicians and raise a question as to whether doctors must adopt a new ethic. Managed care seems to call for the greatest good for the greatest number so far as the budget allows. Dr. Edmund D. Pellegrino objects to this as distributive justice. Dr. Jerome P. Kassirer, former Editor of the *New England Journal of Medicine*, says "intentionally providing minimally acceptable care to some for the benefit of others in an arbitrary group—let alone for the benefit of the bottom line is wrong." He goes on, "When patients are sick and vulnerable they expect their physicians to be their advocates for optimal care, not for some minimalists' standard." Physicians will resist changing to an ethic for a group rather than the individual patient.

Remember, the ethical, empathic, concerned doctor must first meet a professional standard. In its Principles of Professional Conduct, the Medical Society of the State of New York says: "The prime object of the medical profession is to render competent medical service with compassion and respect for human dignity." A doctor can't be ethical if he is not a good doctor.

What is bioethics?

It is a rapidly growing field of study and application of ethics to human biology, health and research. Participants include professionals, doctors, lawyers, priests, ministers and representatives of other disciplines, including philosophy, religion and sociology. Bioethics is becoming a specialty in many schools. Many universities have bioethics or health care ethics centers. Full-time careers in bioethics are developing. An accreditation program does not exist as yet, however, and at present, anyone can call oneself a bioethicist. That will change as standards become clearer. The American Society for Bioethics and Humanities has developed guidelines for competency. A National Bioethics Advisory Commission is also at work.

An important movement is deep or global bioethics dedicated to help the world stay together in the third millennium. Advocates propose control of world population by reducing its rate of increase; support of sustainable agriculture, forestry and fishing and protection; and restoration of the natural environment. They hope to curb the capitalist drive to exploit free markets system of globalization of economic forces that lack responsibility. Medical bioethics relates to physicians and patients. Global bioethics emphasizes our duty to preserve and support our environment for generations to come.

What is a hospital ethics committee? What do they do?

Most hospitals have set up committees interested in and concerned about ethical matters and dilemmas. Members are lay people, clergy, lawyers, nurses and doctors. Often, the chairman is a medical ethicist. The committee is available for consultation with you, your family and physician. If there is concern about an ethical problem, such as withdrawal of life support, the end of life, ICU problems and other concerns, the committee is available for consultation. Call upon them if you need help. They will meet with you, your family, physician and clergy person. They will not intrude, unless you request their help. Your doctor could also seek their help.

61. What is informed consent? What is the Nuremberg Code? What is an Institutional Review Board? How are clinical trials carried out?

What is informed consent?

Informed consent to medical care is your basic right. Without your approval nothing should be done concerning you, whether an operation, a treatment or a study of you or your record. Not only must you consent but your consent must be informed. You must understand the recommendations, the risks and the options. You must be told if the procedure or treatment is standard and accepted by all, such as an appendectomy, or one that is under development, such as a new minimal heart operation for coronary artery disease. For young children and adults who cannot give informed consent, such as Alzheimer's patients, the next-of-kin must consent, unless it is a life-threatening situation, and the family is not available.

If you have had an operation, you are familiar with the standard consent form stating you understand the nature of the operation to be done and its risks, benefits and alternatives. Many of us review the forms with our patients before the operation. If you do not feel adequately informed, do not sign the form.

The form indicates the surgeon may also perform related procedures if necessary, a provision that may be of use during procedures that at first seem to be routine. Suppose the diagnosis is appendicitis, agreed upon by all the doctors consulted. Our diagnostic methods are not so exact, however, that we can be sure about the diagnosis of an abdominal problem. During operation the surgeon finds a normal appendix but an inflamed gallbladder. The advance consent to related procedures allows the surgeon to remove the gallbladder then and there instead of waiting for specific consent to the cholecystectomy. The necessity for consent to related procedures should be explained to you in advance.

The requirement for informed consent is of recent origin. In his history of the doctrine, Dr. Jay Katz marks October 22, 1957, as the date of its first appearance in case law. In *Salgo v. Stanford U.,* Judge Bray of the California Court of Appeals said "a physician violates his duty to his patient . . . if he withholds any facts necessary to form an intelligent consent by the patient to the proposed treatment." In discussing risk, discretion must be used consistent with full disclosure of facts necessary for informed consent. Justice Bray's opinion on informed consent came verbatim from a brief submitted by lawyers of the American College of Surgeons. Then, in a number of other cases, the concept of informed consent became part of common law.

In years past, as Katz pointed out, that earlier concept of beneficence was the principle for patient care. The related admonitions to physicians cannot be faulted in themselves: to be beneficent, do no harm and do whatever they could for the good of the patient carefully and selflessly. The Hippocratic Oath states: "I will come for the benefit of the sick, remain free of intentional injustice, and free of all mischief."

With that principle for care, doctors did what in their view was best for patients without asking for their help in making decisions (Chapter 4). In fact, patients would on occasion say: "Don't tell me about it, go ahead and take good care of me." This is now a different time, and many aspects of technology require patients to participate in decisions. The principle for care now is patient autonomy. In a lecture known to many doctors "The Care of the Patient," the Harvard Medical School physician Frances Peabody said, "One of the essential qualities of the clinician is his interest in humanity, for the secret of the care of the patient is caring for the patient." Katz changed the last word in Peabody's sentence to read, "The secret of the care of the patient is caring for the person." My wife, Rosemary, developed this theme in writing about ethical situations in *The Patient as a Person*. It is an important principle for you to recognize and for all physicians to support.

D. J. Nyman and C. L. Sprung describe elements of informed consent: 1) disclosure of information, 2) competency, 3) understanding, 4) voluntariness, and 5) decision making. They state "informed consent protects patients, encourages rational decision making, helps prevent duress and encourages the medical profession to scrutinize itself. The physician must consider the patient as a person and also their moral, ethical, religious and ethnic background" (Chapter 13).

The lawyer George J. Annas believes 1972 court opinions firmly established the current requirements for informed consent: "after obtaining the patient's consent to treatment, the physician provides the patient with basic information so the patient, not the physician, can make the final decision about proceeding." The basic information includes descriptions of proposed treatment, potential risks and benefits, alternative treatments and their risks and benefits, the likelihood of success as best as can be determined and potential problems in recuperation, and complications. You have the right to refuse treatment if you are medically competent. Informed consent is more difficult to obtain in emergency wards where procedures are done rapidly for resuscitation and in the interest of saving a life. The mere presence of the patient must serve as consent enough, unless family is there to provide it. Consent for procedures in ICUs can be obtained, unless the patient is comatose.

Is informed consent for medical research different?

Informed consent to participate in a medical research project has not always been required. See Chapter 59 for one sad example in American research with the notorious Tuskegee study. In the late 1940s and early 1950s, U.S. government physicians tricked parents of retarded children at the Fednald School into giving permission for their children to participate in a science club where the children ingested radioactive isotopes that posed significant risk. Radiation experiments were also conducted on humans by several agencies of the government between 1944 and 1974.

In 1947, Nazi doctors were tried in Nuremberg for the horrible crimes they had committed in the name of medical experimentation against victims in concentration camps. Sixteen were found guilty, seven sentenced to death by hanging, five to life imprisonment, two to imprisonment for 25 years, one to imprisonment for 15 year and seven were acquitted. One upshot of the trial was the Nuremberg Code, developed with the help of several American judges and physicians to reinforce the Hippocratic Oath and prevent heinous medical crimes in the future.

The Nuremberg Code

1. The voluntary consent of the human is absolutely essential. This means the person involved should have legal capacity to give consent; should be so situated to be able to exercise free power of choice, without intervention of any element of force, fraud, deceit, duress, overreaching, or other ulterior forms of constraint or coercion; and should have sufficient knowledge and comprehension of the elements of the subject matter involved to enable him to make an understanding and enlightened decision. This latter element requires before the acceptance of an affirmative decision by the experimental subject there should be made known to him the nature, duration, and purpose of the experiment; the method and means by which it is to be conducted; all inconveniences and hazards reasonably to be expected; and the effects upon his health or person which may possibly come from his participation in the experiment.

2. The experiment should be such as to yield fruitful results for the good of society, unprocurable by other methods or means of study, and not random and unnecessary in nature.

3. The experiment should be so designed and based on the results of animal experimentation and knowledge of the natural history of the disease or other problem under study that the anticipated results will justify the performance of the experiment.

4. The experiment should be conducted to avoid all unnecessary physical and mental suffering and injury.

5. No experiment should be conducted if there is an a priori reason to believe that death or disabling injury will occur; except, perhaps, in those experiments where the experimenting physicians also serve as subjects.

6. The degree of risk should never exceed that determined by the humanitarian importance of the problem to be solved by the experiment.

7. Proper preparations should be made and adequate facilities provided to protect the experimental subject against even remote possibilities of injury, disability, or death.

8. The experiment should be conducted only by scientifically qualified persons. The highest degree of skill and care should be required through all stages of the experiment of those who conduct or engage in the experiment.

9. During the course of the experiment the human subject should be at liberty to bring the experiment to an end if he has reached the physical

or mental state where continuation of the experiment seems to him to be impossible.

10. During the course of the experiment the scientist in charge must be prepared to terminate the experiment at any stage, if he has probable cause to believe, in the exercise of the good faith, superior skill, and careful judgment required of him, a continuation of the experiment is likely to result in injury, disability, or death to the experimental subject.

The Nuremberg Code focuses on human rights of research subjects whereas the later Declaration of Helsinki focuses on the obligations of physician-investigators to research subjects. Federal regulations emphasize the obligation of research institutions that receive federal funds. Every medical institution or hospital seeking to do clinical trials must obtain approval from its Institutional Review Board (IRB). With physician administrators, lay individuals, ministers or lawyers from the community as members, the IRB reviews a written explanation of the project, with an explanation of how the investigators will obtain informed consent. The committee insists, and rightly so, on knowing in detail exactly what the patients will be told and how the form they must sign elicits informed consent. These forms are kept on file by the IRB. Proposals to review patient records, which are confidential, must be reviewed and approved by the IRB.

In the past, I reviewed records of our patients to determine complications and results of operations. To do this, I submitted an application to the IRB indicating my intent and declaring that I would not name or otherwise identify any individual patient and would refer only to groups.

Research with people as subjects will not be accepted for publication in a medical journal without a statement from the investigators that they have received the approval of their IRB and protected the rights of the subjects. They must have the right to withdraw from a trial, and physicians must stop an experiment if harm is being done. Many other protections are provided by the Nuremberg Code.

Michael D. Lemonick and Andrew Goldstein describe how clinical trials are supposed to work:

Step 1: Basic Research. Step 2: Animal Studies. Step 3: Proposal. Step 4: Recruit Patients. Step 5: Inform Patients.—In order to participate, each patient must sign an informed-consent form. These detail the potential risks and benefits and can run 30 pages long. Step 6: Phase I—to determine if a new treatment is safe. Step 7: Phase II—More patients—Researchers add a control group so they can look for signs that the therapy is having some effect. This step can last several years. Step 8: Phase III—The last step before approval involves up to thousands of patients and lasts up to five years. New therapy is tested for effectiveness by comparing it with existing treatments and/or a placebo.

Investigators must indicate their financial ties or support from the company doing the research. Step 9: FDA Approval—If a treatment proves safe and effective, the FDA gives its blessing, and a new drug is born. The testing continues; in Phase IV, the manufacturer is required to report any unexpected reactions, for up to 10 years (Chapter 55). This phase broke down recently when the Pfizer drug company allegedly did not report findings of increased heart and stroke problems with VIOXX, a pain reliever of the Cox-2 category. Other such drugs have now been implicated as well.

Problems arise when research is being done on severely injured patients or ICU patients. Informed consent remains the same as described by Nyman and Sprung. Waiving consent, deferred consent and surrogate consent have been suggested as ways to circumvent the problem. Deferred consent means that the patient, if possible, signs permission at a later time or a family member signs later. Deferred consent or surrogate consent is much better than waiving informed consent. It is not a perfect solution to the problem but sometimes life-saving research is important and should go on. The FDA has set forth many criteria to fulfill for an exception to informed consent, listed by T. A. Santora, et al. They run contrary to the Nuremberg Code and Declaration of Helsinki. Are controlled trials ethical in children and particularly critically ill children? They must be done to determine the benefit to children but must be done carefully with full consideration for the welfare of the child and family.

Your primary care doctor should never ask you to participate in a research study. He or she is too close to you, to avoid the charge of unfair coercion. You should be approached by the researchers doing the study and should feel free to participate or say no thanks.

Protection of research subjects in federally-funded research is secure, but is not necessarily the case for privately-funded research. The National Bioethics Advisory Committee recommended the Federal Office of the prevention of Research Risk (OPRR) be removed from the NIH elevated to a position in the DHHS and given authority to protect all subjects of human research. This has been done with the Office of Human Research Protection which has authority to stop human research at any institution if they believe safety and proper controls are not in place. They have done this a number of times. Certain diseases occur in specific communities such as ethnic, racial, occupational or religious groups. These require study but again the community must be protected by informed consent and consultation.

Questions you should ask the investigators about trials:

1) What is the purpose of the trial: to help cure patients or advance medical knowledge?
2) What phase is the trial—I, II or III? The earlier the phase, the more experimental the procedure or treatment.

3) What are known risks? What can the doctor tell you about potential side effects?

4) Is the doctor's center the only one conducting the trial, or are others involved? If other centers are further along in the trial, ask for a synopsis of the experience of those patients.

5) What are procedures for reporting problems, ill effects or sudden changes? Is the contact person available 24 hours a day by cell phone or pager?

6) What is the track record of the primary investigator? How long has he or she been conducting trials? (Chapter 55)

New treatments and drugs must be studied to be sure they are safe and effective before they are approved for general use and prescribed by your doctor. If you would like to participate in a trial, do so but be fully informed before you consent. Clinical research trials require careful monitoring and the prompt reporting of adverse events. Guidelines were reviewed by Michael A. Morse, et al.

Remember, occasionally clinical trials, particularly those with toxic drugs or genes, have resulted in deaths.

BILL OF RIGHTS. PRIVACY ACT.

62. What is the National Patients Bill of Rights? What is the Health Insurance Portability and Accountability Act? Why can't I sue an HMO for denying me care that I need? Isn't that my right?

Despite talking for years about the need for a patients' bill of rights, Congress has so far failed to pass one. In 2002 both the Senate and the House passed patients' bill of rights legislation but when they failed to convene a House-Senate conference on the bill it died. "Democrats and Republicans could not compromise over the issue of liability," according to kaisernetwork.org. "Democrats generally want to give patients a broader right to sue their health insurers in disputes over coverage and treatment. Republicans often favor a more limited right to sue. That has stopped agreement before and did so again this time."

The movement for a patients' bill of rights dates back to 1973 with a bill from the American Heart Association outlining 12 rights described by George Annas as "vague in general." They included the right to receive respectful care, to be given complete information about diagnosis and prognosis, to refuse treatment, to refuse to participate in experiments, to have privacy and confidentiality maintained and to receive a reasonable response to a request for services.

In 1996 a Federal Appeals Court ruled Medicare patients are entitled to immediate hearings and other protection when they are denied care by HMOs. Robert Pear in his discussion of this pointed out "this decision about Medicare is significant because it holds that its beneficiaries have rights rooted in the Constitution, not merely in statues or regulations subject to change by Congress and the President." This was the result of a class actions suit in Arizona for nearly six million Medicare patients against HMOs around the country.

The Health Insurance Portability and Accountability Act of 1996 (HIPPA) gives the DHHS power to make rules for privacy regarding your protected health information. Every hospital and health care provider must provide you with a notice of privacy practices. This includes: 1) Uses and disclosure of your health information. 2) Other uses and disclosures. 3) Your health information rights. 4) Change to the notice and complaints. 4) Complaints can be made to the office of Civil Rights, U.S. DHHS, 200 Independence Avenue, SW, Room 509F, HHH Bldg, Washington, DC 20201.

Some hospitals go beyond the requirements of the act with their own rules on advanced directives and patients' rights. The Yale New Haven Hospital in Connecticut gives each patient a brochure describing their rights, responsibilities and ethical decisions. Rights include respect, privacy, a full explanation of care, identification of who is taking care of you, confidentiality, emotional support and informed decision making.

In 1997 President Clinton appointed an advisory commission for protection and quality in the health care industry, and the commission produced an outline of a national patients' bill of rights. In his State of the Union message, in 1998, Clinton proposed a National Bill of Rights in Health Care. He said, "You have the right to know all your medical options, not just the cheapest. You have the right to choose the doctor you want for the care you need. You have the right to emergency care, wherever and whenever you need it. You have the right to keep your medical records confidential."

Clinton's proposals, along with the appellate court decision, indicate that the key provisions of a national bill for patients' rights should be:

1) The right to treatment information.
2) The right to privacy and dignity.
3) The right to refuse treatment.
4) The right to emergency care.
5) The right to an advocate.

These rights are important for everyone and should be established.

In one departure from its lack of involvement in health care issues, Congress has taken on the managed care concept of limiting hospital stays after childbirth by mandating coverage for a specific period of two days minimum, depending upon the patient and the physician. To fill the gap left by congressional failure to enact a patients' bill of rights, some states have enacted bills of their own. However, the state laws apply only to patients not in employer-sponsored health plans, which are subject to regulation by federal laws.

A number of organizations continue a wide-ranging public discussion of a patient's bill of rights. The AMA is a strong supporter of a patients' bill of rights. The National Committee for Quality Assurance has drawn up a document on members' rights and responsibilities. Kaiser Permanente, the group health plan for Puget Sound, has set forth 18 principles for consumer protection. The Health Insurance Plan, the AARP and Families USA have offered proposals. In what some people say is putting the fox in charge of the hen house, the American Association of Health Plans (AAHP), the HMO and health insurance organization, has produced a proposal or recommendation for a patients' bill of rights titled "Putting Patients First." Some insurance groups oppose a patients' bill of rights. Why don't they want you to have rights? Could it cut down on their profit?

Why can't I sue an HMO for denial of health care that I need? Isn't that my right?

If you are in an employer-sponsored health plan, it is not your right to sue an HMO for denial of benefits. Federal law regulates such plans, and a federal law, the Employee Retirement Income Security Act of 1974 (ERISA), makes it difficult to sue on those grounds. The Democratic Party advocated legislation to give you the right to sue. The Republicans would not support it. State laws apply to patients in plans that are not employer-sponsored, however, and a number of states have passed laws meant to help resolve coverage disputes for those patients.

Now state and local public employees and Medicare/Medicaid recipients can sue their HMOs for denial of benefits on the grounds of negligence. While a series of court rulings have made it easier for you to sue for negligence, it is unfortunate you do not as of now have easier legal recourse for denial of coverage for health care. Sad cases of denial of coverage have led to death of patients. Health plans should be legally accountable for their decisions on medical treatment decisions. You deserve better accountability from your health plan.

A cousin of mine had a rapidly growing cancer of the lung that his HMO doctors did not accurately and expeditiously diagnose. He had to go out of the network for an accurate diagnosis and treatment, and shortly after beginning treatment he died. His HMO refused to pay for his outside care. Only the threat of exposure and litigation made them pay.

An article in USA TODAY said, "Pressure mounts against a law cheating patients of power. Without fear of lawsuits HMOs are free to scrimp on services." ERISA should be amended to make managed care organizations (MCO) responsible for their medical decisions. The Attorney General of CT recently sued an MCO for cutting off a patient's prescription benefits. At least six bills have been introduced in Congress to protect you and give you rights to obtain health care through your MCO. None has been enacted. The MCOs are afraid of an increased number of lawsuits that would cause rates to go up. The political maneuvering in Washington over health care issues is full of twists and turns.

63. What is the Human Genome Project (HGP) and how does it affect me? Will my genes predict disease by genetic testing? What is genetic profiling? What is genetic counseling? What about gene therapy?

The HGP began in 1990 as a coordinated international effort to study and map the entire human genome, the complete set of deoxyribonucleic acid (DNA) in the chromosomes—the genetic code for human life—as well as to identify all of the genes in the DNA. Comprising 3.5 billion letters, the genetic code has been called the "Book of Life," "the instruction book for human biology," its mapping the breakthrough of the year and the best medicine of the century.

While the end of the project was celebrated two years ahead of schedule in 2003, with the sequencing of human chromosomes complete, work continues on the identification of genes, under the auspices of the International Human Genome Sequencing Consortium, led in the U. S. by the National Human Genome Research Institute and the Department of Energy. The exact number of the genes encoded by the genome remains unknown.

Every cell in our body contains a nucleus with our genetic material on 46 chromosomes, 23 from each parent. Defined by R. J. Sternberg as "microscopic strands of genetic material," chromosomes determine what we are and what passes on to our children. Chromosomes contain the complex chemical DNA, and the units of DNA are genes, paired nucleotide bases that determine gene function. The genes are precise sequences of the chemicals adenine, thymine, guanine, and cytosine, or, as used in representations of the gene code, A, T, G, and C. Here, for example, is a very short section of the DNA that codes for the fragile X mental retardation protein (FMRP): GACTTACGGCAAATGT. According to Hadad et al, the human genome contains about three million base pairs of chemicals that code for the genes.

Genetic material takes the form of two tightly coiled strands of DNA, a double helix most recently estimated to hold 20,000 to 30,000 genes, far fewer than the 140,000 previously though necessary to "make, maintain and repair" a person. *Human Genome Project Information* notes that the lower gene count came as a shock to many scientists "because counting genes was a way of quantifying genetic complexity. With about 30,000, the human gene count would be only one-third greater than that of the simple roundworm . . . at about 20,000."

In describing the double helix structure of DNA and its components of nucleic acids in 1953, the future Nobel Laureates James Watson and Francis Crick made the HGP possible. Dr. Francis S. Collins, Director of the U.S. National Human Genome Research Institute, directed the U.S. and British effort for the HGP. Collins and Craig Venter of Celera Genomics Company combined forces to complete the project.

Collins and Dr. Victor A. McKusick describe research opportunities and make forecasts about the genetic approach to diagnosis and treatment of disease. They agree that the HGP is at a point, stated by Winston Churchill at the time of defeat of the Germans in North Africa, "Now this is not the end. It is not even the beginning of the end. But it is, perhaps, the end of the beginning."

How does this affect me? What is next?

Fairfield, in the *New York Times*, compared the great importance of this project to that of the Hubbell space telescope, the Apollo moon program, high energy physics research and the Manhattan Project to build the atomic bomb. The HGP is exciting scientifically with great promise for the future but with no immediate effect for you. A lot of work remains to be done before the information can be applied to human disease.

Implications of this project for human health include: 1) identification of hereditary disorders potentially correctable by genetic testing, (personal risk assessment); 2) potential gene and drug therapy; 3) potential cloning of normal human genes to develop new drugs and treat diseases; 4) better understanding of the genetics of cancer. Other potential benefits include prenatal therapy and help with autoimmune diseases such as rheumatoid arthritis.

On the other hand, the project presents the potential of some difficult problems: unethical genetic testing, threats to the privacy of genetic information and discrimination by health care insurers or employers on the basis of genetic information and your medical history. Your privacy must be maintained and the information not used against your will. Other problems include information overload, the need for legal protection and problems with gene therapy. Conflicts will arise over who owns the information and what can be patented.

The genomes of plants and species of animals are being sequenced as are bacteria. The organism causing cholera—the vibrio cholera—has been sequenced. Many predict the HGP will revolutionize the way medicine is practiced and disease is identified, prevented or treated. Thus, a lot of "hype" attends each discovery.

Others urge caution. Drs. Neil A. Holtzman and Teresa Marteau do not accept this "hype." They believe "the new genetics will not revolutionize the way in which common diseases are identified and treated." Their doubts stem from 1) incomplete penetrance of genotypes for common diseases (they are not caused by a single gene but by a combination of many); 2) the limited ability to tailor treatment to genotypes; and 3) the low magnitude of risk brought on by various genotypes. They emphasize differences in social structure, life style and environment as accounting for a much larger proportion of disease.

The technologies for mapping the human genome and knowledge of proteins gained from the process may help develop important new drugs. Particularly needed are new antibiotics for infection caused by antibiotic resistant bacteria.

Will my genes predict disease by genetic testing? Are there problems with this?

Genetic testing for a number of diseases is possible and many more are under development. We know the chromosomal location of many genes responsible for genetic diseases. A DNA screening test can determine a mutation on a gene. About 4,000 genetic diseases are known to exist. Genes indicating increased likelihood of a disease include BRCA-2 and BRCA-1 for breast cancer. More study is needed of anti-estrogen therapy or prophylactic mastectomy in women at high risk because of a family history of breast cancer and BRCA-1 or BRCA-2 abnormalities.

Other possible disease indicators include the HD gene for Huntington's Disease, the APO4 gene for Alzheimer's disease, the MSH-2 gene for colon cancer, the LD receptor gene linked to bad cholesterol, the EPO gene to form oxygen carrying red blood cells and genes for cystic fibrosis, Parkinson's Disease and Wilms tumors. A deadly genetic disease called Canavan Disease destroys the central nervous systems. A mutated gene results in polyps of the colon and cancer, the adenomatous polyposis coli gene. Many other genetic diseases have been identified.

Most illnesses, however, are produced by several or more genes acting or failing together, and it is difficult to sort out the effects of multiple genes, with depression and schizophrenia as two examples. Testing for multiple gene effects is not possible now. Genetic tests, as described by Haddad et al, do not predict getting the disease in a yes-or-no fashion. Not everyone with "an inherited susceptibility," a single gene mutation linked to a disease, will get the disease. How many will or won't is not known. The presence of a mutated gene indicates an increased tendency towards the disease but test results may be difficult to interpret. No clear-cut standards exist.

False negatives and false positives can be a problem. You may be told a test is positive when it was falsely positive. Should the test be repeated to be sure? Results could lead to depression if psychological support is not given.

In any event, while we may identify potential development of a disease, we may be unable to do anything to prevent it. Thus, genetic testing may be hard on patients. If it reveals an inherited tendency towards a disease, it may cause a lot of worry, particularly with respect to children. Should children be tested for the possibility of developing an adult disease that cannot be prevented? How would the child be helped by that? Wouldn't it only increase anxiety?

Genetic testing for the general population would be too filled with ambiguities to be worth the expense. Ethical and moral problems would arise with widespread genetic testing or profiling. Who would get the information? Would HMOs and employers use it to deny coverage for health care? Would it change the way to treat or associate with people with genetic defects? A ban on the use of genetic information by anyone other than the patient is being considered.

Sullivan& Frost, marketing consultants to the genetic testing industry, maintain that an individual's genetic information should be generally available but this would be acceptable only if use of your information does not identify you by name. Currently, genetic testing is recommended only for individuals and families at high risk for development of a certain diseases. If such people seek genetic testing, they should have professional counseling and education before the test and medical and psychological support afterward.

Holtzman believes the HGP has engendered "genohype," creating greater expectations for genetic testing than are actually warranted. The Clinical Laboratory Improvement Amendments of 1988 includes regulations to control genetic testing. Donna Shalala, former head of Health and Human Services, set up a Task Force on Genetic Testing. Controls to assure privacy in genetics research have been strongly recommended by the Privacy Workshop Planning Subcommittee set up by the National Action Plan on Breast Cancer of the NIH (*barbaraf@exchange.nih.gov*)

Other questions arise with the practice of "pre-implantation genetic analysis." In a family with a known severe genetic disease, such as Fanconi anemia, sperm and eggs from the parents may used for in-vitro fertilization. After a few days some growing and dividing cells are removed for genetic analysis. If they are free of the genetic defect, the growing embryo is implanted in the mother's uterus. What if the genetic defect is present? Do you destroy the embryo? We live in wild scientific times.

What is genetic counseling?

Trained counselors, knowledgeable about genetics, testing and counseling, work in medical school hospitals or children's hospitals and also for testing companies so proper interpretations are made of the results. The American Board of Genetic Counseling has a web site, *www.faseb.org/genetics/abgc/ abgcmenu.htm*, as does the National Society of Genetic Counselors, *www.nsgc.org*. These counselors help you in deciding whether you want to be tested, how to interpret results, how many in your family should be tested, and who should get the information from the test. They also provide psychological and emotional support to deal with the results. Unfortunately, there are only about 1,000 such trained counselors in the U.S.

Is gene therapy on the horizon?

Enthusiasts think it will be successful momentarily. I think it will be a long slow process despite recent successes in Italy and England in treating an inherited immune disorder called Severe Combined Immunodeficiency (SCID), which causes an unusual susceptibility to infections. Only a few patients have been treated so far. Two years ago, a report described the development of a leukemia-like syndrome in two children after their successful gene therapy for SCID. Prevention of this so-called insertional mutagenesis requires the development of safety features.

SCID patients also were the subjects of the earliest clinical experiment in gene therapy 15 years ago in this country. At the National Institute of Health researchers inserted a normal copy of the broken gene into two girls' white blood cells. Since then the girls have done better than would have been predicted but the result was ambiguous since the girls also received a new drug treatment that could be helping. The successful Italian and English trials, however, seem to be conclusive.

Nonetheless, in spite of positive results in animals, clinical trials of gene therapy in patients so far have largely failed or produced equivocal results. In a clinical trial at the University of Pennsylvania, an 18-year-old male volunteer died from a reaction to the gene therapy. It may have caused other deaths as well.

As a result most gene therapy trials were shut down while scientists went back to the laboratory to do more research. The FDA and NIH found that some investigators had not been following the rules to protect subjects and took steps to enforce compliance. Eventually, clinical trials resumed.

More than 100 protocols for clinical trials have been approved by the Recombinant DNA Advisory Committee and the FDA. These include 56 protocols for cancer therapy, some for cystic fibrosis and AIDS and several for Gaucher's disease, familial hypercholesterolemia and rheumatoid arthritis. Some of these trials are ongoing but don't expect early or dramatic results. We have much to learn about the basic principles involved. Most of the positive results of gene therapy so far are anecdotal experiences, representing a few individuals who were not in recognized clinical trials. The FDA will not approve a drug or treatment for general use in patients unless it has undergone clinical trials (Chapter 55).

We can alter an abnormal gene producing a disease in two ways. We can add normal genes to the cells hoping the new genes will take over from the abnormal genes or transfer genes directly to an organ. We can also promote DNA repair by stimulating cells' natural restorative power. The body, however, may suppress gene expressions or destroy them. It is difficult to get genes into the millions of cells where they are needed.

Gene therapy for cancer requires a different approach. Genes could be introduced which make malignant cells susceptible to antiviral drugs. This is under evaluation in patients with brain tumors. Another approach induces malignant cells to destroy themselves by a process called apoptosis. Such trials have aroused great expectations.

Initial trials in hemophilia are encouraging as do some with immune deficiency diseases. A gene for Factor IX, defective in hemophilia, was given in a virus vector to six hemophiliacs, reducing the number of injections of Factor IX they required. In-utero gene therapy will be evaluated in animals. More work is needed.

Some researchers, even though based in medical schools, have started commercial companies or receive support from them. This is a serious conflict of interest. A scientist involved with a company conducting a clinical trial should not take part in the trial.

One alternative to gene therapy is to inject cells from similar normal tissues into damaged tissue. This has been done in a few patients with dead heart muscle after a myocardial infarction (heart attack) by injecting normal muscle cells from the leg.

Additional information can be obtained from:

National Center for Biotechnology Information. Online Mendelian Inheritance in Man. *www.ncbi.nlm.gov/omim/*.
The National Human Genome Research Institute, *www.nhgri.nih.gov.*
Celera Genomics—*www.celera.com*
A visual progress report on the federal effort. *www.ncbi.nlm.nih.gov/genome/seq*
Articles, graphics and primers about decoding of the human genome—*www.nytimes.com/genome.*

64. What is cloning? Is it ethical? What about cloning people? What's wrong with using human embryo tissue in research? What are stem cells? Is it ethical to do research on them? What is genetic engineering? Are genetically modified foods safe? Isn't that a health problem?

What is cloning? Is it ethical?

In animals, cloning, or reproductive cloning, is the development of a new animal with cells genetically identical to those of a single parent. DNA cloning is the production of many identical copies of a specific DNA fragment, for use in genetics. Therapeutic cloning, or "embryo cloning," is the production of human embryos to harvest stem cells for use in research. Of the different types of cloning, however, for most people the term means the reproductive cloning technology that created the famous lamb Dolly, cloned from cells of the mother's mammary gland and born in 1997 in Edinburgh, Scotland, in Dr. Ian Wilmut's laboratory.

Cloning is not easy. Dolly's birth was the single success out of 276 attempts in Wilmut's laboratory. In fact, so extraordinary was that success that initially its legitimacy was questioned because no one was able to repeat it. Then in 1999 Dr. XianqzhongYang, at the University of Connecticut, reported the birth of a calf, Amy, cloned from cells removed from the mother's ear, the first such cloning in this country.

Dolly was the first mammal cloned from the cell of an adult animal, rather than from embryonic cells. David Healey has described the sequence of events for Dolly:

> "Nuclear transfer from an adult cell to an enucleated oocyte (egg) after the adult nucleus had been 'starved' into the Go phase of its cell cycle; reprogramming of the nuclear DNA in its new environment activates cell cycles (electrical pulses and other conditions were not fully described) to initiate division as if the oocyte were a fertilized egg. Cell division and development of the activated bioengineered oocyte occurs as an embryo (a blastocyst)— not as differentiated mammary tissue. Implantation of the blastocyst into a ready uterus was done (using established technology of *in-vitro* fertilization) for growth into a fetus and then an adult."

Since the creation of Dolly, cloning has been done hundreds of times in animals. Sheep, cows, goats, chickens, rabbits, mice, dogs, cats, and now pigs and even a few nonhuman primates—monkeys—have been cloned. Pigs are an interesting subject because their organs resemble those of humans so closely that their tissues or organs could be used for transplants in patients (called xenotransplanation—from one species to another). Before that happens, however, genetic changes must be produced to eliminate the rapid rejection of an organ from another species. Means must also be found to prevent the transfer of the pig endogenous retrovirus to patients.

Wilmut sees enormous hurdles before cloning becomes practical, much less profitable. Many people argue that this research is expensive, takes a long time with many failures and provides no immediate use or applicability. Also, cloned animals often don't do well. Millie, a cloned cow, died at nine months of age. However, others have produced calves, and Dolly a lamb.

Cloning of animals doesn't pose ethical problems for most people. They don't object to production of better cows for more milk to nourish the world or genetically modified pigs to provide organs for transplantation. According to C. Cho et al., "it does not violate any fundamental moral precepts or boundaries but does raise questions." How about trying to clone a favorite pet or a dead child? South Korean scientists have now cloned some 30 human embryos and grown them in the laboratory for a week to extract stem cells for further research. They did not implant the cloned embryos in uteri

What about cloning people? Is that ethical?

Most of us-doctors, scientists, lay people-believe it is not ethical to clone people now, if ever, on moral and religious grounds. Wilmut, the pioneer in the field of animal reproductive cloning, is opposed to human reproductive cloning. First, it would be a long difficult process with many failures. We should not subject human tissue to such failures. Richard Seed, a physicist, made headlines by announcing he was going to clone people, but I believe he is a publicity-seeking phony. Healey describes Seed's position as "Kevorkian-like disdain of the social and ethical concerns" of many people.

In a review of ethical issues of human cloning, Hessel Bouma III gives reasons why it might ever be considered: to provide an alternative assisted-reproductive technique for the childless or infertile couple, production of tissues and organs for transplantation, or a copy of a particularly desirable person such as Albert Einstein or Elvis Presley. Set against these are the problems of safety, loss of embryonic or fetal tissue, the loss of human dignity, diminished individuality, altered sense of family, the moral status of the unborn and fetal tissue, and total opposition from Judeo-Christian religions and perhaps others as well.

In 2005 the UN voted to approve a *non-binding* ban on both reproductive and therapeutic human cloning, used for embryonic stem-cell research. This was a compromise after two years of debate. Over 60 countries, including the US, wanted a binding ban on both kinds of human cloning while over 20 other countries, led by Belgium, wanted to proscribe only reproductive cloning. With a non-binding ban, stem-cell research may continue. Theoretically, reproductive human cloning might also proceed, but in fact Britain and all European countries banned the practice on their own. Now is the time for the U.S. to do the same.

In spite of the opposition, Dr. Inda Verma of the Salk Institute said, "If something can be done, people will do it." The world has seen a long history of eugenics proposals to better the human race by getting rid of alcoholism, feeblemindedness, criminality and other unacceptable traits. The Nazi eugenics program of race laws, enforced sterilization, and selective euthanasia was a shocking example. We are reminded of Aldous Huxley's 1932 novel *Brave New World* in which fertilized human eggs are cloned and shocked to produce members of the three lower castes, the gammas, deltas and epsilons, with lower intelligence and smaller size than that of the alphas and betas—a terrifying society where genetic manipulation is the norm.

England granted patent rights for human embryos to a U.S. company. I doubt if this will hold up. A private company, Clonaid, announced it will clone a person after receiving $500,000 from a couple to clone their dead infant. Can anyone do anything they wish? Fertility experts, Severino Antinori in Rome, Panayiotis Zavos in Lexington, KY, and Ben Abraham in Israel have drawn widespread condemnation from the scientific community in announcing they will clone a person in Israel or an Arab nation. Dr. Rudolph Jaenisch, of the Whitehead Institute, Cambridge, MA, said: "They want to use humans as guinea pigs and this is absolutely preposterous." The National Bioethics Advisory Commission (NBAC) has reported that human cloning is "morally unacceptable."

Why study embryos? What are stem cells?

Stem cells come primarily from embryos and can grow into any form of specialized cells and thus serve as a valuable source of transplant or repair tissues. Two types of cells from embryos are being studied, human embryonic stem cells (ESC) and embryonic germ cells (EGC).

The AAMC has provided this description of the production of embryonic stem cells: "Somatic Cell Nuclear Transfer (SCNT) or therapeutic cloning involves removing the nucleus of an unfertilized egg cell, replacing it with the material from the nucleus of a "somatic cell" (a skin, heart, or nerve cell, for example), and stimulating this cell to begin dividing. Once the cell begins dividing, stem cells can be extracted 5-6 days later and used for research." Many scientists believe SCNT should be allowed.

Excess fertilized eggs from fertility clinics are another source of embryonic stem cells. In-vitro fertilization requires fertilization of more eggs than might be implanted in the uterus of the mother-to-be. Those remaining are kept frozen at a charge for use in case the couple wants more children. If they do not, the embryos are destroyed but, if the couple approves, they could be donated to a laboratory for research instead. Many couples are donating unused eggs. Many of us believe this is ethical because the embryo cannot live on its own to become a person and if thawed out will live only two days anyway.

Research on embryonic stem cells offers important possibilities for treatment of human disease. They include growing nerve cells to treat spinal cord injuries; brain cells for Alzheimer's disease and stroke; glial cells from nerves for multiple sclerosis; pancreatic islet insulin-producing cells for diabetes; skeletal muscle cells for muscular dystrophy; cartilage cells for osteoarthritis; bone cells for osteoporosis; heart muscle cells for heart attacks, heart failure and heart valves; blood cells for cancer, leukemia, and other blood diseases; liver cells for cirrhosis and hepatitis; skin cells for burns; and eye cells for macular degeneration and the cornea. Aggressive lymphomas have now been treated in patients with high dose chemotherapy and stem cell support.

Adult stem cells have been used for over 40 years with bone marrow transplantation to stimulate development of blood cells. Bone marrow and umbilical cord blood transplantation has been used with some success in patients with various malignancies, including leukemia. Injection of bone marrow into the heart muscle of patients with severe coronary artery disease and heart failure has led to some improvement in their condition.

It was thought tissues other than bone marrow did not have undifferentiated stem cells capable of both self-renewal and differentiation into one or more mature cell types. Now brain and muscle have been found to contain stem cells, and other tissues may contain them as well. Adult stem cells, however, may not possess the capabilities or usefulness of embryo stem cells. They are harder to grow and may not grow into all kinds of tissues.

In 2001 President Bush announced he would allow the Federal Government to fund stem cell research but would limit the research to some 60 to 64 ESC lines established or currently available, as identified by the NIH. No embryos could be used. The NIH, however, seriously overestimated the supply. Knowledgeable scientists say only 34, and not 64, cell lines may be available, ready and viable for research. Other lines are immature, premature or unavailable. The Swedes say they don't have as many established cell lines as the NIH said they have. A number of key lawmakers are saying President Bush's policy is too restrictive and will limit valuable research. The debate on this subject by the White House, the Congress, the National Bioethics Advisory Committee, and many others in society is not over.

Meanwhile, private laboratories are developing stem cells from embryos. Seventeen new human embryonic stem cell lines have been developed by Cowan, et al., in private laboratories without NIH support. In 2004 voters in California approved a ballot measure to spend $3 billion on stem-cell research, and the New Jersey ballot for the 2005 may include a bond measure for $230 million for such research. The AAMC supports on-going research into SCNT and has endorsed legislation that would allow such research to flourish.

Many of the present stem cell lines have been patented by the Geron Company. Investigators would have to buy these lines from the company. The science, technology, and ethics of stem cells were reviewed in a series of articles in *Science*, volume 287, page 1417-1446 in 2000. Harold T. Shapiro, former chairman of the NBAC and President Emeritus of Princeton University, calls for national and local oversight of human stem cell research. This recommendation is critical with the emergence of web sites that auction human ovarian eggs.

What's wrong with using human embryo tissue in scientific research?

"Surely every medicine is an innovation, and he that will not apply new remedies must expect new evils."

Francis Bacon (1561-1626)

Some people believe that it is wrong to destroy a living embryo to get cells and oppose all research on human embryos. Shapiro said "For those who believe that the embryo has the moral status of a person from the moment of conception, any activity that would destroy an embryo is unthinkable."The late Pope John Paul II was the leading proponent of that point of view. He said, "A free and virtuous society, which America aspires to be, must reject practices that devalue and violate human life at any stage from conception to natural death."

The United States is, however, an ethically and religiously pluralistic country. Some Jewish and Protestant Christian groups have spoken in favor of embryonic stem cell research. Michael Kinsley said, "Are we really going to start basing social policy on the assumption that a few embryonic cells equal a human being?" Robertson, in debating the pros and cons of stem cell research, says, as quoted by M. J. Friedrich, the "early embryo lacks capacity to be born, lacks capacity to have interests and, destroying it to get cells does not harm it or wrong it in any way." The U.S. Constitution provides no grounds for recognizing fertilized eggs or early embryos as persons.

What is genetic engineering?

Isn't that a problem for health? Are genetically modified foods (GMF) safe?

For well over a century, since the time of Gregor Mendel, Luther Burbank and William Beal, crops and plants have been improved by making genetic changes in plant breeding, or hybridization, resulting in higher yields and better resistance to insects, viruses and fungi. Traditional breeding methods, although slow, still yield dividends such as new corn developed by Dr. Evangelina Villegas and Dr. Surinder K. Vasal in Mexico that boosts harvests with more essential amino acids. Hybridization has never been controversial.

During the last 25 years, scientists have developed a new technology that is really no different from conventional techniques of plant breeding but is more precise and controllable.

They have learned how to move genes from one species to another. DNA from a donor plant is removed from cell nuclei, purified and treated with enzymes to break it into small fragments of a single gene. These copies are introduced into the DNA of a plant or animal which, as it multiples and grows, will exhibit a new trait. Tinkering with a crop's own genes may work as well as introducing foreign genes.

Such genetic engineering is used all the time to produce medicines: insulin, growth hormone, vaccines, antibodies, and antihemophilic factor, among others. Now it is used extensively in the "green revolution" in agriculture. In 1998, about 45 million acres of farm land in the world were planted with genetically engineered crops. The FDA approved genetically altered corn, potatoes, soybeans, squash, tomatoes and canola oil, called transgenic crops or genetically modified (GM) foods. Transgenic pest-protected plants reduce the use of chemical insecticides. Most soybean crops contain a gene that make them resistant to an herbicide used to control weeds. Hybrid rice with greatly increased yields and more pro-vitamin A, or beta carotene that could greatly alleviate starvation in the world is undergoing evaluation in China, India and the Philippines. Three billion people eat rice daily, most of them dependant on it for food.

The potential for GM crops is enormous. They are the answer to feeding the world with crops that resist infection, use nutrients more efficiently, are easier to cultivate and produce higher yields, according to Peter Raven, Director of the Missouri Botanical Gardens in St. Louis. He describes them as the sustainable agriculture friendlier to the environment.

According to Brown, the public seems unaware of GM crop potential value. He cites a recent survey that only 8 percent of respondents thought they would help feed the poor and hungry whereas 73% were in favor of such foods if they reduced pesticide use.

Are genetically modified foods safe? Isn't it a health problem?

In spite of all the publicity and opposition to GM foods, particularly in Europe, these foods are safe. Jane Henney, former Commissioner of the FDA, has said, "We have seen no evidence that bioengineered foods now on the market pose any human health concerns or are in any way less safe than crops produced through traditional breeding." She went on, "If a bioengineered food is significantly different from its conventional counterpart—if the nutritional value changes or it causes allergies—it must be labeled to indicate that difference." She believes the health of the American public is well protected by current laws and procedures through the FDA, the U.S. Department of Agriculture, and the EPA.

Why, then, is there so much opposition?

Opposition to GM foods is greatest in Europe and has spread to countries that need more food, such as India and the Philippine Islands. Part of the reason for it is fear and panic about new technology, aversion to change and the tendency to quickly conclude that something is good or bad, safe or dangerous. GM foods do involve the potential hazard of spreading new allergens. Controls are needed but so far there is no reason for fear.

Some have called GM foods "Frankenfoods," and Greenpeace has set the goal of a moratorium against all such foods and plants. Their goal is not to inform but to eliminate biotech foods completely—a very shortsighted approach that would harm the poor and starving of the world as in Africa, which seems to be getting poorer and hungrier. Some people believe the real target of opposition is multinational agriculture companies and their potential for worldwide monopolies. I agree that they are a problem but opposition to GM foods is not the answer.

A recent report of the NAS indicated GM foods are safe but this report led to more controversy. Barry Palevitz and Ricki Lewis describe the opposition particularly in Great Britain "to a combination of media catalyzed fear of the unknown and global sociopolitics." Many jokes about genetically modified foods describe outlandish products like odorless fish, caffeinated oranges (a perfect one-step breakfast), Viagra peas (he will never know), genome-specific salad dressing, ibuprofen tomatoes, boneless rabbit, and multi-vitamin lamb shank.

The National Academy of Sciences (NAS) says, "putting the brake on GM foods would be an enormous disservice to the vast majority of people in the world who are starving." Michael F. Jacobson notes that genetic engineering has cut pesticide use on cotton farms, reduced water pollution by toxic pesticides and increased yields of papayas, potatoes, rice and cotton, but must not be misused. He writes "there is no evidence that GM foods have harmed a single consumer or the environment." I agree. In all of my studies and reading I found no evidence that present GM foods are unsafe.

What is the answer to this controversy?

The answer is education—education of the public to the science and safety of GM foods, by public forums, responsible citizens groups and other forms of communication. The public may not be aware of the potential value of GM foods. Unfounded concern has arisen that weed control will eliminate food for birds and butterflies and introduce other ecological problems. Recently there was a big flack over unapproved biotech corn getting into some taco shells. The only thing it could have caused, in addition to a lot of publicity, was the possibility of a few allergic reactions. The question is whether consumer groups have done more harm than good on this issue.

For more information:

American Association for the Advancement of Science Report—Stem Cell Research: *www.aaas.org/spp/dspp/sfr//projects/stem*
NIH fact sheet on stem cell research: *www.nih.gov/news/pr/apr99/od-21.html*
Ethical issues in human stem cell research: www.bioethics.gov/pubs.html

Section L

Recommendations About Health

A HEALTHY LIFESTYLE, EXERCISE.

65. What is involved in a healthy lifestyle? How much exercise do I need?

A healthy lifestyle includes regular exercise, a healthy diet, weight control, stress control, avoidance of tobacco, moderate alcohol consumption, prevention of injury and a positive outlook. The *Harvard Health Letter* lists 17 things you can do today to enjoy better health tomorrow, among them: start an exercise program (strength training is ok); choose healthy foods; stay safe during a storm; eat more fish; make sure your vision is good; avoid preventable diseases like tetanus, influenza, and pneumococcal infection; keep your teeth intact; get rid of heartburn; eat five servings of fruits and vegetables a day; raise your good cholesterol; check for diabetes; plan to survive a heart attack by getting to a hospital within an hour; and visit the Harvard Health Publications website (*www.countway.harvard.edu/publications/ health-publications*).

Breslow says "great advances will occur when people fully realize the external physical environment has been replaced by personal behavior as the major influence on health. It is up to you and me." He cites the relationships between smoking and lung cancer; drinking and driving and fatal accidents; consumption of alcohol and cirrhosis of the liver; and overeating and coronary artery disease.

How much exercise do I need?

It is never too late to begin exercising. Some people think that if you didn't exercise when you were younger, it could be dangerous to start when you are older. This is not true unless you have an illness. You can benefit greatly from regular exercise. Exercise can help you lose fat, preserve muscle and keep off excess weight after you lose it. It can also help you sleep, reduce the risk of gall stones, colon cancer, diverticular disease, arthritis, anxiety, depression, heart disease, diabetes, osteoporosis, falls and fractures. It can help reduce blood pressure and prostate trouble in men.

Encouraging everyone, particularly the elderly, to walk will benefit their health. Moderate exercise may help decrease the incidence of breast, uterine and ovarian cancer by reducing estrogen levels, although the evidence for this is suggestive and not well established. Hu et al found walking reduced the risk in women of stroke and coronary heart disease. Hakim et al found in older, nonsmoking, retired, physically capable men, regular walking was associated with a lower mortality rate. Jogging is not necessary and can be bad for your knees.

Blair et al found in 9,777 men that those who maintained or improved their physical fitness were less likely to die from all causes particularly cardiovascular disease than unfit men who did not exercise. According to Myers et al, exercise capacity is a more powerful predictor of mortality among men than other risk factors.

Moderate exercise contributes to a healthier life but vigorous exercise is better if you can do it. It takes vigorous exercise to help you live longer. While Paffenbarger found fewer cases of colon cancer in 17,900 Harvard alumni who exercised at a moderate to high level than in their less active classmates, only vigorous exercise reduced the risk of dying during the study period. The study described vigorous activity as walking four to five miles an hour for 45 minutes five times/week, playing one hour of tennis singles three times/week, or swimming laps for three hours, cycling for one hour four times/week, jogging six or seven miles an hour for three hours/week or rollerblading for two and a half hours/week. In women vigorous walking and exercise reduces the risk of type 2 diabetes and of osteoporotic fractures from falling. Exercise is also good for people with arthritis. Arthritis should not reduce your activities.

Aerobic exercise such as walking, running, cycling, cross-country skiing, dancing, rope skipping, rowing, stair climbing, swimming, or skating are all good for cardiovascular fitness and muscle tone.

Vigorous exercise can involve risks. We read about athletes dying after vigorous exercise from heart problems. This is called the paradox of exercise. It is good for you but the consequences can be severe if you overdo. If you have been sedentary, see your doctor before you begin, get an ECG, a stress test if you can, and begin slowly. Walk once around the block, then twice around and each week increase the distance and listen to your body. Stop and get help if anything bothers you.

Guidelines from the Harvard *Men's Health Watch* include: get a medical checkup before beginning a formal exercise program, make exercise a part of daily life, make aerobic exercise a priority, warm up first, use strength training, do it regularly and safely, listen to your body and watch for warning signs like chest pain or pressure, shortness of breath, or lightheadedness. Comparable studies, reports and recommendations have now been made for women. The NIH and CDCP developed guidelines on exercise from a Consensus Development Panel on Physical Activity and Cardiovascular Health published in JAMA in 1996, volume 273, pages 241-246. Check out the Surgeon General's Report on physical activity and health at *www.cdc.gov/nccdphp/sgr/ sgr.htm.*

As described in the *Harvard Health Letter*, resistance exercise strengthens muscles and limbs. Weight training can also be good for you. Exercises for the back, arms, chest, abdomen, hips and legs are easy. For the your abdomen, do a partial curl-up, arms folded, knees facing the ceiling with legs pulled up and elbows touching the knees. This is better for your back than sit-ups or leg-raising while you are lying down. Knee extensions while sitting, lateral leg-raises while standing, hip extension by bending over a chair and heel raises and dips are good. On the other hand deep knee bends, toe touching, leg lifts and sit-ups can be harmful. Stretching before any exercise helps to reduce injuries.

USA TODAY (January 6, 2004) recommends 10 ways to increase physical activity: 1) practice random acts of exercise, 2) move your exercise spaces to where you spend the most time, 3) think of the TV as an activity box, 4) aim to burn 150 calories or more—walking two miles, 5) work in some walking, 6) keep an exercise log, 7) count every step, 8) coach yourself fit—kids teams, etc., 9) play at it with kids and neighbors, 10) walk for convenience.

RELIABLE INFORMATION—A HEALTHY DIET.

66. Where can I get good, reliable information about foodstuffs and diet? What is a healthy diet? Does the public receive information about food that is not true?

One swears by whole meal bread, one by sour milk; vegetarianism is the only road to salvation of some, others insist not only on vegetables alone, but on eating those raw. At one time the only thing that matters is calories; at another time they are crazy about vitamins or about roughage. The scientific truth may be put quite briefly; eat moderately, having an ordinary mixed diet, and don't worry.

Sir Robert Hutchison (1871-1960)
Quoted in JAMA 2000; 284:1533

Hardly a day goes by without an article in the news about dieting, foods, and obesity. As Americans grow fatter and fatter, diets proliferate because everyone wants to get into the act, develop their ideas, sell their books and earn big money. Jane Brody said, "Each time a diet resurfaces it captures the diet book dollars of gullible Americans. Indeed, you might forget buying lottery tickets, writing a diet book with a gimmick is a surer route to riches." The diet industry, comprising books, tapes, videos, pills, powders, spas, and various other programs, brings in as much as $37 billion a year.

My recommendations on diets begin with healthy dietary guidelines gathered from nutrition experts at the USDA and the DHHS, first published in 1980 and updated every five years since. Set forth in *The Wellness Book* by Benson with Stuart, (a Fireside book, by Simon & Schuster, New York), the guidelines are:

1. Eat a variety of foods, covering the four basic food groups.

    a. The milk group: Choose nonfat or low-fat products for calcium, protein, phosphorus and riboflavin. Watch total calories and fat. Eat several servings a day.
    b. Fruit and vegetable group: five servings a day recommended for Vitamin C, other vitamins and fiber.
    c. The grain group: cereals, bread, rice, noodles, millet, barley and oats. Six servings a day recommended as a source of complex carbohydrates (starch), vitamins, iron and fiber.
    d. The meat group: lean poultry, fish, shellfish, nuts, legumes, beans and tofu. Avoid red meat, fat from meat, saturated fatty acids and remove skin from poultry.

2. Maintain a healthy body weight. Check a weight/height table for your ideal weight. Ask your doctor or a dietitian for help—count your total calories. Keeping track for some days of your total intake of calories may help. Estimate this from food labels, the food you eat, and a calorie counter.

3. Select a low-fat, low saturated fat and low-cholesterol diet, with no fried foods or rich foods—no fried chicken, premium ice cream and pastries, bacon and spare ribs. Do not add fats to foods—no butter, margarine, mayonnaise or oils.

4. Eat plenty of vegetables, fruits and grain products.

5. Use sugar, salt and alcohol in moderation. Alcohol is high in calories. The Dietary Guidelines for Americans can be obtained from *www.health.gov/dietaryguidelines* or, for 50 cents, from Consumer Information Center, Department 3786, Pueblo, CO 81009.

For optimal nutrition the Physicians Committee for Responsible Medicine (PCRM) recommends concentrating on the whole grain, vegetable, fruit and legume food groups and eliminating meat, dairy products and fats. Dairy products may produce health problems in children; better sources of calcium include calcium-fortified orange juice, wheat flour, beans and tofu. The food pyramids for healthy Mediterranean and Asian diets limit meat to one serving a month, a healthy Latin American diet to one serving a week. A vegetarian diet contains no meat and eggs only weekly.

Most legitimate doctors, nutritionists and non-profit organizations will, in general, subscribe to the low fat, plant-based diets noted earlier. If you follow such a diet, limit your intake of calories, and exercise, you can lose weight. Limiting total caloric intake to less than you burn in your body is the only way to lose weight no matter what diet you use. The average adult, with normal activities, uses about 2,000 calories a day so the average diet allows for that amount. If you wish to lose weight, you must eat less, exercise more, or both. If you consume more calories than you use up in exercise, you will gain weight. There is no free ride.

Fat contains nine calories/gram and carbohydrates and proteins only four but a low fat diet in itself will not lead to weight loss without control of total calories. If you eat a low fat diet and substitute carbohydrates like sweets, you may gain weight.

The Ornish, Pritikin, Mediterranean and Dash diets (Dietary Approaches to Stop Hypertension) (Chapter 72), all center on fruits, vegetables and grains and in doing so can claim some success in preventive medicine. Dr. Dean Ornish, who runs the Preventive Medicine Research Institute in California, has written *Fat-Free Living, Reversing Heart Disease* and *Eat More and Weigh Less*. With exercise, his low-fat diet does offer protection against heart disease. Nathan Pritikin, founder of the Pritikin Longevity Center and Spa in California, is given credit for lowering cholesterol in people who follow his plant-based diet. The Mediterranean Diet, a good heart-healthy diet, is rich in fish with omega-3 fatty acids, fruits and vegetables. Olive and canola oils are the main fats.

The *Complete Scarsdale Medical Diet*, by cardiologist Herman Tarnower, offers this sound advice: "You will learn to eat better by eating less." He recommends a balanced diet with less fat and carbohydrates, reducing fat in your diet from 40%-50% to 23% and carbohydrates from 40%-50% to 34%, and increasing protein from 15% to 43%.

In all healthy diets, the portions are smaller, as Brody points out. When my wife and I go to a restaurant, the entrée often is more than I wish to eat, and we are often content to share an appetizer and an entrée. I suppose the restaurant thinks they cannot charge $20-$30 for an entrée unless it is a large portion, but often portions are too large. No restaurant is too fashionable for me to ask for a doggie bag. Some restaurant meals contain enough meat, bread and calories for an entire day. Allan Whaler, in the weight loss program at Green Mountain at Fox Run in Ludlow, VT, says: "When you learn to be satisfied with less, you really will be a success." *Volumetrics: Feel Full on Fewer Calories,* by Barbara Rolls, Ph.D., and Robert A. Barnett, explains how to maintain the amount of food you usually eat while lowering the "energy density," or number of calories in each portion. Soup at the beginning of a meal helps by producing a feeling of satiety that makes it easy to cut back on calories in the rest of the meal. Perhaps the French fondness for soup helps explain the "French Paradox:" that people who like to eat so much still manage to stay so thin.

Bran flakes are good with low fat milk as are berries, salsa and low-fat frozen desserts. Whole fruit will make you feel more satiated than will fruit juice. Water is better than sugar-sweetened soft drinks, which, although loaded with calories, quench thirst but do not satisfy hunger.

The Tufts Letter recommends Anne M. Fletcher's *Thin for Life* for ways to lose weight and keep it off. Andrew Weil's *Eating Well for Optimum Health* is a very good guide to food, diet and nutrition.

For his chronically overweight heart patients in the Miami Florida area, the cardiologist Dr. Arthur Agatston, developed the popular South Beach Diet which became a craze in Miami and then spread. Agatston describes the diet as not low carb or low fat but as limited to the right carbs and fats. South Beach dieters may lose 8 to 13 pounds in the first two weeks by following a very strict diet with no bread, rice, potatoes, pasta or baked goods; no candy, cake, cookies, ice cream or sugar; no beer or alcohol; and initially no fruit. Only fat free or low fat cheeses should be eaten. Boiled ham is okay, but not honey-baked ham. Avoid the bad fats, saturated and trans fats. Good fats are unsaturated, non-trans fats found in olive oil, canola oil, fish and nuts. Many people lost weight on this diet and swear by it.

Dr. Steven Pratt has written a book on superfoods, 14 in all. They include blueberries, pumpkin, wild salmon, soy, beans, broccoli, oats, oranges, spinach, tomatoes, turkey, walnuts, tea and yogurt. Certainly these are all generally healthy foods that won't hurt you. Whether they are super is another matter.

In the *New York Times Book of Health*, Jane Brody asks, "Can one diet help prevent heart disease, cancer, high blood pressure, obesity and diabetes? Will people eat it, enjoy it and leave the table satisfied?" She says the answer appears to be yes. Such a miracle diet is readily available in grocery stores, relatively low in fat, loaded with fruits, vegetables and grains, and two or three daily servings of low-fat or nonfat dairy products, modest amounts of lean meat and poultry, (two or fewer three ounce cooked servings a day), fish, dried beans, nuts and seeds (four to five servings a week). Brody sees no need for exotic foods, supplements, or herbal concoctions. Andrew Weil also gives sound advice about a healthy diet in his book *Spontaneous Healing*.

A vegetarian diet with little or no meat is very heart-healthy, producing no deficiencies of iron, protein or vitamin B12. Some studies show a longer life, heart benefits, lower cholesterol and hypertension and gallstones, better diabetes management and good bone building. Soy may prevent bone loss. A vegetarian diet must strike a proper balance among various fruits, vegetables, grains and legumes to provide enough calcium, minerals, protein and vitamins.

My recommendations on diet books definitely do *not* include *The New Diet Revolution,* by Robert C. Atkins, M.D. In the first chapter, he states "Almost all obesity exists for metabolic reasons. Most studies have shown the obese gain weight on fewer calories than people without a weight problem." I say the only reason this can happen is if they exercise less. Next he states "the problem with obesity is hyperinsulinism and insulin resistance." This could happen if you eat a lot of sugar and a lot of sweets. Next, he states "This metabolic defect involving insulin can be circumvented by restricting carbohydrates. When you restrict it, you avoid the foods that cause you to be fat."

Atkins is correct when he says a low fat diet is no good if you load up on carbohydrates. We would all agree with that. His 14-day diet restricts or severely limits carbohydrate intake and allows you to eat as much fat and protein as you wish. A diet of unlimited fats and protein, however, does not add up. Furthermore, the Atkins diet produces ketone bodies in the blood which, while decreasing your appetite, can make you slightly nauseated, lightheaded, and gassy and cause bad breath and body odor. This ketogenic diet poses other risks as well. His book provides no references to supporting evidence for his concept of hyperinsulinism and of more weight gain on fewer calories by obese people than by those who are not obese. Where is the evidence, Dr. Atkins? It seems to be baloney. I know of no scientific evidence for your theory. Jane Brody reviewed the Atkins diet in a *New York Times* column titled "Food, Calories and the First Law of Thermodynamics." The law holds that you can't lose more than you gain unless you exercise; energy taken in equals the energy used or the excess is stored as fat. She says Americans are flocking back to a high protein, high fat, low carbohydrate regimen that failed in the past. The idea that it is carbohydrates, not fat, that make people obese, was first put forward in 1863 by a London undertaker named William Banting and ". . . resurfaces periodically capturing the diet book dollars of gullible Americans." She indicates the low carbohydrate diet works if the carbohydrates you stop eating are cookies, candy, cake, donuts, french fries, pie, ice cream and a host of other high calorie favorites.

Dr. Jules Hirsh, an obesity specialist at the Rockefeller Institute quoted by Brody, states clearly that no diet allows you to eat "all you want" of anything and lose weight unless calories expended exceed calories consumed. Hirsch adds it makes no difference where the calories come from. Brody asks where are the people who have been on the Atkins diet for the 20 plus years since he published his first book *Diet Revolution*. Did they lose the desired amount of weight and keep it off? Were there any long-term ill effects? Atkins provides no evidence in answer to these questions.

I have searched references in Atkins' *New Diet Revolution* book and have found absolutely no mention of any evaluation of the thousands of patients he says he treated. He said millions lose weight and keep it off. Where are the records on them? Why were there no controlled trials? What are the statistics? Why no documentation of how many did or did not lose weight, keep it off and any side effects? The only reference in the book about clinical results is the clinical use of glutamine and clinical results at the Atkins Center. These results were not published in the scientific literature. As best as I can tell, the Atkins *New Diet Revolution* is all hype.

Atkins has a very cozy business. He has sold millions of books. His wife now takes people on cruises. He has "a gourmet chef" writing recipes for his Lo-Carb Program and now sells the Atkins Diet Advantage Bar, the Atkins Diet Shake Mix, the Atkins Diet Bake Mix, and new books the *Vita Nutrient Solution*, nature's answer to drugs, which is said to be a "definitive book on the tremendous value of vitamins, minerals, herbs, etc." and *The Atkins Essentials*. Atkins describes a program for lowering of cholesterol with lecithin granules, chromium, pantothen, niacin, B complex, garlic, vitamin C, borage, primrose or black currant oil, fish oil, and all sorts of other strange ingredients. On the other hand, his diet includes flan, which contains five eggs and cream, hardly consistent with an attempt to lower cholesterol if it is elevated. He calls his cholesterol-lowering essential oil formula, the Atkins Lipid Formula. Atkins is throwing everything, including the kitchen sink, into these formulas. Dr. Pamela Peeke from the University of Maryland Medical School appeared with him on Oprah Winfrey. By most accounts, she won the discussion. She says, "He is a rip-off".

The *Nutrition Action Healthletter*, published by the Center for Science in the Public Interest (CSPI) gave him the back of their hand. They approved of the following diet books: Barry Sears' *The Zone Diet*, *The Pritikin Principle*, *Dieting with the Duchess* (Sarah of York with Weight Watchers), Ron and Nancy Goor's *Choose to Lose*, Rolls' *Volumetrics Weight Control Plan: Feel Full on Fewer Calories*, and Ornish's *Eat More, Weigh Less* by. All of these promote diets that are low in calories and full of fruits and vegetables.

They found unacceptable, however, Dr. Atkins *New Diet Revolution* for endorsing a diet too high in saturated fats and too restrictive of healthy foods, like whole grains, beans, fruits, bananas, carrots. CSPI Director Michael Jacobson points out many of these diets have never been tested. Many people, citing public confusion about diets, urge the NIH to fund studies. The CSPI has asked Congress to ask the NIH to study obesity.

Two studies in the NEJM have compared low carbohydrate, Atkins diets and low fat diets. Both studies were small, many of the randomized subjects dropped out and follow-ups took place only six months in one and a year in the other. The low carbohydrate diet produced somewhat greater weight loss at six months but not at a year. The differences were small and the studies not definitive. Differences may be due to restriction of calories not reduction of carbohydrates.

When shopping for foods, look out for the real meanings of food labels. "Natural" does not necessarily mean the food is healthy. The label "light" or "lite" and/or "cholesterol free," may indicate an excess of other fats. The labels "lean," "diet" or "dietetic" usually means low sugar or sodium content. Look out for "sugar free" or "sugarless" foods; other sweeteners, honey or corn syrup may be used with equal or more calories. If the label says "no preservatives," see if it lists other additives, thickeners or emulsifiers. Beware of an ad for "a vegetable that kills pain, a fruit that gives you energy, a food that cures disease, a vitamin that improves your sex life and an herb that could be the fountain of youth." Problems such as acrylamide in foods are taken up in chapter 85.

Fast foods are *fat* foods; a burger and fries may give you 40% of calories from fat with a minimum of fiber and other nutrients. Eric Schlosser in *Fast Food Nation: The Dark Side of the All-American Meal*, describes unsanitary practices in the meatpacking industry that contaminate fast food burgers with *E. coli* and other pathogens. He deplores the pursuit of children by the fast-food industry, intruding into their lives while leaving them susceptible to obesity and disease. At the very least the fast food industry certainly has contributed to the obesity epidemic.

It is awful that McDonald's restaurants are open for business in some 30 hospitals, including, as reported by the *Washington Post* for December 14, 2004, children's hospitals in Los Angeles and Philadelphia. As reported by the *Post*, the Cleveland Clinic is among hospitals that have severed ties with fast food outlets. The celebrated heart clinic has succeeded in ousting Pizza Hut and is trying to do the same with McDonald's, a move that began after cardiology department chairman Eric Topol asked in a staff meeting how the clinic could in good conscience expose their patients to such unhealthful food.

"I can't tell you how many patients found this repulsive," said Dr. Topol. "How can the Cleveland Clinic, which prides itself on promoting health, have the audacity to have a McDonald's in the main lobby?"

In *Restaurant Confidential*, Michael F. Jacobson and Jayne Hurley of Center for Science in the Public Interest, describe the astounding fat, calorie and salt content of foods offered by favorite American restaurants, the "shocking truth about what you're really eating when you're eating out." Two slices of Pizza Hut stuffed crust pepperoni-lovers pizza contain 2700 mg of sodium, 18 grams of saturated fat, 42 grams of total fat, and 840 calories—wow! That's more than a day's supply of each of them. Think a chicken Caesar salad is perfect for your diet? Think again. It contains 46 grams of fat. Choose a tuna sandwich over the roast beef sandwich? Wrong! It contains four times the amount of fat and twice the amount of saturated fat. The $105 billion fast food industry is now facing a clamor for nutritious food. Salads are being added, burgers, fries, and sweet soft drinks may become dining-out dinosaurs.

Here are Ten Mega Trends in Diet and Health as noted by The *Nutrition Action Healthletter*: (1) the fattening of America—the increase in overweight and obese people; (2) a positive trend—progress in reducing heart attack and stroke rates by better diet, lower cholesterol and treatment of hypertension; (3) turning the tide on cancer—the trends of declining rates of lung, colon, breast and prostate cancer due to diet, physical activity and earlier detection;. (4) Serving-Size Spread—the more for your money theme of McDonalds; (5) a nation on drugs for hypertension and high cholesterol; (6) escalation in the use of dietary supplements, some good, but many not needed. (7) the mixed bag on food safety. While many foods are safe, epidemics of food poisoning caused by E. Coli, Campylobacter, Cyclospora and Salmonella still occur. Now a new strategy called Hazard Analysis and Critical Control Points (HACCP) may help prevent these. (8) eating out. More people eat out and in so doing eat foods with more fat, unsaturated fat, sodium, refined carbohydrates and calories and less calcium. Restaurants, offering large portions, also encourage overeating. (9) the problem of TV, computers, passive entertainment—couch potatoes and lack of exercise. (10 the food-marketing madness we all encounter.

Jacobson says "Twenty corporations pay for nearly three-quarters of all food advertising in the U.S. and spend it to promote highly processed foods soft drinks, cookies and convenience foods. The budget of the National Cancer Institute of $1 million/year to promote eating more fruits and vegetables is equal to what McDonalds spends every 12 hours to promote greasy burgers and fries." The advertising budget of McDonald's is $1 billion/year, that of Coca-Cola Co. $770 million, and that of General Mills $598 million. Giving the NIH more money to promote healthy eating goes against interests of the meat, dairy, soft drink, and fast foods industry. Is our government more responsive to big business than public health? It seems so.

Jacobson points out the hazards of criticizing food companies. He describes law suits filed against critics by big food companies. Texas ranchers sued Oprah Winfrey for saying she would never eat another hamburger. She has now spent about a million dollars in her defense. Many states have food-disparagement laws or "veggie-libel" laws to silence consumer groups. Do companies fear exposure of real health hazards? A campaign is being launched against these laws by CSPI with the American Civil Liberties Union.

Is diet important in health promotion and disease prevention?

You may improve your general health by following a low-fat, plant-based diet, taking plenty of exercise, and avoiding toxins like tobacco, excess alcohol, and industrial and environmental contamination. The PCRM says "Last year a million people left the same suicide note: "Shopping List: butter, eggs, mayo, potato chips, ham, bacon." A Surgeon General's Report on Nutrition and Health declared that of the over two million Americans who die each year, two-thirds of them die in part due to a poor diet. Foods containing saturated fat and dietary cholesterol cause heart disease, stroke, diabetes and even some cancers. Red meat should be avoided except in small portions no more than one to two times a week because of the saturated fat it contains. Even lean meat contains considerable saturated fat.

Caffeine, a drug that may affect many systems in your body, should be used in moderation. Brewed coffee contains more caffeine than instant coffee. All colas contain caffeine, and so does tea. A small amount of caffeine is fine but large amounts may interfere with a number of things in your life. A food may be low in calories but high in sodium. Pickles are an example, there being no such thing as a low-salt pickle

The risk of osteoporosis is decreased by use of calcium and vitamin D supplements. Some diet or supplements may reduce the risk of some cancers but the evidence is less certain. While we must be very careful about the evaluation of specific dietary items, the value of a healthy diet is undisputed.

Does the public receive information about food that is not true?

Even academic institutions can be compromised by money. That is why organizations like the CSPI are important. Unlike some special-interest organizations with names that make them sound altruistic, CSPI is truly independent, non-profit and dedicated to representing the interests of consumers.

CSPI 's *Nutrition Action Healthletter* accepts no advertising and no government or industry funding. Founded in 1971, CSPI advocates honest food labeling and advertising and promotes healthier foods for restaurants and policies for health-safe food additives. Their booklet "Healthy Foods" rates vegetables, fruits, beans, grains, meat and poultry and cereals for contents of sugar, saturated fats, vitamins, calories, minerals and fiber. I benefit from reading and using this health letter and recommend it to you. You may reach them at Suite 300, 1879 Connecticut Avenue NW, Washington, D.C. 20009-5728, 202-332-9110, www.cspinet.org.

In *Nutrition Action Healthletter,* Jacobson exposed the funding behind some high-sounding fronts in the food industry. The American Council on Science and Health says they are a "non-profit consumer education organization" but their funding comes from Pepsi Co., Coca-Cola, Dow, Exxon and others. Despite its objective-sounding name, the International Life Sciences Institute and the International Food Information Council gets its backing from big food companies. The American Dietetic Association publishes "nutrition fact sheets" that defended the fake fat Olestra, fast foods, starch-filled baby foods and sugar, giving it a clean bill of health. Sponsors were McDonald's, Proctor and Gamble, Gerber and the Canadian Sugar Institute. Georgetown University Center for Food and Nutrition Policy defended over-consumption of soft drinks and refined sugars as a partner of the Grocery Association of America and a recipient of grants from the Sugar Association. Jacobson cites other examples. There may be many more.

Another good source of independent information is the *Harvard Health Letter,* published by the Harvard Medical School in Boston (Harvard Medical School Publications, 164 Longwood Avenue, Boston, MA 02115, www.countway.harvard.edu/publications/).

The University of California Berkeley publishes a wellness letter on nutrition, fitness and stress management. Their outspoken assessment of a claim for a dieting supplement: "This claim is completely bogus." Address: 48 Shattuck Square, Suite 43, Berkeley, CA 94704-1140. The Tufts University *Diet and Nutrition Letter* (800-274-7581) is reliable. The Mayo Clinic and other medical schools and clinics also publish diet and health letters. (Chapter 56)

I also recommend *Health News,* published by the NEJM, and The American Diabetic Association's *Complete Food and Nutrition Guide.* Their hotline is 800-366-1655 and *www.eatright.org.*

PCRM offers excellent publications on food: the "Vegetarian Starter Kit," "Foods that Fight Pain," "The Medical Costs Attributable to Meat Consumption," "Racial Bias in Federal Nutrition Policy," "Eat Right, Live Longer and Food for Life." Contact information: 5100 Wisconsin Avenue, Suite 404, Washington, DC. 20016, (202)686-2210, fax (202)686-2216, *www.PCRM.ORG.*

Some excellent health-smart cookbooks:

1) *The American Heart Association Cookbook.* New York. David McKay Company, 1984.

2) *The American Heart Association Low-fat, Low-Cholesterol Cookbook.* New York: Times Books, 1989.

3) Brody, J. *Jane Brody's Good Food Book.* New York: Bantam Books, Inc.,1985.

4) Connor SL and Connor WE. *New American Diet.* New York: Simon and Schuster, 1986.

5) Goor R and N Goor. *Eater's Choice.* Boston: Houghton Mifflin Company, 1987.

Section M

Disease Prevention and Health Promotion

67. Is obesity really a big problem in the U.S.? Is it a genetic problem? How can I keep from getting fat? If I need to lose weight, how can I do it?

"You can't gain more weight than that of the food you eat"
Attributed to Calvin Trillin's father.

"Obesity, like smoking, kills," reads one headline. Obesity soon will surpass the use of tobacco as the top cause of preventable deaths in this country, partly the result of 30-year increase in caloric consumption, most of it carbohydrates, as reported by The Centers for Disease Control and Prevention (CDCP). It is estimated that some 300,000 US adults die each year of causes related to obesity. A study by HHS under Secretary Tommy Thompson showed a 33% increase in deaths due to excess weight over the past ten years. Without any doubt, most of the population is getting fatter. More than half of women and men in the U.S., 120 million people aged 20 and older, are now considered overweight and nearly one-quarter clinically obese, with an increased risk for heart disease, diabetes, and cancer. WHO and other officials have declared an epidemic of obesity in the U.S. and around the world, which is ironic since hundreds of millions of malnourished people don't get enough to eat to maintain health, much less enough to get fat.

Disease burdens associated with obesity include cardiovascular disease, type 2 diabetes, hypertension, stroke, high cholesterol, osteoarthritis, gallbladder disease and cancer. Up to half of the deaths from breast cancer in older women may be laid at the door of obesity. It contributes to high lipid levels, which are bad for your heart, blood pressure, and blood sugar and may contribute to early onset of diabetes. An epidemic of diabetes in children is clearly linked with obesity.

Eugenia Calle et al conclude the risk of death from all causes increases with both men and women of all ages who are moderately overweight and is higher still for those severely so. It is greater for whites than for blacks. Upper body obesity, particularly in the chest and abdomen, is more dangerous and more frequent in men than lower body obesity of hips and thighs, more common in women. Obesity and low cardio-respiratory fitness, as measured by a maximal exercise treadmill test, increased mortality in men. The Institute of Medicine (IOM) says fat people are costing citizens more than $70 billion annually in both direct health care costs and indirect ones, such as lost productivity.

What about just being pleasantly plump? In a report on the 2000+ men in the Framingham Heart Study by Robert Garrison and his National Heart, Lung and Blood Institute (NHLBI) colleagues, Garrison said "Being slightly overweight carries a risk for a lot of people. This has been found in other trials and studies as well." The evidence is clearcut that it's safer to be skinny.

Lowest mortality rates are found in women with Body Mass Indexes (BMI) less than 19. Your BMI is your weight in kilograms divided by the square of your height in meters. You may easily find your BMI by using the calculator on the website of the National Heart, Lung and Blood Institute (NHLBI) at *www.nhlbisupport.com.*

The BMI of the average US woman now is about 26. Risk of death increases 20% for BMIs from19 to 25; 60% for BMIs from 27 to 29; and more than 100% for BMIs of 29 and higher. Heart disease risks showed a similar trend in a health study by Dr. JoAnn Manson and colleagues of 10,000-15,000 young and middle-aged female nurses followed for 14 to 16 years. Ingrid Wickelgren in *Science* indicated the modern medical case against obesity began in 1959 when the Metropolitan Life Ins. Co. published tables based on hundreds of thousands of policyholders showing risks of premature death increased steadily as body weight increased above the so-called desirable weight. Desirable weight was 126 pounds (57 kg) for a 5'4" woman and 154 pounds (70 kg) for a 5'10" man. These are standards for leanness that 80% of American men and women do not meet.

Why has an obesity problem arisen now?

Environmental factors promote overeating. Dr. Kelly Brownell, a Professor of Psychology, Epidemiology and Public Health at Yale, believes the reason we are getting fatter is the pressure to eat. Food is available everywhere all of the time, and portions are larger. The fast food industry contributes immensely by pushing super portions and high fat foods, to children as well as adults. Food experts suspect childhood obesity starts with early consumption of hot dogs, sweetened sodas, french fries, pizza and candy.

Brownell asks whether Joe Camel was any different than Ronald McDonald in encouraging children to adopt habits bad for their health. Americans are being seduced by "our toxic food environment," he says, a diet high in fat and calories, delicious, widely available, and low in cost—foods that should be regarded as potential disease-causing agents like alcohol. In Brownell's opinion: "Junk food advertisements should be regulated and excise taxes imposed on high-fat foods just as on other toxic products." He says, "Don't blame Americans for being fat. Blame the American Dream. We've built our land off milk and honey and now it's doing us in."

Ali H. Mokdad et al say the spread of the obesity epidemic requires a higher public health policy for weight reduction and maintenance. Health care professionals who should be advising many obese patients to lose weight are failing to do so. As Americans export fast foods everywhere, WHO plans to try to regulate fast food advertising and promote healthy food. Nutrition experts recommend that the food industry stop bombarding children with junk fast foods and soft drinks; that fast food chains stop pushing large portions; that schools offer healthy food; that celebrities stop hawking fast foods; and that Disney stop using their cartoon characters to brand sugar foods.

Is obesity a genetic problem?

"It is not inconceivable to me that individuals who have greater conscious ability to consume less food might have slightly different neural circuitry or more powerful neural connections that might ultimately be visualized through mapping studies," said Jeffrey M. Friedman in a piece on the regions of the brain that control food intake, in the Howard Hughes Medical Institute (HHMI) newsletter.

In 1994, along with other HHMI investigators, Friedman discovered leptin, a protein that helps control weight by regulating appetite and energy expenditure and serves as the signal in a negative feedback loop. As BMI increases, leptin levels rise, telling the individual to stop or slow down on eating. Leptin levels tend to be high in obese and low in lean people, with considerable variation. In obese and lean mice leptin fusion decreases the desire to eat. The same result may be unlikely in obese people but clinical trials are underway.

Friedman explains: "A possibility is obesity results when the body is less responsive to leptin than normal." That might mean a failure of leptin to connect with the leptin-receptor neuropeptide Y from the GI tract, which jacks up appetite and slows metabolism. A deficiency of the fragment peptide yy3-36-pyy may contribute to obesity. Pro-opiomelanocortin (POMC) is a pre-cursor of beta-endorphin, a nervous system morphine-like substance, and alpha-melanocyte stimulating hormone (a-MSH) that affect food intake and fat storage. POMC gene deficient mice, so-called chubby mice, are obese, with altered skin color and little adrenal gland tissue. If a-MSH is injected they return to normal. Children identified with this gene abnormality are obese, have red hair and adrenal gland failure. Defective melanocortin 4 receptor genes are associated with binge eating and obesity.

Drugs to block Melanin-concentrating hormone (MCH) may be future candidates for anti-obesity drugs. A recently discovered hormone, ghrelin, may increase hunger. Rising before meal time and with weight loss, it is a potential target for appetite control. Another hormone, PYY3-36, from gut cells shuts down hunger feelings in rats. A number of these hormones may be inter-related and inter-reactive. The genetics of weight control is a complex subject and a great deal more is being learned. In the meanwhile, obese people should not wait for a shot or pill to cure their problem but go ahead with what is available to decrease risk of death from obesity. Increases in obesity in the last two decades can't be due solely to changes in genetic background.

How can I prevent obesity?

Inactivity and obesity go hand in hand. Increasing physical activity decreases the risk of various diseases, particularly heart disease. Seriously obese patients will live longer if they lose weight. For those with smaller increases in weight, the evidence is not as clear-cut so many experts believe that the best approach to obesity is to prevent it from happening in the first place. Health professionals, policymakers and the general public must recognize the serious threat of obesity to health and alter the environment to prevent it.

The NEJM editors J. P. Kassirer and M. Angel recommend prevention as the best public health approach to obesity. In "Losing Weight-An Ill-fated New Year's Resolution," they argue that attempts at weight loss are futile. They indicate, however, that progressive fattening of the population is not inevitable. Promotion of a healthier lifestyle, exercise and improved diet will go a long way towards decreasing the obesity epidemic. Kassirer says, "Preventive measures are better than beating on obese people who really can't do anything about it." The emphasis should be on avoidance of substantial weight gain during early adulthood. Exercise sociologist Glenn Gaesser of the U. of Virginia writes in NEJM, "We should heed one of Hippocrates' more insightful aphorisms: 'Do not allow the body to attain extreme thinness, for that too is treacherous, but bring it only to a condition that will naturally continue unchanged whatever that may be.'"

Unfortunately, many young children are obese now. In JAMA, Thomas N. Robinson raises the question: "Does television cause childhood obesity?" Studies suggest a significant correlation between obesity in children and television viewing, with snacks. Anderson et al also found a statistically significant correlation between adiposity and television viewing by children. Children need help with this.

Altering the environment to encourage behaviors to prevent obesity may seem an insurmountable challenge. Changing the environment to reduce cigarette smoking must have seemed equally insurmountable in the 1960s. The same is true with control of HIV. It will take a lot of work and government programs and education but it can be done. Many recommend a national war on obesity. How about work incentives to lose weight, cafeteria reforms, and taxes on fats like the attack on tobacco? Individual physicians can play a major role.

Should I be taking a dietary supplement to get rid of fat?

Anti-obesity drugs could take four possible forms: 1) appetite suppressors 2) inhibitors of fat absorption 3) enhancers of energy expenditure 4) stimulators of fat mobilization.

No available drugs enhance energy expenditure. All of the other agents involves some problems and potential side effects. Two dietary supplements already have been withdrawn from the market because of serious side effects: Fenfluramine or Fen-Fen, which damages heart valves, and Dexfenfluramine or Redux. The makers of these drugs may be forced to set up a trust fund of billions of dollars for damaged patients. The maker of Fat Trapper has had to refund $10 million to customers to settle deceptive advertising claims and add a disclosure that eating less or exercising more is necessary to lose weight. The FDA urges consumers to avoid Triax metabolic accelator.

The drug orlistat, or Xenical, reduces fat absorption by inhibiting the pancreatic enzyme lipase that breaks down large fats. Approved by the FDA, Xenical caused weight loss but also produced side effects of diarrhea and gas. Phentermine and sibutramine are still available as appetite suppressors. In some trials, sibutramine (Meridia) assisted in weight loss. Others seek its ban because they believe it has been associated with 29 deaths and other adverse events. In another clinical trial, an anti-epileptic drug, Zonisamide, may help with weight loss. Such drugs should be considered only in consultation and review with your physician.

Dietary supplements to get rid of fat probably won't help you any if at all and can be expensive. No pill or medicine can get rid of fat. Some dietary supplements are said to prevent storage of calories as fat, to bind with fat, to burn more calories or to put on muscle not fat. Evidence for all of these claims is either zero, limited or the result of inadequate studies. They cite no references but claim that doctors recommend them. Which doctors? Not this one! The FTC warns against weight loss scams. If it sounds too good to be true, they say, it's probably not true.

James Hill, Director for Nutrition at U. of Colorado Medical Center said of Fat Trapper and Exercise in a Bottle, "This ticks me off. They've taken a little bit of data and blown it way out of proportion." He is surprised the FTC has not stepped in. David Schardt of the *Nutrition Action Health Letter* said, "They have so exaggerated the research—the claims far exceed what the research shows and misrepresents the safety of the products." How about ads that say "lose weight while you sleep" or "melts away fat" or "revs up metabolism." RS-FIVE ads read "Eat all the foods you love and still lose weight (the pill does all the work)." You don't believe that, do you?

So-called fat burners include:

Ultra Burn all natural	Thin-Thin
Fat Burners	Hydroxy citric acid (citrimax-citrin)
All Natural weight loss plan	Fat trapper (Chitosan)
Super Fat Control	Conjugated linoleic acid
Pyruvate Punch	Ephedrine—Diet Fuel (may be dangerous)
Pyruvate C	Provate 1—Pyruvate
Thermogenic Ultra Lean	Cellasene—to remove cellulite
Fat Magnet	Exercise in a Bottle.

But as Dr. David Katz of Yale said, "We'll never find an ultimate solution to weight control in a pill bottle".

How can I lose weight?

There seem to be as many weight reduction books and diets as there are stars in the sky. *In Bottom Line Personal* Anne Fletcher, former Editor of the Tufts U. *Diet and Nutrition Letter* and author of a number of books about healthy eating, recommends drinking a glass of water before meals, kicking the red meat habit by thinking of meat as a condiment rather than as the main course, eating low-fat and fat-free foods, keeping track of what you eat and not letting exercise become boring.

Lawrence J. Cheskin, M.D., Director of the Johns Hopkins Weight Management Center, discusses the psychological reasons for eating too much in *Bottom Line Personal.* "Most people fail at dieting because they don't correct permanently the basic psychological behavior that leads to overeating," he says. He lists learned behaviors at fault: 1) Food as a comforter. "I am feeling lonely so I need to eat something." 2) Food as a stress reliever. "I am really busy at work and I don't have time or energy to eat healthy right now." 3) Food as reward. "I finished a project today. Let's have dinner and celebrate." 4) Food as boredom-reliever. "There is nothing to do so I'll just snack." 5) Food as social facilitator. "Sure I'll eat something if you are eating, too." 6) Food as habit. "It's 6:00 p.m. so I'll eat dinner even if I am not hungry."

Many are discouraged about weight loss because it is often futile. Many have extreme difficulty in taking off weight and then keeping it off. Remember the only way to do it is by reducing calorie intake or by engaging in physical activity at least 150 minutes or more a week or preferably both. The National Weight Control Registry monitors individuals who have successfully maintained weight reduction for at least a year, showing that it can be done.

More physicians are specializing in obesity and can help you. You may reach them through the Center for Obesity Research [CORE] in medical centers such as the U. of Colorado, U. of California at Los Angeles, Mayo Clinic, Minnesota Obesity Center, Northwestern U., Pennington Center in Baton Rouge, Beth Israel Deaconess in Boston and St. Lukes-Roosevelt in New York or through a medical school or large hospital in your community.

George Blackburn, M.D. of Beth-Israel Deaconess at Harvard is described as a five star general in the war against obesity. He emphasizes using encouragement, suggestions, empathy, compassion and respect to help obese patients. In reviewing fad diets, Katherine Greider reports that most fail in the long run because they abuse your body, are difficult to stick with for long and do not center on eating less and exercising more.

Bender et al. studied the effect of age on excessive mortality in obesity. Obesity-related excess mortality declined with age at all levels of obesity so beyond the age of 75 it was not an increased risk factor. My question for him is "How many obese people are alive at the age of 75?" I don't know many.

For families with obese children, nutritionists emphasize a family program. Don't single out or stigmatize the child; treat diet as a family problem. Cut back or eliminate sweet and salty items, fried foods, sweet beverages, and fast foods like burgers and fries. Prepare tasty meals with modest portions lower in calories and fat. Plan low calorie snacks: fruit and vegetables, low fat milk and ice cream. Parents must watch what children eat and encourage moderation. Encourage active play and decrease TV time. Help is available for kids at *www.eatright.org*, *www.committed-to-kids.com* and *www.cdc.gov/nccdphp/dnpa*.

Animal studies show that calorie restriction, 30% less than controls, increases longevity by 50%. Many studies have confirmed this finding. Studies of decreasing food intake in primates show a lowering of blood pressure and cholesterol levels. Hayflick argues, however, that it is not caloric restriction that increases longevity but ad lib feeding that decreases longevity. Anyway, animals that eat less live longer. Does this apply to humans? Who knows? I do know that very few obese people reach their 80s. Most elderly people are slim and trim.

For the morbidly obese, with life-threatening obesity, gastric stapling, banding or bypass banding can reduce the size of the upper stomach so the individual cannot eat as much and gets full faster. This bariatric surgery, also known as a duodenal switch, leads to considerable weight loss, a high cure rate of diabetes and sleep apnea, and improvement in hypertension and osteoarthritis. Gastric bypass reduces the biochemical markers of inflammation suggesting that obesity is an inflammatory condition. This procedure can now be done as a "minimal" operation (laparoscopy). It is referred to as bariatric surgery.

Advice to eat less begins with using a smaller plate, taking smaller portions, beginning with salad or soup in going from light to heavy, planning some 300 calorie meals, thinking in terms of the "b" words—boil, broil, barbecue, braise or bake—using cooking oil sparingly, eating lunch, curbing the urge to splurge, planning snacks, moving foods out of sight and cutting calories.

When dining out, take nutritionists' advice: 1) downsize your sandwich, 2) see red-tomatoes, 3) pass on the bread basket, 4) order soup then split an entree, 5) watch for clues of fattening foods in descriptions like batter, breaded, deep fried, etc., 6) order veggies, 7) wrap up any excess and take it home, 8) skip or split dessert, 9) order a kid's portion, 10) choose an appetizer for a main dish.

FAT—CHOLESTEROL

68. How much and what kind of fat should I eat? What is cholesterol and why is it important? Why is it bad? How can I lower my cholesterol? What are cholesterol-lowering drugs? What about eggs? What about sugar and chocolate? What about fast food or junk food?

Saturated fats include all animal fats from meat and dairy products and some highly saturated tropical plant oils like palm and coconut oil. Saturated animal fats like butter and lard are solid at room temperature. Unsaturated fats include oils from olives, peanuts, corn, soybeans and other plants, and, in general, are liquid at room temperature. Trans fatty acids or trans-unsaturated fats start out as liquid unsaturated vegetable oils but become solid after saturation through hydrogenation, a food-processing technique that produces soft substances for baking or spreading on toast. All fats are alike in comprising chains of carbon, hydrogen and oxygen atoms with a carboxyl group at one end (fatty acids) but they differ in the number of atoms, structure, and effect. Saturated fats contain the most hydrogen atoms.

Lipases break down fats in our intestines, and after absorption the resulting fatty acids are incorporated into cell membranes and adipose, or fat tissue, our body's insulation, cushion and energy reservoir. Fatty acids also carry the fat soluble vitamins A, E, D and K to be absorbed from foods. Dietary side effects vary greatly, however. Diets high in saturated fat and trans fatty acids increase the risk of coronary artery disease. Diets high in monosaturated fats and polyunsaturated fatty acids decrease that risk considerably. Modifying diet by lower fat intake is important to reduce the risk of heart disease.

Whenever possible, substitute safflower, corn and other such vegetable oils for butter. Cut down on other sources of saturated fats, including meat, cheese, ice cream, whole milk and cream, pizza and most cakes, pies and pastries, all regarded as primary bad actors in elevating cholesterol and the risk of heart disease. Better yet avoid these unhealthful foods altogether. Saturated and monounsaturated fats can be made in the human body and are not necessary in the diet.

Worst of all are trans fatty acids, which, although called polyunsaturated, actually contain more saturated fat than untreated saturated fats and are thus more harmful. Trans fatty acids are found in stick margarine and many other processed foods like salad dressing, sausages, microwave popcorn, ice cream, cakes, cookies, french fries, baking mixes, vegetable shortenings like Crisco and milk shakes. Hard stick margarine is worse than butter. Soft tub margarine is a little better as are semi-liquid margarines. Trans fats are the hidden killer responsible for thousands, perhaps tens of thousands, of deaths each year.

Choose fats that are healthful in reasonable amounts. They include monounsaturated or Omega 9 fatty acids in hybrid sunflower, hybrid safflower, canola and olive oils and Omega 6 fats in regular sunflower, regular safflower, corn, and soybean oils. Best of all are Omega 3 polyunsaturated fats in fish and vegetables. Omega-3s reduce inflammation, help maintain the lining of blood vessels and inhibit blood platelets to decrease risk of heart attacks. They may strengthen the immune system and reduce irregularities of the heartbeat. The Omega 6 and Omega 3 families include two essential fatty acids that the body cannot make: linoleic acid and alpha linolenic acid, respectively (polyunsaturated fatty acids or PUFAs). They are important in maintaining the membranes in the body and for making prostaglandins. You may obtain them from some of the above oils as well as fruits, vegetables, nuts and seeds.

What is cholesterol and why is it important?

Cholesterol is a fat that circulates in the body, transported in the blood plasma as a component of lipoproteins. It is synthesized in the liver and produced partly by the body but mostly absorbed from foods, primarily dairy products, egg yolks, meat (organ meat, fatty and prime cuts), poultry, especially the skin, and shellfish, especially shrimp. Closely related to homocysteine (Chapter 69), cholesterol is both good and bad. It is important in many body functions, in building and repairing cells, producing estrogen and testosterone, and aiding in the digestion of fat. But too much cholesterol can form plaques in arteries that produce arteriosclerosis, narrowing and blocking arteries to the heart and elsewhere. If total blocking of the vessels occurs suddenly, it will produce a heart attack. Elevated cholesterol is a major factor in coronary artery disease.

The density of lipoproteins indicates their cholesterol content, with the lower the density, the greater the fat content. Commonly known as the "bad cholesterol," low density lipoprotein (LDL) cholesterol causes arteriosclerosis by becoming oxidized by oxygen free radicals. The higher the LDL blood level, the greater the risk of coronary artery disease.

Three foods will elevate LDL cholesterol: saturated fat, transfat and cholesterol. Monounsaturated fatty acids like oleic acid, found in olive and canola oil, protect against LDL but linoleic acid, a major polyunsaturate, does not.

High density lipoprotein (HDL) lowers the risk of coronary artery disease. The *Harvard Health Letter* indicates that in its role as the "good cholesterol" HDL can be likened to a garbage collector that picks up cholesterol from blood vessels and delivers it to the liver where it is hauled away. Trans fatty acids like hard margarine reduce HDL.

Should I have my cholesterol checked?

It is a good idea to have it done, but not frequently. If you have heart disease, a family history of heart disease, lipid disorders, high blood pressure, or diabetes or if you smoke cigarettes, get a basic lipid profile. If it is normal, you don't need another one for five years. Routine testing in males 35 to 65 and women 45 to 65 is recommended by the American College of Physicians (ACP) but the American Heart Association (AHA) recommends beginning at age 20 in males.   ·

A baseline value will help you decide on your diet in conjunction with your doctor or a dietician or nutritional professional. The AHA recommends beginning a non-drug therapy program if your cholesterol is greater than 200 mg/dl, lowering your saturated fat intake to 7% or less of total calories and your cholesterol intake to less than 200 mg/day and losing weight if you are overweight. Engage in regular physical activity according to your fitness level. If your LDL is greater than 130 mg/dl, it is unlikely non-drug therapy will reduce it below 100; a cholesterol lowering drug may be necessary. The desirable or undesirable cholesterol numbers are shown in Table 1. The Harvard Health Letter (HHL) reports a normal level of 200 mg/dl may be too high for patients who have had heart attacks. (Table 1)

How can I lower my cholesterol?

The National Cholesterol Education Program, part of the National Heart, Lung and Blood Institute (NHLBI) recommends major effort by all of us to control or reduce our cholesterol or hyperlipidemia (hypercholesterolemia or hypertriglyceridemia or both). You may do so in three ways only: through diet, exercise and medication. Exercise daily (Chapter 65), maintain or go to an ideal body weight (Chapter 67), control hypertension and follow a diet low in saturated and trans-fats. With such a program you may not need cholesterol lowering medication. However, more and more studies include a statin drug to reduce the risk of heart disease and stroke.

Many reports describe lifestyle modifications that reduce the risk of heart disease and improve lipid values. These were effective in randomized clinical trials in patients with high blood lipids and other more normal individuals. About 35% of the decline in heart disease and deaths in the United States over the past two decades has been due to cholesterol reduction. The bottom line message is that it is important to reduce the risk of heart disease, stroke, and other health problems by avoiding fatty foods and those with saturated and trans fatty acids and reducing total fat intake. The benefits are great for patients without heart disease and are critical for patients with coronary artery disease and other arteriosclerotic manifestations. A moderate to low fat diet is better for your overall health and helps to prevent cancer and to decrease the risk of arteriosclerosis, coronary artery disease and heart attacks. An extremely low fat diet is only necessary if one has bad coronary artery disease. For everyone else the diet should include a maximum of 26% of dietary calories as fat, which means no fast foods and fat-rich delights.

Emphasize consumption of mono and polyunsaturated fats (omega 9, 6 and 3). Good evidence shows that omega-3 contributes to your health. Eat fewer animal products, drink skim milk and cut out packaged baked goods, snack foods, French fries and crackers while eating plenty of fruits, vegetables, whole grains and legumes. Avoid fried foods. Eggs are another problem. An egg yolk contains 220 mg of cholesterol so a low fat diet necessarily limits consumption of eggs. I no longer eat them, even though I love Eggs Benedict. A recent study suggested one egg a day has little impact on risk of heart disease in healthy men and women. Note the word "healthy." If you have high lipids, heart disease or a family history of heart disease, avoid them.

Look for salad dressings low in saturated fat, calories and sodium and for light cheeses with reduced total or saturated fat. Include in your diet soy bean oil, nuts, cereals and other fruits and vegetables containing plant sterol esters and stanol esters that block absorption of cholesterol from food and help reduce blood cholesterol levels. Benecol and Take Control are substitutes for butter and margarine but these "functional foods" may also lower blood levels of carotenoids which protect against cancer, heart disease and eye problems. Thus, be careful in their use (Table 2). A low fat diet such as the DASH diet (chapters 66) will lower blood pressure. An oat bran called Nu-triam lowers cholesterol due to B-glucans-soluble fibers. A recent prospective, double-blind, placebo controlled trial found no affect or benefit of garlic on cholesterol, contrary to popular belief. The Ornish, Pritikin and DASH diets are very low fat diets and are important for people with heart disease. The Mediterranean diet is low in fat but has a higher unsaturated fat content. (Chapter 66).

The fat substitute, Olestra, has been approved but has not caught on. Its efficacy and safety have not been adequately tested. It may cause abdominal cramping, gas, loose stools and anal leakage. It also takes with it vitamins and carotenoids.

What are cholesterol lowering drugs?

Evidence indicates that middle aged people with only slightly elevated cholesterol levels should, in addition to a diet and exercise program, take a cholesterol-lowering drug, or statin. Statins are taken once a day with few side effects. Over a half dozen are available, including Lovastatin (Mevacor), Simvastatin (Zocor), Atorvastatin (Lipitor), and Pravastatin (Pravachol).

Statins have revolutionized treatment of high cholesterol and heart disease with proven reduction of total cholesterol and LDL in well carried-out studies. Statin drugs reduce stroke risk in some studies by 29% and mortality by 22%. They may have anti-inflammatory actions. Recently, Lipitor has been found to lower death rates by 28% from all causes. Cholesterol drugs may ease the damage of Alzheimer's disease and help maintain and build bone in osteoporosis. Other statins available may be just as good but have not been compared to the older drugs and may vary in potency and ability to lower LDL. One statin, Baycol (cerivastatin), was taken off the market because it was associated with fatal muscle damage but that problem has not arisen with use of any of the other statins at usual doses.

For years investigators thought triglycerides did not influence heart disease risks; now, recent studies suggest high levels of triglycerides, the fatty acids absorbed from foods, may increase the risk of heart disease in women. Atorvastatin is known to also reduce triglycerides. Other statins may do that as well. If you are given medication to reduce cholesterol and LDL, have them checked periodically and keep in touch with your doctor.

After menopause, women's levels of LDL tend to increase while HDL decreases. Hormone replacement therapy may reverse this but statin drugs may be better. Be careful about agents or advertisements of drugs to reduce cholesterol other than statins. Check with your doctor. Some people have pushed recently to make statins over the counter drugs available without a prescription. An FDA panel rejected this because the drugs are not needed by many, are expensive and involve a few complications and side effects. The health guidelines of the National Cholesterol Education Program now recommend tighter control of cholesterol and more frequent use of the statins, a move that worries people whose health care premiums could be increased. Also, doctors worry that we will take pills rather than adopt healthy habits.

What about fast foods? Why are they bad?

The McDonalds, Burger Kings, Wendys and other drive-throughs serve exactly the opposite of a healthy diet. Their foods and drinks are high in calories, fats, saturated fats and salt. They are popular because the service is fast, the food inexpensive and the portions large, as in a Big Mac or a Whopper. Kids like the food and the gimmicks to hook kids like toys with a meal and playgrounds. Fast foods contribute to the epidemic of obesity and diabetes. In *Fast Food Nation*, Schlosser writes that "The executives who run the fast food industry are not bad men. They are businessmen. They will sell whatever sells at a profit." I have difficulty with the ethics of the fast food and tobacco industries. Their products are unhealthful. We are told we can refuse them, and we should.

Fast foods are a "mine field of fat and salt," according to Hurley. A double Whopper with cheese contains 1020 calories (a half day's requirement) with high sodium, saturated fat and cholesterol. A Big Mac contains 590 calories with high sodium, saturated fat and cholesterol. A large order of French fries at McDonald's contains 450 calories, 22 grams of fat, and salt. On the other hand, a baked potato contains 220 calories and is fat free. The huge advertising budgets of McDonalds ($1.1 Billion) Coca Cola ($866) dwarf the Government's efforts to promote healthy diets. Jacobson said, "For all practical purposes the American diet is determined by market forces, not health concerns." Recently, the fast-food places have introduced salads and some more healthy foods. They have a long way to go, however.

The HHL and the *Nutrition Action Health Letters* tell you how much fat is in the fast foods of all the different chains. Calorie-counting books in your book store do the same.

What about sugar and chocolate?

Basic sugar is glucose in the blood produced by the breakdown of sugar and carbohydrates and used by body cells for food. White table sugar from sugar cane combines glucose with fructose, the sugar from vegetables, fruits and honey. Fructose and glucose are stored in the liver as glycogen. Lactose, the main sugar in milk, is glucose plus galactose. Starch is a series of glucose molecules forming polysaccharides.

The HHL recently asked, "Is sugar bad for you?" and replied, "After fat and cholesterol, nothing in our diet is as notorious as sugar. It rots our teeth. It makes us fat. American craving for sugar and starch has led to obesity and diabetes."

Too much sugar may cause diabetes by decreasing the ability of the pancreas to produce enough insulin and by contributing to insulin resistance in body cells. Sugar plays a major role in obesity by providing excess calories, encouraging overeating and not curbing appetite. A low fat diet won't help if you load up on sugar-carbohydrates. Sugar will squeeze more healthy foods out of the diet. The USDA recommends limiting added sugars to six teaspoons a day.

Refined or added sugars from sugar cane, sugar beets, corn and other sources add 20 teaspoons or more to the average diet each day. Added sugar is not included in Nutrition Fact Labels but should be so you know how much you are eating. Be careful of frozen desserts; go with low calorie, low fat yogurt, sorbet and sherbet, cookies and fruit bars. Even McDonalds now offers a low fat fruit and yogurt parfait.

Soft drinks and sweet baked goods are the biggest sugar culprits. Sweetened soda adds greatly to sugar intake. It is a trap because most people don't think of all the sugar calories in a large Coke at McDonalds. The Atkins low carbohydrate diet limits sugar intake but is effective only if you also limit total calories (Chapter 66).

Is chocolate good for me?

Supposedly, chocolate helps prevent cancer, protects the heart, doesn't make you fat and fits into a healthy diet. None of these claims are true. They cannot be proven. The Chocolate Manufacturers Association supports the idea that it is "a wonder food." Chocolate contains some antioxidants which are good but it is no health food. A "dose" of M&Ms contains 399 calories, 11 grams of saturated fat and 46 grams of sugar—all bad. The Consumer Reports on Health says, "It makes little sense to consume chocolate for its health benefits". Chocolate should be savored in moderation, as a treat for the taste buds, not for the heart. A craving for chocolate may occur because of hunger between meals. A piece of chocolate rapidly satisfies this, which Rolls says may reinforce the craving. I know of no evidence for chocolate addiction.

Table 1

Understanding the Numbers

Test	Desirable	Borderline	Undesirable
Total cholesterol	Below 200	200-240	Above 240
LDL cholesterol	Below 100	130	Above 130
HDL cholesterol	Above 40	35-45	Below 35-40
Triglycerides	Less than 150	200	Above 200

Levels given in milligrams per deciliter.
*From the Harvard Health Letter, January 1998, page 3.

Table 2

Fats

Good Fats	Found In	Good Fats	Health Effects
Monounsaturated fat	Olive oil, canola oil, olives cashews, almonds, avocados	Monoun	Lowers LDL, raises HDL — hints of protection against cancer — may be the effect of the Med. Diet
Polyunsaturated fats— Omega-3—essential fatty acids	fish, flexseed oil, walnuts, canola oil	Omega-3	— little effect on cholesterol — lowers risk of arrhythmias — lowers triglycerides (blood fats) — might help depression
Omega 6-fats	corn, soybean, and sunflower oils	Omega-6	— lowers LDL, raises HDL — may reduce risk for heart disease and diabetes
Bad Fats			
saturated fats	red meat, whole milk, cheese butter, ice cream, chocolate chocholate, poultry skin coconut and palm oil	Bad Fats Sat Fats	— raises LDL and HLD — modest increase in heart disease — ? prostate disease cancer
Worst Fats			
Trans fatty acids	many margarines, cookies crackers, fast foods, french fries, vegetable shortening— Crisco	Worst Trans.	— raises LDL—lowers HLD — Linked to an increased risk for heart disease

Harvard Health Letter, January 2004

Homocysteine

69. What is homocysteine and what does it have to do with arteriosclerosis?

Authorities once believed that arteriosclerosis was all due to cholesterol and not at all to homocysteine, an amino acid circulating in the blood and serving as a carrier of LDL (low density lipoprotein commonly known as bad cholesterol) as homocysteine aggregates. These aggregates are precursors of plaques in arteries, formed with cholesterol, and may damage the endothelium or lining of arteries and trigger an increase in smooth muscle cells, thereby promoting clogged arteries. Other complex mechanisms have been proposed.

When the pathologist Dr. Kilmer McCully threatened the belief in cholesterol as the sole source of arteriosclerosis by describing the role of increased homocysteine levels, he was told by Harvard Medical School and the Massachusetts General Hospital (MGH) that there was no place for him. He was virtually driven out of Boston. The NIH no longer gave him support. He came under a cloud and, even when he looked for jobs elsewhere, Harvard allegedly made poison phone calls. Finally, he became a pathologist at the Providence VA Medical Center in Providence, Rhode Island, where he remains.

Now, the true story of homocysteine has come out and its great importance in cardiovascular disease is recognized. Increased levels of homocysteine are associated with heart disease and stroke. Soon, measurement of homocysteine levels in older individuals will be routine. Only more than 30 years after his groundbreaking discoveries is McCully receiving the acclaim he is due.

In 1969 McCully reported on the occurrence of coronary artery disease in several children with homocystinuria, a congenital abnormality producing abnormal levels of homocysteine in the blood. McCully did other studies on the links between homocysteine, arteriosclerosis and coronary artery disease and the importance of folate or folic acid and vitamin B6 in preventing problems with homocysteine, all dismissed at the time.

McCully's sad experience as a pioneer indicates that many experts were so close to their own work they could not see the possibility of something new and different, particularly if not in agreement with their own theories. I have seen this many times in physicians and scientists. Moreover, cholesterol dominates the heart disease debate because it represents big money in cholesterol-lowering drugs for pharmaceutical companies. Thomas James said, "This multi-billion dollar industry has a huge stake in fanning the flames of cholesterol." The present chief of pathology at the MGH, Robert Colvin, indicates "McCully was so far advanced in his thinking about the biochemistry of arteriosclerosis and the NIH is not very good at funding really innovative or creative research. They are better at funding natural extensions of existing theories."

The easiest and best way to reduce homocysteine levels in the blood is to take folic acid (vitamin B-12) or pyridoxine (vitamin B-6). A daily intake of 400 micrograms of folate and 3 milligrams of vitamin B-6 is recommended to minimize cardiovascular mortality and morbidity. In a recent study in JAMA, Ridha Arem et al found that intake of folate and vitamin B6 above the recommended dietary allowance seems important in primary prevention of coronary heart disease in women. Some authorities recommend 1 to 2 milligrams per day of folic acid since it produces no side effects and costs very little.

Peter B. Berger, in the American College of Cardiology journal, says among patients with homocystinuria in whom the highest levels of homocysteine were found, vitamin therapy to lower homocysteine levels is the standard of care and is crucial to reduce morbidity and mortality from vascular complications. He adds, "Clinical trials are under way to demonstrate the effectiveness of lowering homocysteine on stroke and heart disease. Until such clinical trials are completed, definitive recommendations about the need to screen all patients and identify those with an elevated homocysteine are not possible." Increased homocysteine levels have been found in critically ill patients. The clinical significance of this change has not been determined.

Important natural sources of these B vitamins are leafy vegetables, dried beans, enriched whole grain cereal, orange juice, chicken liver, cooked broccoli, uncooked spinach, sweet potatoes, bread, peanuts, and strawberries. The FDA requires folic acid fortification in enriched foods such as breads, flours, pasta and rice and many of the breakfast cereal makers add folic acid to their products.

Folic acid also reduces the risk in the fetus of neural tube birth defects such as spina bifida, a disabling birth condition resulting from failure of the spinal cord to close. It *may* reduce the risk of colon cancer, a theory currently under investigation. Folic acid is needed for production, growth, and repair of cells throughout the body and for the formation of DNA, the genetic code that controls life. See Chapter 70 for references for folic acid and other vitamins.

SUPPLEMENTS

70. What is important about proteins, vitamins, minerals and antioxidants? Should I take supplements? If so, what kind?

What about proteins?

Among other important functions, proteins serve as the structural components of the body in bones, muscle, and other tissues; in their role as enzymes they carry out chemical reactions in cells; and as antibodies they protect the body against infection. These large molecules comprise hundreds of amino acids in some 100,000 different complex folded or twisted structures. They contain nitrogen, which distinguishes them from fat and carbohydrates.

Unlike fats and carbohydrates which are stored in the body, fats as triglycerides in fat tissue and carbohydrates as glycogen in muscle and liver, proteins have no stores. All proteins turn over daily, breaking down and rebuilding. Of the twenty different kinds of amino acids, the body can make eleven; you must obtain the other nine from food. The average person loses about an ounce of protein a day and should consume two ounces. Dietary protein should amount to about 15% of total daily calories.

The typical American, however, consumes more protein than needed, particularly from meat and dairy foods. Nuts, legumes, poultry, and fish are, on balance, more healthful sources of protein, and a vegetarian diet can provide all you need, in nuts and legumes. The medical costs attributable each year to meat consumption come to billions of dollars. Savor a steak only now and then. Vegetarians are healthier.

The Atkins' high protein, low carbohydrate diet is not healthful.

Vitamins, minerals, antioxidants. What should I eat?

Vitamins help enzymes release usable energy from the breakdown of proteins, carbohydrates and fats but, unlike those foodstuffs, provide no energy on their own. Your body benefits from functions of the following vitamins: beta carotene, biotin, folic acid, niacin, pantothenic acid, riboflavin, thiamin, Vitamins A, B_6, B_{12}, C, D, E and K. Unable to produce vitamins itself, your body must obtain them from food, where they are widely available.

Vitamin C, E, and beta-carotene are anti-oxidants, needed to decrease the likelihood of arteriosclerosis and other degenerative diseases. Vitamin C, ascorbic acid, plays an important role in a number of body functions, including the provision of immunity. It is no wonder drug, however. It may moderate symptoms of colds but does not prevent them. It may decrease GI inflammation but does not prevent cancer. Some people take 1000 to 2000 mg/day for its antioxidant effect but unnecessary mega doses like those either go unabsorbed or cause iron overload or kidney stones. The Recommended Daily Allowance (RDA) was 60 mg/day now raised to 90 mg/day for men and 75 mg/day for women. Ample amounts are found in fruits and vegetables.

Vitamin E, or alpha tocopherol, is of critical importance. Deficiencies are unusual but if present cause anemia, fragile red blood cells and neurological abnormalities. Besides helping to prevent heart disease, Vitamin E may reduce the incidence of GI and lung cancer, help the immune system retard aging and help prevent cataracts, type 2 diabetes and neurologic diseases. Evidence for all of these alleged benefits is still being evaluated.

Vitamin D helps develop muscles as well as bone, may improve walking and joint function, and prevents hip fractures, osteoarthritis and osteoporosis. It is best obtained from milk or a vitamin pill (Chapter 9) but most seniors over 65 need vitamin D supplements, particularly in winter. Most Americans get 10% of vitamin D from food and 90% from sunlight but not the elderly. They are less likely to get adequate exposure to sunlight and in any event their skin is less capable of synthesizing Vitamin D from sunlight.

The *Nutrition Action Healthletter* reports that B12 is critical for blood cell function and nervous system development. While sources include milk, poultry and eggs, people over age 55 should take a supplement of 25 mcg/day to play it safe. B12 deficiency can cause anemia, memory loss, mental confusion, blurred vision and tingling of the feet. Vitamins B6, E, folate and fiber may lower the risk of heart disease.

Many foods are rich in vitamins, minerals and other beneficial foods, as noted in the following list: oranges: vitamin C and folic acid; watermelon: vitamin C and carotenoids; cantaloupe: vitamin A and C; broccoli: vitamin C, carotenoids, and folic acid; spinach and kale: vitamin C, carotenoids, and calcium; whole grain bread: fiber and a dozen vitamins; sweet potatoes: loaded with vitamin C, carotenoids, potassium and fiber; beans: rich in protein, folic acid and fiber; bran: fiber; salmon, and other fatty fish: omega-3 fats. If you follow a balanced diet perhaps you don't need vitamin supplements.

Good evidence indicates too much vitamin A (retinal-Vitamin A) found in supplements contributes to osteoporosis and hip fractures. Do not take vitamin A pills.

Important minerals are calcium, iron, magnesium, phosphorus, potassium, selenium, sodium, sulfur and zinc. Some evidence indicates that, if you do not get an adequate amount of magnesium, the deficiency can contribute to the incidence of diabetes, high blood pressure, osteoporosis and arteriosclerosis.

The proof, however, is suggestive and not confirmed. As with most substances, you probably get adequate magnesium from natural foods, particularly green leafy vegetables, whole grains, nuts and legumes. In many studies, associations of deficiencies with health or disease do not as yet prove a cause-and-effect relationship. It may not be known if adequate supplementation would prevent a certain disease.

Zinc offers well-demonstrated benefits but contrary to popular belief these do not include prevention of the common cold. While zinc lozenges are available over the counter, they are not recommended. In fact, large doses of zinc may impair the immune system. Selenium, another anti-oxidant, may offer protection against heart disease and cancer. The best source is a supplement. Good sources of potassium are bananas, milk, dry beans and chicken.

Calcium may cut the risk of colon cancer and prevent osteoporosis. The best sources are low-fat milk, cheddar or cottage cheese and calcium-fortified orange juice. The maximum safe dose per day is 1500 to 2500 mg. Some iron is necessary for blood cell development but too much may increase the risk of heart disease, cancer and liver damage.

Not recommended are supplements containing beta-carotene, Echinacea, yohimbe, ginseng, creatine, lecithin, coenzyme Q, DHEA and the dangerous ephedra (now off the market) and gamma butyrolactone.

Many of us take multi-vitamins for extra anti-oxidants and to play safe on other vitamins and minerals. Dr. Andrew Weil, author of the best-selling *Spontaneous Healing,* takes an antioxidant formula to reduce the risk of cancer and heart disease, retard aging and protect against toxic injury. He takes mixed carotenoids (25,000 IU), vitamin E (800 IU), selenium (200 mg) and vitamin C (2000 mg) vitamin supplements in addition to following a healthy diet as a natural preventive of illness.

Dr. Isadore Rosenfeld recommends extra vitamins for those who don't or can't follow a balanced diet, people over age 50, women who are pregnant or of child-bearing age, women with calcium deficiency and women who are menstruating with iron-deficiency anemia. Other markers include a family history of colon or prostate cancer, heart disease or Parkinson's disease; elevated levels of blood homocysteine; cancer; a weight reduction diet, or an intestinal condition. Vegetarians may need vitamin supplements.

In selecting a multivitamin supplement, ignore iodine, manganese, molybdenum, chloride, boron, nickel, silicon, tin, vanadium and lutein. They are not needed. Obtain potassium from fruits and vegetables only. You don't need alfalfa, pumpkin seeds, barley grass or watercress. Descriptions such as "high potency," "ultra, mega, maximum for men, women and seniors" are marketing ploys.

The *Harvard Men's Health Watch* cautions that "testimonials and anecdotes, however well intentioned, don't convey scientific facts." In spite of this, testimonials and anecdotes help the marketers of multiple vitamins, Vitamin C, B3-niacin, selenium, zinc and other vitamins and minerals do a multi-billion dollar business.

The Rodale Press pamphlet "Vitamins: A Prescription for Healing" makes dubious claims for use of vitamins and minerals in the treatment of illness. On the other hand, it does provide an excellent list of food sources for vitamins and minerals and for trace minerals, describes some hazards with excessive intake of a certain vitamin or mineral and indicates natural food sources are often adequate and even better than supplements. Charts are available which list foods with the most vitamin C, folate (Folacin), B_6, beta carotene, potassium, calcium, magnesium, selenium, zinc, fiber and others. This pamphlet may interest you.

Be careful about information and recommendations about vitamins from those selling their own special preparations. Dr. Mathias Rath in full-page advertisements states he "is the world's most renowned vitamin researcher." I have never heard of him. I wrote to him for information about his breakthroughs and received an unsigned letter asking for a method of payment, a product list of two books and 11 vitamin combinations from $18 to $42 plus volume discounts, an application to be a consultant, etc. Is he real or a phony? Do his products have any special benefits or is it all hype? Again, he provides no evidence, no studies, and no documentation. If he has done such great research, why didn't he publish it? If he did publish it, where?

Do we need more antioxidants, thought important in the prevention and treatment of disease, than we can get from eating fruits and vegetables? While healthy people probably do not, patients with coronary artery disease or at high risk of it, should very likely take supplements of Vitamin E and perhaps Vitamin C. Cardiologists recommend 400 to 800 U of Vitamin E and 500 to 1,000 mg. of Vitamin C daily for those patients. Losomczy, et al., in a study of over 11,000 elderly U.S. people, found fewer coronary artery disease events in those who took Vitamin E than in those not taking it. It may take a year or so for Vitamin E to have any effect. Routine use of beta carotene does not seem beneficial.

Vitamins C, E, beta-carotene and the mineral selenium are not the only sources of antioxidants. As with all living species, the human body produces antioxidants to control production and disposal of free radicals, or reactive oxygen species. Very toxic, free radicals contain an odd number of electrons from reduction of molecular oxygen during a number of cellular processes. These toxic molecules may leave their parent cells to attack neighboring cells or membranes but they also perform a necessary function. Their production is what gives white blood cells, or neutrophils, the ability to kill bacteria they have ingested. Free radicals are produced in a variety of tissues including white blood cells, the cells lining blood vessels and blood platelets and all other cells during the use of oxygen.

Other antioxidants are the carotenoids, salicylates, the xanthine oxidase inhibitor, Allopurinol, N acetylcysteine, Probucol, a lipid-soluble cholesterol-lowering agent, and calcium channel blockers. The oxygen radical absorbance capacity test (ORAC) measures antioxidant action in foods. Tomatoes test high in containing an antioxidant lycopene, which helps decrease risk of heart attack and perhaps prostate cancer. Lycopene is present in both raw and cooked tomatoes. Berries contain high levels of antioxidants.

Widespread use of antioxidants has led to overuse. High doses of antioxidants may lead to diarrhea, bleeding and toxic reactions. To avoid toxicity from overdoses of vitamin C, take no more than 2000 mg/day. Vitamin E in a dose of 200 IU/day is sufficient, but large doses seem safe, up to 1500 IU; selenium from 55 mcg/day to a maximum of 400 mcg/day and carotenoids—no limit now.

Interactions of antioxidants and statin drugs complicate the picture. In a trial of the statin Zocor and niacin in patients with clinical coronary artery disease, the statin-niacin was very beneficial. Addition of the antioxidants Vitamins E, C, beta-carotene, and selenium, however, worked against the statin-niacin.

Melatonin, sold as an over-the-counter dietary supplement, is secreted by the pineal gland in our brain, which helps regulate sleep and wake cycles. Melatonin levels in the body rise at night and fall by day. Known as the "darkness hormone," it is used for jetlag and insomnia, perhaps unwisely so. The *Wellness Letter* of the University of California at Berkeley says that while melatonin may promote sleep, the evidence is not definite and that long-term effects of its use are unknown. "Hormones are powerful substances and can produce unexpected results, so we don't recommend melatonin," says the *Wellness Letter*.

The latest push is for flavenoids or polyphenols, compounds found only in plants as part of their defense system. They are antioxidants concentrated in the leaves and fruits of plants. So far evidence indicates little benefit for you.

FIBER

71. What is fiber and why is it good to eat foods that contain fiber?

Fiber is the non-digestible part of plant foods that passes through the small intestine and colon virtually unchanged, without absorption by the body. Composed of carbohydrate and lignin, fiber adds bulk to the stool and helps the colon to function. The *Harvard Health Letter* provides evidence that diets high in fiber help lower cholesterol, reduce risk of heart disease, and prevent constipation and other bowel problems. In softening the stool enough to prevent pressure on the colon, fiber may ward off diverticulosis and diverticulitis, hemorrhoids, and irritable bowel syndrome. The fiber-diet trials found still other benefits: a reduction in heart disease, diabetes and high blood pressure. Evidence indicates that diabetics eating fiber can better control their blood sugar levels. It also may prevent phlebitis in the legs.

You may obtain fiber primarily from oats; wheat; bran; whole grain cereals; beans, potatoes, peas and other vegetables; and apples and other fruits. You will also find an excellent source of dietary fiber in foods containing the recently developed fat replacement Nutrim, which comes from cooking oatmeal and putting it through a sieve. Rich in beta-glucans, Nutrim is more effective than whole oat bran in lowering cholesterol and replacing fat in the diet. It is digestible in contrast to the fat substitute Olestra, which passes untouched through the gastrointestinal tract.

For some time it was thought a low-fat diet decreased the likelihood of colorectal cancer but recent evidence suggests this is probably not true in both men and women. It is the reduced intake of animal or saturated fats that makes the difference. Fatty meals and dairy products may increase the risk of colon cancer. Fruits, vegetables and calcium may help decrease it. A. Wolk et al. found evidence supporting the hypothesis that higher fiber intake, particularly from cereal, reduces the risk of coronary heart disease in women. Beans are a good source not only of fiber but also of phytochemicals (folate) and potassium, protein, magnesium, B6, zinc, copper and iron. Beans are low in fat, and you can prepare a low sodium variety by washing and soaking them. A high fiber diet may involve one drawback: A switch to it may result in bloating and gas. Increase the amount of fiber slowly and drink a lot of water.

A study by David S. Ludwig, et al. indicated high-fiber diets may protect against obesity and cardiovascular disease by lowering insulin levels. Another observational study, "What did you eat?" by E. B.Rimm et al., indicates men, particularly from 45 to 64 years of age, who followed a high-fiber diet experienced a reduction in risk of coronary deaths or non-fatal heart attacks. Dietary fat should also be controlled. Thus, increased intake of vegetables, fruits and cereal fiber is good for your heart.

The Tufts U. *Health and Nutrition Letter* warns about the misleading labels of some non-whole-grain foods that suggest they are in fact whole-grain. For example, despite their names multi-grain bars and whole wheat waffles are not whole-grain foods. Fiber medications such as Metamucil provide good fiber, stool bulk and protect against diverticulitis. I recommend them.

Good Sources of Fiber

Beans	Bran Cereals
Flaxseeds	Fruits
Oat Bran	Peanuts, walnuts
Psyllium seeds	Rye crisp crackers
Vegetables	Wheat bran
Wheat crisp crackers	Whole grain bread
Whole grains	Wheat berries
Barley, buckwheat	Rye, bulgar
Whole wheat pasta	

DIETS AND THE HEART

72. If I have coronary artery disease, can diet help me? Are there special diets for people with heart disease and high cholesterol?

Please see Chapters 66 and 68 for information on several excellent such diets.

In 1998 Dean Ornish, M.D., described a study of 45 patients with partially clogged coronary arteries. After five years 20 patients who made intensive dietary and lifestyle changes experienced less blockage. Fifteen patients who made smaller changes experienced less change and 2.5 times more heart attacks or other heart events. Ten patients dropped out. In a second study, more than 300 people with severe coronary artery disease were able to make the intensive changes required by Ornish's program including: (1) a diet, very low in fat, with whole grains, fruits and vegetables; (2) aerobic exercises such as at least a half an hour of brisk walking a day; and (3) stress management training, stretching, meditation, relaxation, psychological support by friends and family, participation in religious and spiritual activities. Smoking is not allowed. Ornish agrees he cannot say how much of the program's success is due to the diet as opposed to the exercise and stress management and all may be related; however, there was improvement. Table 1 contains the perfect 10 of Ornish's menus from his book *Eat More, Weigh Less*. It is essentially a vegetarian diet. Table 2 contains a menu from the DASH (Dietary Approaches to Stop Hypertension), a diet low in fat but high in unsaturated fat.

Medicare will now pay a number of patients to try the Ornish plan rather than undergo cardiac surgery. It is accepted that treatment of lipoprotein disorders can slow progression of heart disease, reduce clinical events and result in some small degree of arteriographic regression of coronary narrowing. Also detailed tests of lipoproteins (LDL) and others will help treatment. New components are being evaluated such as apolipoprotein B, small dense LDL, LDL subclass B and intermediate density lipoprotein which increases risk and apo A-1, apo A-II and HDL subclasses which reduce risk.

The *Harvard Health Letter* describes three studies in patients with coronary artery disease. The Lyon Heart Study tested a Mediterranean diet limited to fish, vegetables, grains, fruits and reduced-fat olive oil, which reduced the risk of heart problems by 73%. A Diet and Reinfarction Trial (DART), a low-fat diet with a higher proportion of fish, produced a 16% decrease in heart attacks. A trial in India of a diet of vegetables, fruits, vegetables and fish saw a 41% decrease in heart attacks. A total vegetarian diet is good if you wish to do it but you must choose low-fat dairy products and get protein from beans and tofu.

A less extreme approach is the full Mediterranean diet of grains, beans, vegetables and fruit with small amounts of yogurt and cheese daily and fish, eggs and poultry only a few times a week. Olive is the only oil allowed, following from the observation that heart disease was less common in people along the Mediterranean where olive oil is the main cooking oil and table fat. They also eat more fish. Olive oil is a monounsaturated fat which may lower LDL and not HDL (chapter 66).

The Pritikin diet is a very low-fat diet with a lot of fruits, vegetables, whole grains and beans which will lower cholesterol, if you follow Pritiken's advice to exercise and lose weight as well. Some nutrients are good for one organ but a problem for others. Such is the case with alpha-linolenic acid, an omega-3 fatty acid from vegetable products (flax seed oil, canola oil, soy bean oil). It is good for the heart but may contribute to the incidence of prostate cancer.

In the *Nutrition Action Healthletter*, April 2004, David Schardt reviews supplements that help the heart: fish oil, psyllium (Metamucil), niacin (vitamin B-3), phytosterols, aspirin, folic acid and B-12. He notes that beta-carotene is a problem and describes as worthless the supplements garlic, guggul, tucotrienols, isoflavones, red yeast rice and policosols.

The best way to prevent heart attacks is not a stent or bypass but avoidance of smoking, control of blood pressure, a low level of cholesterol, and prevention of blood clotting. Big meals increase the risk of heart attack by temporarily raising blood pressure, which could trigger a blood clot.

Table 1

A Perfect Ten

What does a vegetarian, plant-based, whole-foods diet with no
more than 10 percent of calories from fat look like?
Here's one day's menus from Dean Ornish's
Eat More, Weigh Less (1997, Harper-Collins, New York, $6.99).

BREAKFAST
>Cold cereal
>Nonfat yogurt
>Fresh fruit or juice
>Whole-wheat toast
>Preserves
>Warm beverage

LUNCH
>White beans, greens, and sun-dried
>   tomato crostini
>Red potato soup with garlic and
>   wild greens
>Tossed green salad

DINNER
>Roasted quesadillas with
>   Chiquita bananas
>Pico de gallo salsa
>Vegetarian chili
>Spanish rice
>Tossed green salad
>Broiled pineapple with
>   cinnamon and rum

*From the *Nutrition Action Healthletter*, June 1999, p. 7.

Table 2

The DASH Diet

Dietary Approaches to Stop Hypertension

Each component of this diet has a role in combination high blood pressure, while providing adequate nutrition. The diet is rich in fruits, vegetables and lowfat dairy foods but low in saturated and total fat. It is also low in cholesterol, high in dietary fiber, potassium, calcium and magnesium and moderately high in protein. Serving plan is based on 2,000 calories and the number of servings may vary with caloric needs.

Food Group	Servings*	Examples	Significance
Grains and grain products	7 to 8	Whole wheat bread, English muffins, pita bread, bagels, cereals, grits, oatmeal	Major sources of energy and fiber
Vegetables	4 to 5	Tomatoes, potatoes, carrots, peas, squash, broccoli, turnip greens, collards, kale, spinach, artichokes, beans, sweet potatoes	Rich sources of potassium, magnesium and fiber
Fruits	4 to 5	Apricots, bananas, dates, grapes, oranges, orange juice, grapefruit, grapefruit juice, mangoes, melons, peaches, pineapples, dates, strawberries, tangerines	Important sources of potassium, magnesium and fiber
Low-fat or nonfat dairy foods	2 to 3	Skim or lowfat milk, low-fat buttermilk, nonfat or low-fat yogurt, lowfat mozzarella, nonfat cheese	Rich sources of protein and magnesium
Meats, poultry and fish	2 or fewer	Only lean meats, with visible fat trimmed away; broiled, roasted, or boiled, not fried; poultry with skin removed	Rich sources of protein and magnesium
Nuts, seeds and legumes	4 to 5 a week	Almonds, filberts, mixed nuts, peanuts, walnuts, sunflower seeds, kidney beans, lentils	Rich sources of energy, magnesium, potassium, protein and fiber

FRUIT—VEGETABLES

73. How much fruit and vegetables should I eat? How can I eat the recommended 7-8 servings of fruits and vegetables a day? Is garlic good for me?

All healthful diets should include large portions of fresh fruits and vegetables and some cooked fruits and vegetables, to assure adequate intake of fiber and vitamins and minerals. A diet high in fruit and vegetables with five to seven or even eight to nine servings per day decreases risk of heart disease, stroke, cancer, hypertension and obesity. A vegetarian diet has been associated with lower blood pressure perhaps related to intake of fiber, potassium, antioxidants, vitamins, folate, or moderating homocysteine. In 832 men, ages 45 to 65, free of cardiovascular disease at the time of entry into the study, intake of fruits and vegetables was associated with a decrease in stroke. One hypothesis is that increased consumption of fruits and vegetables may decrease consumption of other harmful foods or alcohol.

Two other studies show decreased risk of stroke with consumption of fruits and vegetables, particularly cruciferous vegetables—broccoli, cabbage, cauliflower—green leafy vegetables and citrus fruit and juice. Some evidence indicates that the risk of cancer of the gastrointestinal and respiratory tracts is lowered by consumption of fruits and vegetables. Tomatoes, rich in the antioxidant lycopene, help cut the risk of heart attack. Choose brightly colored plant foods whenever possible, like strawberries, blueberries, blackberries, carrots, oranges, kale and spinach. They can absorb the most oxygen radicals and thus serve as antioxidants that can help fight cancer and heart disease. (Table) Seaweed, described as a wonder vegetable, includes agar-agar, dulse, kombu, nori and wakame, all great in soups and salads. Consumption of fruits and vegetables doesn't do everything, however. It does not decrease the risk of breast cancer.

How in the world can I eat seven to eight servings of fruits and vegetables a day?

In all recommended healthy diets, portions are smaller. As Jane Brody points out, eight to ten servings of fruits and vegetables a day may sound formidable but a single serving is only half a cup of cooked fruit or vegetables, half a grapefruit, a medium apple or an orange, a small banana, six ounces of fruit or vegetable juice, a quarter cup of dried fruit or one cup of raw leafy greens. One slice of bread, a half cup of rice, pasta or dry or cooked cereal are each a serving. One glass of milk in cereal, a container of yogurt, an ounce and a half of low-fat or nonfat cheese gives you three servings and enough calcium for the daily requirement.

Brody gives a sample dinner menu from the DASH diet, designed to protect against systolic hypertension: three ounces of baked cod, one cup of rice, one-half cup of broccoli, one-half cup of stewed tomatoes, a very small spinach salad, one small whole wheat dinner roll, a teaspoon of margarine and a half cup of melon balls. This adds up to these servings: one of fish, three of grains, four of vegetables and fruits and one and a half of fat. The DASH diet confines dairy foods to low-fat or non-fat products, limits consumption of meats and excludes added fats and oils. It is low in sodium. (Chapter 72) The diet is a good one for maintenance of general good health, weight control and lowering blood pressure.

Isn't garlic good for me?

The claims that garlic helps your health are not backed up by scientific evidence. It does not lower blood cholesterol. Evidence that garlic prevents blood clots, heart attacks and strokes is lacking. It does not help intermittent claudication, pain in the legs with walking because of narrowed or blocked arteries. It does not decrease blood pressure, blood sugar or decrease risk of breast or colon cancer or other tumors. A few reports associate decreased incidence of colorectal and stomach cancer with garlic intake of six or more cloves a day but these studies are not well documented. Many brands of garlic release only small amounts of the active ingredient, Allicin.

Table 1

The Color of the Diet

	CONTAINS	BETTER FOR
RED—tomatoes, grapefruit, cranberries	Lycopene Anthocyanins	Prostate, Blood pressure
WHITE—white onions, leeks, garlic	Allicin	Cancer and heart
BLUE—blackberries, purple grapes, eggplant, plums	Anthocyanins Phenolics	Cancer and heart disease Aging
YELLOW—apricots, squash, carrots clementines, lemons, pineapples	Beta-carotene Bioflavonoids	Less cancer, heart disease Less cancer, better skin
GREEN—broccoli, green peas, spinach brussel sprouts, cauliflower, kale	Lutein Indoles	Better vision, heart, vessels Less breast & prostate cancer

Each of these has certain benefits (See Consumer Reports)

HCAs

74. What Are HCAs And PAHs? Are They Bad For Me? Why?

HCAs are heterocyclic amines produced when meat, poultry or fish are cooked at very high temperatures. "We know these compounds probably cause cancer in humans," said Elizabeth G. Snyderwine, Chief of the Chemical Carcinogenesis Section at the National Cancer Institute (NCI). "What we don't know yet is how significant a problem they are in the American diet." In the meanwhile it makes sense to avoid them. Meat should be cooked thoroughly, given the hazard of bacterial infection, but not at a high temperature.

Beef, pork and chicken produce most of the HCAs because they contain the most amino acids and creatine that are converted into HCA's. Seafood produces much less and plant foods almost none. Grilling, barbecuing, broiling and pan frying are more likely to produce HCAs than baking or roasting because they generate more heat. A propane gas grill set on high can reach 640 degrees F. while a typical roasting temperature is 350 degrees.

Pre-cooking or marinating reduces HCAs. Before grilling meat or poultry, cut it into small chunks, precook it in a microwave for several minutes, throw away the juice and marinate it, to reduce HCAs by 90 percent. Sausage casings and hot dog skins seem to prevent HCAs. Fewer HCAs are found in fast food burgers because they are cooked so quickly.

According to the *Nutrition Action Newsletter*, "cooking with liquid—boiling, steaming, poaching or stewing, for example, generates no HCAs because the temperature never tops the boiling point of water. The same is true for microwaving so long as the food is not overcooked or dried out."

PAHs are polycyclic aromatic hydrocarbons formed when fat drips on a flame, a hot heating element, or hot coals. The PAHs come up in the smoke and land on the food. They can also form directly on food when it is cooked to a crisp as in grilling a hamburger with fat dripping off and flames and smoke shooting up. Proof that these substances cause cancer in man is still elusive but they do so in a large number of animal species. Twelve of 18 PAHs cause cancer in animals.

To avoid these substances, it is best to cook lean cuts of meat and poultry, use fish or shellfish, try tofu or veggie burgers, and grill or broil vegetables or fruit. Frozen meat or poultry should be thawed in the refrigerator before cooking so that high temperatures are not needed. Try a gas grill set on low; use hardwood charcoal; don't build a huge bed of coals and spread the coals evenly across the bottom of the barbecue; rake them to one side, instead, and cook the food on the opposite side. Avoid eating blackened or charred food and take the food off of the heat as soon as it is cooked. Prevent fat from dripping on the heat source.

HCAs and PAHs are like smoking guns; we are suspicious of them but can't be positive. People who eat more meat are at greater risk for colon and prostate cancer but is this because they consume more saturated fat and fewer fruits or vegetables or is exposure to HCAs and PAHs the cause? Some studies suggest people with breast, colon or stomach cancers ate more fried or well-done meats. To increase the confusion the levels of HCAs vary greatly in food as do levels of susceptibility in people. The Livermore Labs conclude well-done or very well-done meat is not good for you.

DIET AND CANCER

75. Does diet have anything to do with cancer? Are there new diets that help prevent cancer? What are these scares about cancer? Can infection cause cancer? What does too much sun do?

The overall incidence of cancer is decreasing due to the reduction in smoking, early detection and treatment. However, the incidence of certain cancers is increasing: breast cancer, leukemia, melanoma and liver cancer.

Does diet have anything to do with cancer?

The answer is that diet is very important for certain cancers. A diet rich in vegetables and fruits is associated with a decreased risk of cancer in many locations in the body. These plant foods seem protective in their own right, particularly deep green and yellow-orange fruits and vegetables and cruciform or cabbage family vegetables, which contain phytochemicals and isothiocyanates. The evidence for their help is strongest for cancers of the lung, mouth, larynx, esophagus, stomach, colon and bladder.

Bonnie Liebman describes the evidence for the effects of diet, habits, and exercise on cancer in the *Nutrition Action Newsletter* (Dec. 1998), from the report "Food, Nutrition and the Prevention of Cancers, a Global Perspective." The evidence for factors decreasing risk is divided into 1) convincing evidence; 2) probable evidence; 3) possible evidence; or 4) suggestive but insufficient evidence. The same is true for factors which increase risk.

Factors tending to decrease the likelihood of cancer, in general, include vegetables, fruits, carotenoids in food, vitamin C in food, minerals in food, cereals or grains or starches, fiber, physical activity and refrigeration of food. Negative factors increasing the risk of cancer include alcohol, tobacco, fatty foods particularly from animal sources, high meat intake, salt and salty meat, eggs, cholesterol, milk and dairy products, sugar, coffee contaminants and obesity.

Vegetarians run about half the cancer risk of meat eaters. Certain cancers are influenced by diet, exercise and body size.

This report (760 pages), by a panel chaired by John Potter, is available from the American Institute for Cancer Research at 800-843-8114 for $35, including shipping and handling. See Table 1 for advice from the panel on how to decrease the risk of developing cancer.

The big four cancers for Americans are lung, breast, prostate and colon cancer. The major risk factors for lung, esophagus, larynx, mouth and pharynx cancer are alcohol and tobacco. For breast cancer and diet, the relationships are not strong. In *The Breast Cancer Prevention Diet*, Dr. Robert Arnot recommends a low-fat, low-cholesterol diet, which is generally healthful, anyway. Many experts believe, however, that the title of his book is misleading. Dr. Mortimer, Director of Clinical Oncology at Washington U. in St. Louis, was quoted by Kristina Sauerwein in the *St. Louis Post-Dispatch* as saying that "the book is totally unfounded." Mortimer went on to say, "It's ridiculous to think somehow you are what you eat and disregard genetic, environmental and other factors involved with breast cancer." For example, she indicated women who menstruate early or have children after age 30 are at a higher risk for breast cancer regardless of diet. Also, there is a genetic basis for many breast cancers.

Some doctors indicated Arnot's use of their research was misleading and, as Sauerwein stated, the Memorial Sloan-Kettering Cancer Institute in New York City asked that references to the Institute be removed from future editions of the book. No scientific evidence as yet supports the claim that a diet such as that proposed by Arnot decreases the likelihood of breast cancer. Obviously, the book is selling well because it raises the expectations of women, even though its recommendations lack substance as yet.

Several risk factors contribute to development of prostate cancer. Dietary fat has been implicated. Excess calcium may be harmful. Diet can lower the risk. Vitamin E may help in prevention of prostate cancer, and now it seems clear that selenium, a trace element in vegetables and grains, fish and nuts, also offers protection. Food seems to be the best source of selenium. Whether supplements are needed by all males is not established. The *Harvard Health Letter* recommends exercise and a diet including whole grains, which are rich in selenium; soybean oil; and tomatoes, for their lycopene content; and reducing fat intake from meat and whole dairy products. Consumption of vegetables and fruits, with adequate physical activity, may decrease the likelihood of colon and rectal cancer. Alcohol and smoking, however, increase the risk, as do consumption of meat, fat, and saturated animal fatty acids, especially grilled and barbecued meat. Diets high in protein and fat are linked to risk for lymphatic cancer (Yale Bulletin, March 26, 2004). Obesity is a risk factor for a number of health problems, such as diabetes and cancer. This includes increased frequency of breast, esophageal, gallbladder, kidney, pancreatic, uterus, prostate, and colon cancer. Even a small reduction in weight may help.

Phytochemicals in fruits and vegetables may decrease the frequency of cancer. Toxins used by plants to fight off insects and other predators, phytochemicals may turn on enzymes that decrease the effects of carcinogens in the environment. However, scientists don't know which factors are important so they cannot put them in a pill as yet. Some evidence indicates that the antioxidants Vitamins C and E and the carotenoids lutein and zeaxanthin are associated with fewer cataracts of the eyes and cases of macular degeneration.

The panel on Food, Nutrition and the Prevention of Cancer does not recommend supplements, believing they are not necessary if one follows a healthy diet. Experts disagree, however, about whether studies of cancer prevention should be done with changes in the whole diet or with use of supplements. There is no easy answer. Some supplements have been called nutraceuticals, isolated or purified food components sold in medicinal forms. Vitamins and other products that may help decrease the likelihood of cancer are beta carotene and other carotenoids, vitamins C, D, E, all of which are found in adequate supply in foodstuffs, as are all phytochemicals. Americans allegedly spent $5.7 billion on vitamin and mineral supplements in 1997.

Information about carcinogens in food and in the environment is available from the American Council on Science and Health, Inc., (ACSH) 1995 Broadway, New York, NY 10023. However, this organization has been criticized for its association and support from various corporations that use possibly carcinogenic chemicals and additives. The reader must be careful.

Are there new diets that help prevent cancer?

Reports in newspapers and on television indicate some foodstuffs or some particular diet can prevent a certain disease as a low-fat high-fiber diet has been said to decrease the likelihood of colon cancer. Then you read later that this has not been proven, and that fiber may not be related to colon cancer at all. Why so much confusion about diet and disease? Why are there on-again, off-again reports?

The major reason is that many studies are based upon a recollection of what individuals think they ate rather than upon an exact record of what they actually ate. Also, individuals' diets change over time. They may go from one diet to another. Finally, a number of factors may confuse the issue. If you increase the amount of fish in your diet, for example, it may be that you cut back on other potentially harmful foods. What is responsible for any beneficial results: the presence of fish or the absence of harmful foods or both? If you begin a diet high in fruits and vegetables, you may also begin to exercise more. The pros and cons of solving the diet and disease puzzle composed the cover story in the May 1999 issue of *Nutrition Action Healthletter*. If you are interested in learning more about the problems related to diet and disease research, I recommend this article to you.

Diet studies fall into three types. A retrospective study compares people recently diagnosed with a disease with other people who were not, to see whether the sick people ate more or less of some foods or nutrients than the others. Advantages include quick answers and clues perhaps to some uncommon illnesses. Limitations include inaccuracies in subjects' recollection of what they ate or took and confounding factors: If people who say they consume more than recommended amounts of fat run a higher risk for colon cancer, what else do they do that puts them at high risk?

A prospective study collects information about diet and other activities of a group of healthy people and then waits a number of years to see who gets what disease, if any. The advantage is lack of a recall bias. The study provides more than one snapshot and covers more than one disease; however, it can involve misclassifications and less variability in diet.

Speaking generally, the most valuable approach by far is a clinical trial that randomly assigns a large number of people with or without a disease to one group or another. One group follows the diet that is supposed to protect against the disease while another group follows an ordinary diet. The investigators wait several years to see if the disease affects more people in one group than in the other. (Table II) This approach involves no misclassifications or confounding and produces less equivocal results. Potential limitations include the possibility that investigators chose the wrong group of people or not enough people or that an individual took the wrong dose or that the trial is too short or too long. Maybe investigators were looking at the wrong diet.

A randomized trial has produced valuable adverse information about the use of beta carotene supplementation with vitamin A. The trial showed that the supplementation failed to decrease lung cancer risk and may have produced adverse effects. Beta-carotene supplementation for 12 years also did not decrease the incidence of malignant neoplasms, cardiovascular disease or death from all causes.

Many of us believe controlled clinical trials are the only way to get reliable information about diet and disease. It is necessary to look at a consistent picture in many of the studies and repeat all of them. The dietary guidelines for cancer prevention are listed in Table III.

There have been big scares about things that cause cancer. What are they and why?

Ames and Swirsky said: "No human diet can be free of naturally occurring chemicals that are rodent carcinogens. Of the chemicals people eat, 99.96% are natural." In its special report "Facts versus Fears: A Review of the Greatest Unfounded Health Scares of Recent Times," ACSH deplores the cranberry scare of 1959 in which a weed killer was found as a residue on cranberries. The pesticide caused cancer of the thyroid in rats but only if they consumed an amount that in a human diet would come to 15,000 pounds of berries every day for years. Other unjustified scares about carcinogens centered on DDT, Cyclamates, DES in beef, nitrates, red dye number 2, hair dyes, asbestos in hair dryers, benzene in Perrier and many others. DDT, DES and the other substances pose other risks to health, however. Cell phones are not associated with brain cancer. H.L. Mencken said, "the whole aim of practical politics is to keep the populace alarmed (and hence clamorous to be led to safety) by menacing it with an endless series of hobgoblins, all of them imaginary." A holiday dinner menu lists a number of mutagens and carcinogens which are naturally occurring and are rodent carcinogens but no problem for us. Food additives and preservatives, pesticide residues and the products of spoiled foods pose only slight risks if any at all for cancer.

Can infections cause cancer?

Yes, they can. Both viral and bacterial infections can do it. Both the human papilloma virus and the bacteria chlamydia are associated with cervical cancer. H. pylori infection in the stomach is associated with stomach cancer. Hepatitis C-virus transmitted by blood transfusion can cause liver cancer. It can be treated if found before occurrence of the cancer. Hepatitis B can cause liver cancer and can be prevented by vaccination. Infection has also been associated with cardiovascular disease, asthma, multiple sclerosis and schizophrenia.

What does too much sun do?

Excessive sunning contributes to premature aging, sun damage to skin and skin cancers. The three skin cancers are basal cell cancers, raised growths that usually stay localized; squamous cell cancers, thin flat cells resembling fish scales at the microscopic level that can spread to lymph nodes; and melanomas, irregular pigmented brown to black lesions that can be malignant and spread anywhere in the body. Melanomas are said to be on the increase. A melanoma can be distinguished from a mole by "ABCD" guidelines. It is Asymmetrical, has irregular Borders and edges are notched or ragged, uneven Color and the Diameter is irregular.

Sun exposure is the major risk factor for melanoma. The best way to prevent skin cancer is to avoid the sun and stay in the shade particularly from 10:00 a.m. to 4:00 p.m., the time for the most intense ultraviolet rays. If you must get out in the sun, cover up with sunglasses, hats and long-sleeved shirts and pants. If you must sun yourself, use liberally applied sunscreen which protects against ultraviolet A and B with a sun protection factor of at least 15. Some disagreement has arisen about how effective sunscreens are. Always check your exposed skin carefully for growths.

For further information contact:

American Cancer Society—1-800-ACS-2345 or go to *www.cancer.org*
Harvard Center for Cancer Prevention. *www.yourcancerrisk.com* to find out about
your risk of individual cancers, based on questions about diet, weight, exercise
and smoking habits.
National Cancer Institute—1-800-4-Cancer, *www.cancer.gov* for information about
cancer trials, statistics, treatment, screening, prevention, research, etc.

Table I

1. Plant foods. Choose predominantly plant-based diets rich in a variety of vegetables and fruits, legumes (beans), and minimally processed starchy foods.
2. Body weight. Avoid being underweight or overweight, and limit weight gain during adulthood to less than 11 pounds (five kilograms).
3. Physical activity. If occupational activity is low or moderate, take an hour's brisk walk or similar exercise daily, and also exercise vigorously for a total of at least one hour a week.
4. Vegetables and fruits. Eat five or more servings a day of a variety of vegetables and fruits, all year round (not including potatoes, beans, and other starchy fruits and vegetables, which are addressed below).
5. Other plant foods. Eat more than seven servings a day of a variety of grains, legumes, roots, tubers, and plantains. (Tubers and roots include potatoes, sweet potatoes, beets, parsnips, etc.) Choose minimally processed foods. Limit consumption of refined sugar to less than ten percent of calories.
6. Alcoholic drinks. Alcohol consumption is not recommended. If consumed, limit to less than two drinks a day for men and one for women.
7. Meat. If eaten at all, limit intake of red meat to less than three ounces daily. Choose fish and poultry in place of beef, lamb, or pork.
8. Total fats and oils. Limit consumption of fatty foods, particularly those of animal origin. Use modest amounts of vegetable oils. Total fats should provide 15 to 30% of calories.
9. Salt. Limit consumption of salted foods and salt. Limit sodium to less than 2400 mg. per day. Use herbs and spices to season foods.
10. Food storage. Store perishable foods in ways that minimize contamination with fungi.
11. Food preservation. Use refrigeration to preserve perishable foods.

12. Food preparation. Do not eat charred food. For meat and fish-eaters, avoid burning meat. Consume the following only occasionally: meat and fish grilled (broiled) in direct flame; cured and smoked meats.
13. Supplements. For those who follow these recommendations, dietary supplements are probably unnecessary, and not helpful, for reducing cancer risk.
14. Tobacco. Do not smoke or chew tobacco.

From Food, Nutrition and the prevention of Cancer as cited in Liebman's report.

Table II

Trials Being Conducted

AGENT	DISEASE
Folic acid	Colon polyps
Low fat diet with fruits, vegetables and fiber	Breast cancer
Fruits, vegetables rich in carotenoids	Precancerous cervical lesions
Selenium	All cancers
Low fat diet	Skin cancer
Low fat, calcium and vitamin D	Breast and colon cancer, heart disease, hip fractures
Vitamin C	Heart attacks, stroke, cataracts
Vitamin E	Clogged arteries

Table III

The dietary guidelines for cancer prevention provided in the Harvard Men's Health Watch (November 1998) are:

1. Maintain a desirable body weight.
2. Eat a variety of foods.
3. Choose most of the foods you eat from plant sources, including minimally processed starchy foods.
4. Eat five or more servings of fruit and vegetables a day. Try to eat at least 15 ounces daily.
5. Eat low fat foods such as whole grain products and legumes; eat 20 ounces daily.
6. Eat less fat, particularly from animal sources.
7. Eat less meat and whole milk dairy products; if you eat red meat, limit yourself to three ounces a day.

8.   Limit consumption of alcohol beverages, if you drink at all.
9.   Limit consumption of nitrite-preserved, salt-cured and smoked foods and, of course, no smoking.

SALT—HIGH BLOOD PRESSURE (HYPERTENSION).

76. How much salt should I use. What should I do about my blood pressure? What is my risk of stroke?

Salt (NaCl), already present in many foodstuffs, is part of a healthy diet. Added salt is not necessary but some people salt all their food anyway for taste. The question is: "Is added salt bad for you?" If so, should you be on a low-salt diet?

If you are over 60 with any evidence of hypertension, the answer is "yes, you should be on a salt restricted diet with no more than about 1800 mg. (1.8 grams) of salt a day," as indicated by a JAMA study titled "The Trial of Nonpharmacologic Interventions in the Elderly (TONE). Patients in the study had experienced modest or mild hypertension with a systolic blood pressure of 145 mm. Hg and 85 diastolic and were taking anti-hypertensive medication. The study found that patients who decreased their sodium intake to no more than 1800 mg. a day for three months could be taken off their blood pressure-lowering drugs. After that some overweight patients also lost weight, at least 10 pounds. Subjects who continued to cut down on sodium were 31% less likely to have a relapse of high blood pressure than those that did not. Obese patients who lost weight were 36 to 40% less likely to have a relapse; obese patients who both lost weight and cut back on sodium were 53% less likely.

Bonnie Liebman, in the *Nutrition Action Healthletter*, compared these results to a study by Michael Alderman, et al., Albert Einstein College of Medicine, New York, reported in *Lancet*. Alderman was formerly a consultant to the Salt Institute raising a big question about the study at the outset. His report claimed the death rate was slightly higher in people who reported using the *least* salt. Were they trying to show sodium is not a factor in blood pressure and disease? Liebman said this study was riddled with flaws. Brent D. Opell of Johns Hopkins said, "No good researcher would ever publish unadjusted data as they did" and asked how this "outrageous" study got published in the first place. The controversy aired in the *New York Times*, which did not look closely at the studies. The *Times* seemed to give them equal weight, calling them merely contradictory even though the JAMA study was flawless and the *Lancet* report has been called "junk science".

Is a salt lobby at work to fight restriction of salt intake? The food industry is on record as opposing salt restriction. It would impair their ability to sell high sodium foods, and the truth is that salt sells. The controversy about salt, however, does not provide simple answers.

On the one hand, Feng J. He et al. found a high sodium intake strongly and independently associated with increased risk of cardiovascular disease and mortality in overweight persons. On the other hand, A. Graudel et al. found a meta-analysis of 58 trials did not support a general recommendation to reduce sodium intake, in the Trials of Hypertension Prevention (TOPH) II. Sodium restriction did not produce a beneficial lowering of blood pressure.

So, what is the answer? The major answer is that sodium is not the only factor in blood pressure control. We are complex organisms, and not everyone is affected the same by sodium reduction. Some people who use a fair bit of salt do not develop hypertension.

The Institute of Medicine (IOM) in February, 2004, set a tolerable upper intake level (UL)—a maximum amount that people should not exceed—at 5.8 grams of salt per day, noting that more than 95 percent of American men and 75 percent of American women ages 31 to 50 regularly consume salt in excess of the UL. They found American men's daily median intake of salt to be between 7.8 and 11.8 grams and women's between 5.8 and 7.8 grams. For healthy adults aged 19 to 50 the IOM recommended a daily sufficient amount of salt to be 3.8 grams. In general, humans can survive on 1.5 grams of sodium a day. Other authorities do not accept these restrictions. In Canada, no sodium restriction is recommended for those with normal blood pressure. Sodium restriction does not seem to prevent hypertension. It may be that a low sodium diet is good for some people but is not necessary for others. (JAMA, April 14, 2004)

To control high blood pressure, Jane Brody provides this summary: consume less salt, lose excess weight, eat more fruits and vegetables, eat more low-fat dairy products, don't smoke and exercise regularly. A diet high in fruits and vegetables is also low in sodium. Brody describes societies where little salt is consumed and less hypertension is experienced with aging.

Everyone wants to put salt on food. Fortunately, many salt substitutes—most of them are potassium chloride—taste good. I use them routinely. You might also try spices, herbs, garlic, or onion powder as substitutes for salt. You can also find low-sodium variants of most foodstuffs, such as tomato juice or vegetable juice and soy sauce. The only food high in sodium without a low sodium variant is pickles. Be wary of potato and corn chips, salted pretzels, cured olives, sauerkraut, frozen turkey dinners and Big Macs with cheese. Many canned soups are loaded with sodium. The *Nutrition Action Newsletter* provides the sodium content of many foods in an article titled "High Blood Pressure."

Evidence now indicates a gene mutation leading to early-onset hypertension. It is a salt recycling pathway causing the kidneys to absorb salt and water and return them to the body, which puts salt right in the middle of it. What about controlling salt intake at younger ages to prevent hypertension? This is probably important, but the evidence is mixed. Americans eat too much and add too much salt all through their lives. Does this contribute to cardiovascular disease later on in life? It very likely does but is difficult to prove. The recommendations of the American Heart Association and others are: Control your sodium intake and get rid of the saltshaker.

What should I do about my blood pressure?

First, find out what it is. If it is high, see a doctor and get treatment. Many supermarkets have blood pressure machines but I don't know how accurate they are. The safest way is to have your doctor check it, especially if you are over 50. You can measure blood pressure at home with simple cuffs with stethoscopes, electronic monitors and finger machines. Some people believe a home setting is better because your blood pressure may be higher when your doctor measures it, due to "white coat hypertension." Ambulatory blood pressure monitoring uses a device on your arm to measure and record blood pressure every 30 minutes for 24 hours. Blood pressure changes with activity, tending to go up with heavy exercise, anger and stress and to go down with rest and relaxation. The 24-hour device gives a picture of your blood pressure during normal activities and sleep. It is a good way to monitor blood pressure, in some studies better than conventional measurements, but at about $150 a study, it is expensive.

Normal blood pressure is 120 mm of mercury (systolic) over 80 (diastolic), high normal 130-139/85-89. Systolic pressure measures the effect in arteries as the heart beats and contracts (systole), ejecting blood into the arteries. Diastolic pressure represents the relaxation of the heart (diastole). Blood pressure tends to increase with age as arteries become stiffer due to hardening, or arteriosclerosis. Thus, a high blood pressure of 140/90 is common in older people.

A high blood pressure of 140-159/90-99 represents mild hypertension. Moderate hypertension is set at 160-179/100-109 and severe at 180/100. Pressures from mild on require treatment. Isolated systolic hypertension can be dangerous. Hypertension contributes to strokes, heart disease, peripheral arterial disease and damage to organs such as the kidneys and eyes. It is estimated 50 million Americans experience hypertension, with 60% of Americans over age 60 hypertensive. High blood pressure kills about 42,000 Americans a year and contributes to death in about 210,000. Factors involved in hypertension which you cannot change are your genes (parents or siblings had hypertension), race (more common in African-Americans), sex (more common in men) and age (blood pressure increases with age).

A troubling trend has developed in the effort to control high blood pressure. Improvements have begun to slow with a slight rise in stroke, kidney disease, and heart failure and a leveling off of the death rate from heart disease among U.S. adults. The National Heart Lung and Blood Institute (NHLBI) believe the reason is complacency in individuals with hypertension. They issued still-current guidelines for treatment and prevention of hypertension, and emphasized changes in lifestyle along with diet, as reported in the January 1998 issue of the *Harvard Health Letter.* 1) follow the Dietary Approaches to Stop Hypertension (DASH) Diet; 2) keep daily salt intake to no more than 2.4 grams, about one teaspoon (preferably 1,500 mg); 3) consume potassium-rich food and/or drinks, like spinach, cantaloupes, almonds, orange juice, bananas, potatoes, prunes and yogurt, to get 3.5 grams of the mineral per day (up from an average daily consumption of 2.8 to 3.3 grams for American men and 2.2 to 2.4 for American women); 4) maintain a healthy weight; 5) limit alcohol intake for men to no more than one ounce of pure alcohol, 24 ounces of beer, or 10 ounces of wine per day, and half that for women; 6) 30 to 40 minutes of aerobic exercise on most days; and 7) don't smoke. The DASH diet is low in fat and rich in fruits and vegetables, whole grains and dairy products. (Chapter 72) Only 27% of calories should come from fat with plenty of fruits and vegetables, grains, low fat or nondairy products, and very small amounts of meat, fish, or poultry and nuts. The IOM recommends a higher intake of potassium, 4.7 grams a day.

This eating plan significantly and quickly lowered blood pressure in hypertensive participants enrolled in a multi-center study published in the April 17, 1997, issue of the New England Journal of Medicine (NEJM). A more recent trial of the DASH diet by Dr. Frank M. Sacks et al. showed a larger decrease in blood pressure, particularly for the low-sodium part of the trial.

Thus, a low-sodium diet is not the only answer to hypertension. A healthful diet and weight control are important. For women a diet of fruits, vegetables, fiber and magnesium with weight and alcohol control was helpful. Dr. Andrew Weil suggests six natural ways to manage hypertension: 1) maintain optimal weight; 2) get regular exercise; 3) eat lots of fruits and vegetables and follow the DASH diet; 4) relax; 5) don't smoke and 6) take anti-oxidants.

What should I do if diet, exercise and weight loss do not reduce my blood pressure? Your goal should be a blood pressure of 140/90 or less with medication prescribed by your doctor. Standard medications are diuretics such as hydrochlorothiazide or Lasix (furosemide) which decrease body fluid by getting rid of sodium in the urine, beta blocking agents and angiotensin-converting enzyme (ACE) inhibitors (Table 2). Calcium antagonists and alpha-blockers have caused troubles in some studies. Be careful of them. When taking a diuretic, you must eat foods containing potassium. Low potassium may contribute to hypertension. Your medication program should be carefully monitored by your doctor. Optimal anti-hypertensive treatment described by

Brown should involve drugs that lower blood pressure the most and are symptomatically and biochemically the best tolerated. Diuretics should be the initial mainstay.

What is my risk of stroke?

The risk of a stroke is closely related to risk factors for a heart attack such as lack of exercise, smoking, obesity, high cholesterol, hypertension and a family history of vascular disease. A stroke can occur by the blocking of a vessel to the brain by a blood clot or by rupture of a plaque in a blood vessel. The best defense is prevention: treatment of hypertension, reduction of cholesterol levels, no smoking, moderate alcohol use, weight reduction and exercise. Some people take a low-dose aspirin pill (82.5 mg) each day but the evidence is mixed about how worthwhile this is. The same is true for hormone replacement therapy in women, vitamins and anti-oxidants.

The most important preventive measure is treatment of systolic hypertension, which decreased the incidence of stroke in elderly people. Next on the scale of preventive measures come physical activity; weight loss; eating fruits and vegetables; taking folate, B-6 and B-12; eating seafood; and consuming whole grain and fiber. A drug which lowers blood pressure, Ramipril or Altace may also reduce the risk of stroke by other actions. Other means to prevent strokes are being studied but the evidence is not in yet on anti-oxidants like vitamin E and low saturated fat.

If you suffer a severe sudden headache, unexplained dizziness or falls, sudden dimness or loss of vision, sudden difficulty speaking or understanding, sudden and transient weakness or numbness of the face, arm or leg on one side, seek medical attention. These symptoms may be precursors of a stroke. If such an attack comes and goes, it is called a transient ischemic attack (TIA), and it is a warning. A stroke is an emergency and much can be done to help you if you go immediately to a hospital.

For more information:

NHLBI Information Center, PO Box 30105, Bethesda, MD 20824-0105 or
    www.nhlbi.nih.gov for your guide to lowering high blood pressure.
American Heart Association. *www.americanheart.org*
National Alliance to Reach Blood Pressure Goals. PO Box 27965, Washington,
    DC 20038-7965.
National Council on Aging—*www.ncoa.org.*
American Stroke Association. ·1-888-478-7653 *www.StrokeAssociation.org*
Institute of Medicine of the National Academies. Report on Dietary Intake Levels
    for Water, Salt and Potassium. 1-800-624-6242

Table 1

Sodium Food Labels

Sodium Free	5 mg or less/serving
Very low sodium	35 mg or less
Low sodium	140 mg or less
Reduced sodium	Usual sodium level is reduced by 25%
Unsalted or no salt added	No salt added during processing
Table salt	2300 mg (2.3 grams) of sodium per teaspoon

Table 2

Common blood-pressure drugs

Thiazide diuretics
Beta-blockers
Angiotensin-converting enzyme inhibitors
Angiotensin-receptor blockers
Calcium channel blockers

FISH

77. How much fish should I eat? What are omega-3s? What about contaminated seafood and mercury?

Tuna, crab, oysters, clams, and other seafood give you high quality protein that is usually low in fat and cholesterol. Nutritionists indicate that seafood one to three times a week is part of a heart-healthy diet. Protein from seafood is complete protein, containing all eight essential amino acids the human body cannot make. In the late 1970s, a study showed that Greenland Eskimos experienced a low rate of heart attacks in spite of a diet high in fat but with a pound or so of fish a day, a finding that began the continuing research into the benefits of fish oils.

The important component of seafood is two Omega 3 fatty acids, docosahexanoic acid (DHA) and eicosapentanoic acid (EPA). Another dietary source of these fatty acids is the third Omega 3 fatty acid of nutritional importance, alpha-linolenic acid, found in flaxseed oil, dark green leafy vegetables and other plant sources and converted by the body into DHA and EPA.

Women and men who eat fish have higher levels of Omega 3 fatty acids and less chance of heart disease. Heart-attack survivors did better taking omega-3 supplements. The *Harvard Health Letter* indicates fish oils may hinder the formation of blood clots causing heart attacks and strokes, and may reduce severely high levels of blood triglycerides, a risk factor for heart disease. Some evidence indicates that fish oils may help reduce blood pressure and prevent abnormalities of heart rhythm. According to Andrew Weil, fish in your diet may help protect against heart disease, breast cancer and rheumatoid arthritis. Several studies show clearly that men who consume fish once or twice a week have a lower mortality from coronary artery disease than men who do not eat fish. Eating fish may reduce sudden cardiac death by 50 percent. Women who ate fish two to four times a week had about half the risk of strokes caused by blood clots as compared to women who ate seafood less than once a month.

The American Heart Association recommends two fish meals a week. The Mediterranean diet with fish and vegetable oils is richer in omega-3s. The Nutraceutical industry has jumped in with supplements, Nutra Flax, DHA Omega-3 eggs, Omega-3 enriched cheeses and ice cream. Could we overdose on these products? Fish is still the answer. Fish is better than fish-oil capsules. Eating fish every day is not a problem.

Fish may also decrease the likelihood of dementia with Alzheimer's disease, with only one serving of fish a week effective in doing so. The *Physician's Health Study* reports five or more servings of seafood a week for four years offered no better protection against cardiovascular disease than one or two servings.

Salmon, mackerel, herring and anchovies are higher in fat, whereas cod is a lean fish. (Table) Clams, oysters, mussels and scallops contain little fat and cholesterol. Shrimp, lobster, and crab contain more cholesterol but shrimp doesn't seem to raise cholesterol levels in people. Herring, mackerel and salmon contain the greatest amount of the beneficial long chain omega-3 fatty acids; trout, bluefish and whiting a medium amount, and cod, canned tuna, catfish and haddock the least.

Frying fish in saturated fats, or adding cheese or butter undoes the benefits of omega-3 fatty acids. Be wary of prepared fish products; handy crab cakes and fish burgers, crunchy fish sticks, breaded and Cajun filets may contain added calories, saturated fat and sodium. Study the labels. See the table in the Beyond Fish Sticks reference. Be careful of seafood in restaurants. Broiled or grilled fish, shrimp or scallops may contain excess sodium, calories and saturated fat. A McDonald's fish filet is high in all.

The world's oceans and waterways are over fished, and, with wild fish harder to get, fish farming has become a big industry. Salmon, shrimp, oysters, clams, mussels, catfish and trout are frequently farmed. Farmed fish are fatter but their fat is monounsaturated and their levels of omega-3s are equal to those of wild fish. Overfished species include swordfish, flounder, halibut, lobster, red snapper, Atlantic salmon, sea bass, sea scallops, blue fin tuna, shark, orange roughy and Atlantic cod.

What about contaminated seafood?

Viruses and various bacteria may be present in partially cooked or raw seafood, particularly clams, oysters and other shellfish. You can play it safe by eating only thoroughly cooked shellfish. Shucked oysters, for example, should be boiled for at least three minutes.

Toxins may build up in fish like grouper and red snapper. Mercury may accumulate to high levels in swordfish, king mackerel, tilefish, and some tuna. Mercury poisoning is a particular threat to babies in utero and small children; children and pregnant or nursing mothers and women who may become pregnant should avoid these fish. The rest of us should limit our servings.

Locally caught fish from streams polluted with industrial mercury are most dangerous. The *Harvard Health Letter* recommends obtaining seafood only from reputable dealers and quality restaurants. Light tuna tends to contain less mercury than white tuna. Limit the canned tuna. Four types of fish are unsafe in any amount for pregnant or nursing mothers: shark, swordfish, mackerel and tile fish.

Farm raised salmon have become popular, but contain PCBs (polychlorinated biphenols) which cause cancer in some animals. Perhaps they cause some cancers in people, but the evidence is not strong. PCBs should be avoided by pregnant women because they affect their babies. PCBs in salmon come from the feed—herring and anchovies. Hopefully, this can be controlled.

Table 1

High in Fat (but more protective for the heart)

Salmon
Mackerel
Herring
Anchovies
Sardines
Trout

Lower in Fat (also protects the heart)

Cod
Flounder
Haddock
Sole

More Cholesterol

Shrimp
Lobster
Crab

Low in fat and cholesterol

Clams
Oysters
Mussels
Scallops

SOY

78. Should I be eating more soy or taking soy supplements? What good are they?

Soybeans as a foodstuff have been around in Asia for centuries but while they are a major U.S. agricultural crop, they serve primarily as animal feed in this country. The current interest here in soybeans and health began with the observation some years ago that Asian women, who have low breast cancer rates, follow diets rich in soy. Asian immigrants who come to Western countries and change their diets accordingly experience an increase in the incidence of breast cancer. Extensive research is being done on soy but the evidence is circumstantial with much disagreement. No good evidence, as yet, shows that soy prevents or inhibits breast cancer. Japanese men experience a less severe form of prostate cancer than do men in Western countries, and it was thought this could be due to a high soy diet. Again, this relationship is not clear-cut and not well understood.

Soy protein is the only plant food that contains all essential amino acids, which cannot be made in the body and must come from diet. Like animal products, soy protein is a complete protein; with no cholesterol and less saturated fat than meat or poultry, it is a good substitute for them. Furthermore, its weak estrogen-like isoflavones or phytoestrogens may protect the heart much like estrogens naturally produced by pre-menopausal women or the estrogen pills taken by post-menopausal women. Estrogen seems to allow coronary arteries to dilate. Soy may be particularly good for post-menopausal women as an alternative to estrogen therapy.

In October of 1999 the FDA gave food manufacturers permission to label products high in soy protein as possibly helpful in lowering the risk of heart disease. The FDA said, "A daily diet containing 6-25 grams of soy protein, low in saturated fat and cholesterol, may help reduce the risk of heart disease." Notice they said *may* not *does* and linked it to a diet low in saturated fat and cholesterol. In order to achieve an effect on cholesterol and thus heart disease risk, a diet must include a continuous daily intake of 25 grams of soy protein with a low intake of saturated fat and cholesterol. Forms of prepared soy protein include tofu, soy milk, soy flour, textured soy protein, Tempen, Miso, and soy nuts. Soy milk, however, does not taste like cow's milk, and some people don't like the taste. Improvements are being sought. Soy sauce contains little protein and is high in sodium. A thorough review of soy, soy diets and health is provided by Henkel of the FDA. The *Harvard Men's Health Watch* recommends soy in the daily diet.

In the *Nutrition Action Healthletter*, Bonnie Liebman lists and describes all of the soy and soy supplements in drinks and powders (14) and in foods (14) and pills (6). She writes that while tofu may no longer be trendy, "tofu cured soybean" tastes terrific in stir-frys and when marinated and grilled or right out of the package." Tofu is a source of protein that is good for you and your diet even though it may have little effect in preventing breast or prostate cancer.

In many studies, soy seems to lower cholesterol. The bottom line, according to Liebman: "Roughly 25 grams a day of soy protein with its naturally occurring isoflavones is enough to lower low density lipoprotein (LDL) or bad cholesterol by about 10% in people who start out with an LDL above 160. Total cholesterol also goes down, HDL is not affected." Dr. James W. Anderson et al. report soy protein intake rather than animal protein significantly decreased serum concentrations of total cholesterol, LDL cholesterol and triglycerides. Dr. John R. Crouse et al. obtained similar results with isoflavones isolated from soy protein.

However, isoflavones isolated from soy such as genistein and daidzem and used by women for menopausal hot flashes, could increase the risk of breast cancer in post-menopausal women. To play it safe, women who have had breast cancer shouldn't load up on soy protein or take isoflavone pills. Some experts also warn that excessive soy taken as supplements could be harmful.

More research is needed on the possibility that the soy milk protein genistein may weaken the immune system. Mice fed genistein to levels found in soy-fed babies showed a decrease in the weight of the thymus gland where immune cells mature and in the number of thymocytes or immune cells. It is not known if this happens in babies. Fifteen percent of infants in the U.S. are fed soy-based formulas.

For more information:

American Soybean Association, Suite 100, 12125 Woodcrest Executive Drive, St. Louis, MO 63141, 1-800-688-7692, *www.amsoy.org*.

United Soybean Board, 1-800-TALK-SOY, *www.talksoy.com*
Soyfoods Association of North America, 202-986-5600.
Society for Experimental Biology and Medicine, 162 W. 56th Street, Suite 203, New York, NY 10019, phone 212-541-7855, fax 212-541-7508, *www.sebm.org.*

FUNCTIONAL FOODS

79. What are functional foods and what should I know about them?

Functional foods are natural foodstuffs combined with minerals, vitamins or other additives. In the April 1999 *Nutrition Action Healthletter*, Beth Brophy and David Schardt note that functional foods have been around at least since the 1920s with the addition of iodine to salt to prevent goiters of the thyroid gland. Milk became a functional food with the addition of Vitamin D. The list continues with enriched flour, kava kava snack chips, soups with various additives, teas with added ginseng and gummy bears with added vitamins.

Functional foods now represent one of the faster growing parts of the food industry, on a worldwide basis. The Kellogg Company has announced plans to bring out an Ensemble line of 22 functional foods that include pastas, cereals, frozen entrees and bread made with a natural soluble fiber from psyllium husk, said to help lower cholesterol. Retail sales of functional foods are now over $10 billion a year and growing.

Nutritionists are concerned because functional foods may distract people from choosing healthy diets. The New York University nutritionist Marion Nestle says functional foods are about marketing not health. "Fruits and vegetables are already perfectly adequate to help prevent cancer and heart disease," she said.

Claims about health benefits of functional foods are a real problem. In 1993 the FDA was told by Congress to start approving these so-called "health claims" on labels of foodstuffs. Bruce Silverglade, Director of Legal Affairs for the Center for Science in the Public Interest (CSPI), said "A label can say, for example, a diet low in saturated fat and cholesterol can reduce the risk of heart disease, but only if it has the FDA's approval and only if the food isn't unhealthy."

Since 1993, the FDA has approved only ten health claims, but in 1994, Congress said that dietary supplements could make structure-or-function claims, and the practice has gone wild. Instead of making a health claim that mentions a disease, they indicate that a component of the foods can affect the structure or function of the body and so bypass the FDA. Thus, the structure-or-function claim for psyllium husk in grain products does not mention heart disease but says that this cholesterol-lowering component "promotes a healthy heart." The FDA notified the manufacturer of a soup containing St. John's Wort to stop marketing this functional food as a "dietary supplement." Michael Jacobson predicts that if the FDA does not act to ensure products are safe and claims are true, many functional foods may amount to little more than 21st century quackery.

Advertisements promote Adam and Eve Relaxation Cocktail with kava kava, Golden Temple Herbal Brain Power Cereal with gingko and gotu kola, Robert's American Gourmet Personality Puffs with St. Johns Wort and gingko. Are these additives safe? Who knows? None of them are approved by the FDA. They don't belong in food.

Steven DeFelice, Chairman of the Foundation of Innovation in Medicine, says, "Ninety-five percent of functional foods haven't been tested and make claims unsupported by clinical data." Whose health is the U.S. Congress interested in—ours or that of their industrial supporters?

Joan Gussow, a nutrition educator said, "I want my food to be food. Eating should be a pleasure not an intellectual (or scientific) exercise." Andrew Weil describes functional foods as a mixed bag of groceries and says, "Don't waste your money."

The important questions for functional foods are (1) "Does it work?" and "What is the evidence for a functional food improving health?" (2) "How much of the additive does it contain?" Often it contains very little of the substance mentioned. (3) Is it safe? Does it cause allergic reactions or drowsiness or interact with drugs? (4) Is it healthy or really a junk food? (5) Is it necessary? (See Chapter 42 on alternative medicine and herbal medicine).

The *Nutrition Action Healthletter* reviewed in great detail common food additives, listing them under the categories of **Safe, Cut-backs, Caution,** and **Everyone Should Avoid**. Additives listed under **Cut-backs** are not toxic, but large amounts may be unsafe or unhealthy. **Caution** additives may pose a risk for certain people and require better testing. **Everyone Should Avoid** additives include **Acesulfame potassium** found in artificial sweeteners, which may cause cancer, **Olestra, potassium bromate, saccharin** and **sodium nitrate and nitrite.**

ALCOHOL

80. Are a few alcoholic drinks a day healthy? What are the problems with alcohol?

The use of alcohol has been studied primarily in patients with heart disease. A recent report from the Physician's Health Study by Camargo et al. provides some support for the "alcohol hypothesis." Doctors who consumed one drink a day had a 30% reduction in risk for angina pectoris, and a 35% decrease in risk for a heart attack. The risk for heart disease was lower in those who drank two or more drinks per day, suggesting a 56% reduction in risk for angina pectoris, or chest pain during exercise with inadequate blood flow to the heart muscle, and a 47% decrease in risk for a heart attack. Studies have shown light or occasional alcohol consumption lowers stroke risk by 62% but five drinks daily triple it.

A "standard" drink is 5 oz. wine, 12 oz. beer, and 1.5 oz. 80-proof liquor. While excessive drinking, or more than three drinks a day, may cause heart disease, moderate alcohol intake of up to three drinks a day has been associated with increased levels of the beneficial high-density lipoprotein (HDL) and decreased risk of heart attack and strokes. Alcohol may also act on platelets in the blood. Self-reported moderate alcohol consumption of seven drinks a week in the year prior to a heart attack was associated with reduced mortality. Increasing alcohol consumption to the moderate range was also associated with decreased risk of heart failure among older persons. Dutch researchers found light-to-moderate alcohol consumption cut the risk of developing Alzheimer's disease and dementia over age 55 by about 40%. Other studies suggest maximum benefit from alcohol related to overall good health seems to be at the level of one drink per day.

The dangers of excess consumption are considerable, particularly in producing liver damage. Alcohol abuse can also produce heart trouble, hypertension, intestinal and digestive symptoms, musculoskeletal problems, male genitourinary problems, breast cancer, reproductive disorders, blood and immune system problems. Women with increased risk of breast cancer should avoid alcohol. Others who drink one drink a day may increase their risk of breast cancer.

The *Harvard Health Letter* points out that few studies have followed people without heart disease for some years to determine whether their drinking habits indicate what will happen to their hearts in the future. Such studies might show that modest alcohol consumption is fine. Some studies put that at a glass or two of wine a day but this does not mean that someone who does not drink alcohol should begin drinking. The problem with some of these studies is that wine drinkers tend to be more affluent, fit, health-conscious and likely to develop good habits in diet and exercise as compared with beer drinkers.

Some studies suggest wine, particularly red wine, is healthier than other forms of alcohol. It has been given credit for the French paradox: a low heart disease rate in a country renowned for high fat food. Red wine produces antioxidant activity through resveratrol and polyphenols which slow production of artery-clogging chemicals in the body. Other studies, however, find no difference between red wine and other forms of alcohol. Other chemical explanations have been proposed for the supposed benefits of drinking red wine. Andrew Weil believes they can be obtained from many fruits, vegetables and whole grains without alcohol. Cardiologists have found drinking a pint of purple grape juice inhibited platelets by 84%.

Alcohol is both good and evil. It can improve people's health and prolong their life. It is also a leading cause of death and disability in the U.S. It is the Jekyll and Hyde of preventive medicine. The key is moderation. A little is good but more is not.

Drinking and driving is a major problem. Motor vehicle crashes are the leading cause of injuries and deaths, and alcohol is involved in about 50% of them. Heavy use of alcohol before the accident increases the risk of mortality. Three drinks in one hour produces a blood alcohol level approaching 0.08%, the level that significantly prolongs reaction times. The result may be inability to stop in time at a red light. This is not social drinking. The answer is careful control of driving and drinking. Bars and restaurants should be patrolled. Intoxicated drivers should be identified before they get in the car and sober drivers should be designated. Intoxicated drivers who survive a crash should enter a compulsory rehabilitation program. Drinking and boating also involve a high risk of mortality.

Before you toast your health benefits of moderate drinking, ask yourself these questions:

1) Have you ever tried to cut down on your drinking?
2) Have you ever been annoyed by criticism of your drinking?
3) Have you ever felt guilty about your drinking?
4) Have you ever had a morning eye-opener?

If the answer to any of these is yes, be careful. If you know you have or have been told you have an alcohol problem, see your doctor. Many institutions have withdrawal programs and medications such as Ondansetron can help early onset alcoholism.

Alcoholics Anonymous is a great program and has helped many of my friends and relatives after they have gone through a withdrawal program. It is an international fellowship of men and women who share their experiences to have a satisfying life without alcohol.

81. Is there anything worthwhile about smoking?

S moking offers no redeeming features whatsoever other than what smokers describe as pleasure. While smokers may associate smoking with relaxation and stress relief, they are falling victim to an addiction that damages their lungs and other parts of their body. Why do tobacco companies want to market a product that causes harm? Their defense is that smoking is voluntary. Industry spokesmen say we can accept the harmfulness and enjoyment of smoking, or we can reject it. They say it is a matter of choice. That is not exactly true given the many existing cases of addiction, the efforts to create more cases by upping the nicotine content in tobacco and so increasing its addiction levels, and other plots of the tobacco companies to keep people hooked on cigarettes, cigars, and pipes. The truth is: It's the money. Smoking is a big business that pulls in billions of dollars.

As a thoracic surgeon who was addicted to cigarettes at the age of 14, I know very well the horrors of the addiction. Mine continued even while I was operating on patients with blackened, cancerous lungs. Eventually I did break free by using self-hypnosis but not before causing lung damage that left me with decreased ability to exercise and a lung cancer. Why is it so hard to quit smoking? Nicotine sends false messages to the brain that nicotine is good and in response the brain promotes behavior that delivers more nicotine. According to the cancer biologist Theodore Slotkin, "Addictive behaviors defy reason, not because people are irrational but because invisible factors, at work in their brains, compel them to seek out substances they know are bad for them."

It has been over 50 years since the British cancer epidemiologist Sir Richard Doll revealed to an unsuspecting world that smoking causes lung cancer. For many years tobacco companies vigorously tried to contest this finding, even while shredding their own scientific reports on harmful effects of smoking, but no longer. The relationship between carcinogens in the smoke and lung cancer is now too well established. On its website tobacco giant Philip Morris Co. says, "There is overwhelming medical and scientific consensus that cigarette smoking causes cancer, heart disease, emphysema and other serious diseases."

Premature deaths from smoking in this country ran about 440,000 annually from 1995 to 1999 and continue at about the same rate now. Probably thousands of Americans die each year from lung cancer brought on by exposure to other people's smoke. The annual cost of health—related economic loss from tobacco use is upwards of $157 billion. The *Harvard Men's Health Watch* estimates if smoking was entirely eliminated from American society, the number of cancer deaths would fall by 30% each year.

Slow, progressive self-destruction occurs over years with the use of cigarettes, cigars and pipes. Such damage is inevitable and varies only in the amount of smoking over how many years. The end result is emphysema, chronic obstructive pulmonary disease, and pulmonary failure, the need for an oxygen tank to stay alive, and eventually for a ventilator to support breathing. Problems with smoking not only involve the lungs, mouth, and esophagus, but other organs. Products of smoking and inhaling tobacco smoke get into the bloodstream and contribute to development of cancer of the pancreas, kidneys, bladder and cervix. Mental illness contributes to the likelihood of smoking.

Cigarettes may be deadlier for women. Smoking-lung cancer deaths for women are increasing rapidly and now exceed those from breast cancer, in part the by-product of successful advertising to women. Virginia Slims represented cigarettes as a symbol of feminine emancipation and glamour with the help of the slogan "You've come a long way, baby." Smoking also increases risk of other diseases such as rheumatoid arthritis. Smoking cessation decreases the risk of cataracts in men.

Yet about 3000 teens begin smoking each day. Tobacco use is common in college students. Nicotine allegedly is used in increased quantities in cigarettes to hook young people for good, sometimes within the first few days of smoking.

How many young people can know of the horrors of end-stage lung disease: of people pulling a little wagon wherever they go with an oxygen tank and hose leading into the nose; of their chronic cough and the pain and deterioration of incurable and/or recurrent lung cancer. No one would select such an end for life if they knew or understood what is ahead. What a terrible way to go!

Smoking is industry-assisted suicide, over a long period of time. The great national debate over physician-assisted suicide focuses on a sudden event leading to death in a few minutes. The overwhelming majority of doctors will not assist patients in efforts to commit suicide. However, assisting an individual, mentally competent and not necessarily terminally ill, to end life early by smoking is a problem for physicians and ethicists. Can we, as a civilized society, allow progressive INDUSTRY ASSISTED SUICIDE in perfectly healthy, young and middle-aged people? Do these people truly have informed consent when they decide to smoke? Are you free to destroy yourself even if it takes 30 years? What can we say of companies that sell slow, progressive destruction for profit and maintain that, even if addicted, you can choose not to smoke? Will we allow INDUSTRY ASSISTED SUICIDE as a freedom guaranteed by the Constitution?

We are spreading this tragedy around the world. To big tobacco companies, smokers are a disposable commodity and at the right price governments can be convinced to trade the health of their citizens for a lucrative revenue stream. The Philip Morris Company reminded the Czech Republic that in addition to taxes on tobacco products they get another benefit: the premature death of smokers.

Tobacco companies agreed in 1998 to stop promoting cigarettes to youths aged 12 to 17. Evidence indicates they have not lived up to this agreement. Charles King III and Dr. Michael Siegel found advertising for Camels, Marlboros and Newports increased in youth-oriented magazines since the settlement. Tobacco companies, they say, have a history of lying and subterfuge.

As described in USA TODAY, advertisements show seductive young women smoking Camel cigarettes in *Rolling Stone* and athletic-looking young people choosing Newports in *People*, magazines with a large youth readership. Danny McGoldrick, research director for the Campaign for Tobacco-free Kids, notes: "Tobacco companies lend an image to their product exactly what young people are looking for, an image of cool—an assertion of independence."

I often wonder how much support actors and actresses get from tobacco companies for smoking in films. Brands are often identified. In "My Best Friends

Wedding," Julia Roberts lights up a Marlboro in a scene that makes smoking look glamorous to young people, a bad and dangerous practice. Children exposed to the deceptive glamour of smoking scenes are 2.5 times more likely to begin to smoke.

Lawsuits for damages against tobacco companies by families of smokers who die of lung cancer are becoming more frequent as Connecticut and other states allow such suits to go forward. What should tobacco companies do? Some years ago, they seemed inclined to diversify into food products. Now they seem inclined to stonewall. Perhaps only government regulation and a sufficient number of lost lawsuits will persuade them to stop assisting suicide. The record on government regulation so far, however, has not been promising.

In 1996 the FDA issued a rule making it illegal to sell tobacco products to youths under age of 18. Photographic I.D. was required for anyone under 21. Although many compliance checks were carried out, illegal sales were rampant. The FDA stopped compliance checks after a 2000 Supreme Court ruling that Congress had not given the FDA the authority to regulate tobacco as a drug. Medical organizations like the Society of Thoracic Surgery challenged the Supreme Court decision and urged Congress to act quickly to give the FDA that authority but it has not. More interested in fund-raising and re-election than in your health, Congress has defeated bills to regulate tobacco. In 1998 Philip Morris spent more than $30 million blocking tobacco regulating legislation in Congress. Candidates received $8.6 million in 1999 from the tobacco industry.

Another setback came after the U.S. Justice Department, under Janet Reno, moved ahead with plans to sue cigarette manufacturers for the cost of elderly Americans who got sick from smoking. The governors of five tobacco-growing states opposed the suit because their states could lose money. Now the Bush administration settled the suit for less money. Anti-tobacco forces say the administration gave up.

A parallel suit by 46 states yielded a settlement of $246 billion. The money was to be used for public health and anti-smoking programs but once the states got the money many forgot about health problems. In Niagara County, New York, $700,000 of the tobacco settlement was spent on a sprinkler system for a public golf course. Seventeen states used the money for basic research that had nothing to do with smoking. Also, the attorneys who filed the suits got a big chunk. Many states do little or nothing in the way of smoking prevention programs.

Why doesn't my doctor counsel me about the hazards of smoking?

Doctors were not educated for counseling about smoking. Also, smoking cessation counseling is time-consuming, highly individualized and often unsuccessful. Health plans seldom pay for such programs or for drug therapies.

The U.S. Public Health Service makes specific recommendations to doctors: 1) every patient at every visit should be asked about tobacco use; 2) urge patients to quit; 3) ask if they are willing to try to quit; 4) help the patient with a plan; 5) provide practical counseling; 6) provide social support; 7) help if extra treatment is needed; 8) recommend pharmacologic support; 9) schedule follow-ups. Medical schools are urged to have a core curriculum about smoking cessation.

How do I stop smoking?

In USA TODAY Anne Carey and Gary Visgaitis gave these reasons why smokers can't quit: stress 29%; joy of smoking 12%; craving too strong 12%; spouse/friend smokes 7%; no one thing 7%; addiction habit 7%; weight gain 5%; can't change 5%.

Some people have switched to cigars from cigarettes believing they are safer, but a recent study in the New England Journal of Medicine indicated "regular cigar smoke can increase the risk of coronary artery disease and cancers of the lung and throat." In spite of reduced tar and nicotine, the National Cancer Institute (NCI) has reported that "light" and "ultra light" cigarettes are no safer than regular cigarettes. (Bennet LeBow, CEO of Vector Tobacco, said its low-tar Omni "will not kill them as quick or as much." Now there's a slogan!)

"The truth is that light cigarettes do not reduce the health risks of smoking," said the NCI. "The only way to reduce a smoker's risk, and the risk to others, is to stop smoking completely." Cutting back on cigarettes won't help. Eventually you must quit.

George Avery wrote, "There is no magic formula for kicking the smoking habit," and I agree. Most people try to quit by themselves. Others may want to consult a doctor or therapist for help. Some hospitals offer smoking cessation clinics. Hypnosis and acupuncture may help.

Federal guidelines first endorse an antidepressant Zyban for help with smoking cessation. Sustained release bupropion hydrochloride (Zyban—Wellbutrin) requires a prescription but may help you come off nicotine. The second-line drugs Clonidine and Nortriptyline (Aventyl, Pamelor) also require prescriptions. Precautions, side-effects and adverse effects of each of these are described in the article "A Clinical Practice Guideline."

The guidelines also endorse four nicotine products: nicotine gum, inhaler, nasal spray, and patch. Combinations of these have not been approved by the FDA. Some of you may need nicotine products for some years, and some people report getting hooked on nicotine products. That is better than smoking, however. These products contain a low dose of nicotine and are generally harmless. Tobacco companies have tried to interfere with advertisements for smoking cessation products. Promotion of a nicotine vaccine has not removed a worry that it could encourage smoking.

Some health effects of prolonged smoking are irreversible, as reviewed by Paul Brodish. On the other hand, cessation brings some almost immediate benefits and the long-range statistical outlook is more encouraging, as noted by Dr. David K. Murdock under the auspices of the American Heart Association: Give up smoking for 8 hours and your carbon monoxide levels return to normal. Give up smoking for 24 hours and your risk of heart attack begins to decrease. Give up smoking for 3 months and your lung function increases by 30%. Give up smoking for 1 year and your excess risk of heart attack drops by half. Give up smoking for 5 years and your risk of stroke drops to that of non-smokers. Give up smoking for 10 years and your risk of lung cancer decreases by half. Give up smoking for 15 years and your overall risk of death is the same as that of a non-smoker.

Andrew Weil recommends 10 strategies to stop smoking: 1) break the habit—change habits of when you smoke; 2) get some guidance (quit net *www.quitnet.org* or the American Lung Association book *Seven Steps to a Smoke-Free Life*, John Wiley and Sons, 1998); 3) stay active; 4) breathe deeply; 5) practice safe stress relief (meditation, relaxation); 6) picture yourself smoke free; 7) consider cessation products; 8) be hypnotized and taught self hypnosis; 9) explore acupuncture; 10) reward yourself with the money you save. To this I would add—get angry at cigarettes for addicting you.

Tobacco dependence treatment programs can be quite effective. The U.S. Department of Health and Human Services publishes an excellent book on Treating Tobacco Use and Dependence. Every doctor should get one.

Do tobacco control programs work?

Yes, they do. Florida's Program on Tobacco Control made progress in reducing youth tobacco use. Bans on smoking in households, work places, airplanes, restaurants, public places and now bars help decrease smoking by all. An antismoking group, The American Legacy Foundation, was created from more than a $1 billion settlement with the Lorillard Tobacco Company and seeks to curb smoking through ads. On-line sites may be more effective for teens such as Thetruth.com or tobaccofree.org, a project of Patrick Reynolds, grandson of the founder of the R.C. Reynolds Co., makers of Winstons and Camels. An increase in the price of cigarettes and taxes helps decrease consumption.

The former U.S. Surgeon General David Satcher described six major ways to reduce or prevent tobacco use: 1) school based prevention programs; 2) physicians' advice to patients against smoking; 3) strong clean indoor air regulations; 4) stronger warning labels; 5) increased cigarette prices and taxes; 6) change in the social environment to reduce acceptability of smoking. In his continuing campaign against the tobacco industry, the former Surgeon General C. Everett Koop called it "the sleaziest bunch of lying businessmen that ever existed on this planet." Leonard H. Glantz and George J. Annas believe a separate Tobacco Control Agency is needed.

The WHO and an International Group, the Framework Convention on Tobacco Control (FCTC), seek worldwide tobacco control through international treaties. Members of the Society of Thoracic Surgeons who operate on patients with lung cancer are sponsors of "Kick Butts Day" for tobacco-free kids. Canada requires that 50% of a cigarette pack contain messages along with graphic pictures about hazards of smoking, as a cause of stroke, lung cancer, mouth disease and harm to babies

The government believes the number of new teen-age smokers is dropping. In 2001, fewer teens smoked cigarettes, but use of the drug Ecstasy increased. The number of non-smokers is increasing, and deaths from smoking related illnesses are decreasing. However, tobacco is now a world-wide problem. Three hundred to three hundred and forty million Chinese smoke. In Japan, the tobacco industry is state-run. The U.S. exported death by tobacco for years and Joe Camel is still active in Europe.

ACCIDENTS—GUNS

82. Can accidents and injuries be prevented and, if so, how? What is the big problem with guns?

In recent years the medical community has become increasingly interested in injuries as a public health issue. Doctors taking care of injured people believe prevention of any injury is far superior to the best treatment and economically more advantageous, and they believe in the effectiveness of injury-control interventions. "Most injuries to people and nearly all injuries to children can be predicted and can be prevented," said the former U.S. Surgeon General C. Everett Koop.

Practitioners of injury prevention speak of injuries rather than accidents, to denote the damage caused by chance events instead of those events, according to Dr. Frederick P. Rivara et al. in their definitive report on injury prevention in the New England Journal of Medicine (NEJM). They speak of crashes rather than auto accidents because they may not be chance events, particularly if alcohol is involved.

Injury is the fourth leading cause of death in the United State, behind heart disease, stroke and cancer, and the greatest cause of loss in productivity, with 36 life years lost per death compared with 16 years per death from cancer and 12 years per death from heart disease and stroke combined. Motor vehicle crashes are the third leading cause of loss of potential years of life for people under the age of 35. Crashes with motor vehicles accounted for most fatal bicycle injuries. Many elderly drivers, who drive safely but slowly, die in crashes caused by other drivers.

Rivara et al. report that 150,956 people died from injuries in the United States in 1994. Unintentional injuries caused 61% of these deaths and of those nearly half were the result of motor vehicle crashes, the leading cause of unintentional death. Falls, primarily among the elderly, were the second leading cause. Third came poisoning, classified as an injury, with most due to unintentional overdoses of drugs. About equal numbers of people died from fires, scalding and drowning.

The Rivara article notes that passive prevention strategies that come into play automatically, as with making automobiles safer, are more successful than active intervention strategies, which require people to change their behavior. Active intervention includes preventing activities like driving while intoxicated or treating cases of road rage, now established as a mental illness. Doctors are helping with both passive and active injury prevention strategies, and with mixtures of both.

Dr. Flaura Winston, a primary care pediatrician, and Dr. Dennis R. Durbin, a pediatric emergency physician, are experts in the prevention of motor vehicle occupant injuries to children. They say buckling up is not enough for children in autos. Children should be kept in child safety seats (CSS) until they are four years old and weigh at least 18 kg.; infants should sit facing the rear of the car until they are at least one year of age and over 9 kg. The CSS's harness must fit the child snugly and a seatbelt should hold it securely in place. From age four until age eight or nine, children should sit in booster seats, with a correct safety belt fit. The seatbelt must go across the waist; the shoulder belt should **not** cross the neck or head. Age—appropriate restraining devices reduce mortality and severity of injury in children. In light of that finding the National Highway Safety Administration mandated a child-restraint anchorage system in cars by 2002. Where is it?

Doctors can help with the problem of driving under the influence of alcohol by identifying patients with alcohol problems and referring them to programs that can help. Doctors can also lend their support to community-based programs that encourage responsible beverage service, reduce underage drinking by limiting access to alcohol, increase local enforcement of drinking and driving laws, and limit access to alcohol by zoning restrictions

Driving under the influence of alcohol plays a major role in motor vehicle crashes with fatalities. Many children riding in cars—often unrestrained— innocent pedestrians, bicyclists and other drivers are killed by drinking and drunken drivers. Should drunken drivers who kill someone ever be allowed to drive again? They certainly should not, without evidence of success in a rehabilitation program.

The number of crashes by teenage drivers has been reduced by graduated licensing systems now in thirty-two states. In North Carolina 15 to 17-year-old beginning drivers are allowed to drive only with a designated adult for a year. For the next six months they may drive unsupervised only from 5 a.m. to 9 p.m. and only without passengers; with supervision they may drive at any other time. Then they may receive a full license. With teenage drivers risk of a crash increases with the number of passengers in the car.

A. Myer, in the *Journal of Trauma*, describes the estimated cost of injury in the billions. Huge savings would result from interventions to reduce injury, including a child pedestrian injury campaign, bicycle helmet protection, strict driver education an increase in the age for licensing drivers to 17, motorcycle helmet laws, reduced flammability of cigarette paper, air bags, side crash protection and automatic vehicle lights. The former U.S. Surgeon General David Satcher writes that injury is an overlooked global health concern.

Methods of prevention are listed in Table 1.

What is the big problem with guns? Everybody seems angry about them one way or another.

The big problem with guns is that they are available to almost everyone in this country. In 1995 guns accounted for an estimated 34,990 deaths and 1.3 million rapes, robberies or aggravated assaults. The year before, guns were involved in 72 per cent of homicides. You have read about the school shootings in Arkansas and Colorado. It is estimated one in five teenagers is armed. Where do those children get guns? They get them from the homes of parents and grandparents, from gun stores, and from others selling guns.

The problem of death by gunshot is so immense the medical profession is running an active campaign for gun control as a public health issue. Dr. C. Everett Koop, former Surgeon General, and Dr. George D. Lundberg, former editor of the JAMA, note that safer roads and cars, stricter licensing and drunk-driving laws have led to a dramatic decline in auto death rates. They believe a similar decline in shooting deaths could be achieved by gun controls. Doctors are urged to counsel patients about the problems posed by guns.

Doctors Against Handgun Injury (DAHI) is working actively for hand gun control. They advise parents to not leave the keys lying around where kids can get them and to store guns and ammunition separately in locked containers. Geoffrey A. Jackman et al. report that many boys aged 8 to 13-years-old who find a gun lying around will handle it and pull the trigger.

In England, where handguns are outlawed, there have been almost no deaths from firearms until recently. Most English policemen, or bobbies, do not carry guns. Guns for hunting require an application and a permit. Now some people fear the rise of a gun culture in England with the smuggling of illegal weapons from Eastern Europe and the USSR into the country. Guns have become a "fashion accessory" for some teenagers. Recently firearm murders have been on the increase but the number is still small compared to that for the U.S.: 62 firearm related murders in 1999-2000 in England as compared with 7950 in 1999 in the U.S. The police now have armed response units.

In the U.S. the National Rifle Association (NRA) and other groups say that the Constitution guarantees everyone the right to have a gun. When the Constitution was written, all guns were loaded with powder and shot and were stored unloaded. There were no shells and virtually no hand guns or assault weapons. Rowland T. Berthoff reviews the writings of Don Higginbotham and Michael Bellesiles who explode the myth of a historical American gun culture. The Second Amendment provision for the right to bear arms represents a desire to assure their availability to state militias, not to support individual ownership of guns. In colonial America only one in six people owned muskets or rifles; most members of militias did not. At that time four-fifths of murders were carried out by means of knives, axes, poison, beating or drowning—not guns—and the murder rate was very low.

Mass production of guns began after 1840, Union soldiers were allowed to take their guns home, and "the government succeeded in arming America." In their advertising gun manufacturers stressed the importance of owning a gun. They said: It is your Constitutional right to have a gun for family security. In the 1870s the NRA was born. Then and only then did an American gun culture fall into place.

Some people insist on keeping guns, no matter what tragedies they bring about, but why? The NRA says we need guns for self-defense but the evidence shows that guns kept in homes are more likely to be involved in fatal or nonfatal accidental shootings, or suicide attempts rather than self-defense. The answer to home safety is a burglar alarm connected to the police station. The NRA believes carrying a concealed gun helps protect people from attackers but can produce no evidence that it does.

The evidence is clear: In the U.S., the number of injuries and deaths due to firearms and crimes committed with firearms is much greater than in any other industrialized country. It is estimated "Every hour, guns are used to kill four people and to commit 120 crimes in the U.S." In spite of this, the former U.S. Attorney General Ashcroft defends the gun lobby.

Philip J. Cook and Jens Ludwig estimate gun violence costs Americans $100 billion a year, half of that borne by taxpayers. In a year, Minor reports, firearms killed 0 children in Japan, 19 in Great Britain, 57 in Germany, 109 in France, 153 in Italy and 5285 in the United States." How does the NRA explain the magnitude of the U.S. problem compared with the small number of gun-related deaths in other countries?

The roll of school shootings in this country includes one in 1997 by a 14-year-old and two 16-year-olds; four in 1998 by an 11, 15, 17 and 18-year-old; four in 1999 by a 12, 13, 15 and two 18-year-olds (in the Columbine Colorado High School tragedy 15 dead and 23 wounded and in Georgia 6 wounded) two in 2000 and one in 2001. In 1999, 7 were shot dead in a church in Forth Worth, 5 were wounded in a Jewish Community Center in Los Angeles and 12 shot dead and 12 wounded in an Atlanta suburb.

Many people fault the parents of the shooters for not supervising them and helping them with emotional problems, and for not storing guns safely. They fault schools for not recognizing bizarre behavior and allowing cliques to torment outsiders with rejection, humiliation, and bullying, making them want to get even. They note that such children may come from broken, loveless families, suffer from depression or develop pre-occupation with violence and hate. There is conjecture about the contribution of publicity in the use of guns and killings. If a kid learns that another kid in another school shot a bunch of people he did not like, his reaction might be "I can do that, too." Some years ago news of a domestic hijacking of an airliner seemed to prompt a rash of copycat hijackings.

Nonetheless, the common denominator in these terrible events is guns. The causes of gun violence are many and complex, but the first and foremost cause is the availability of guns. The NRA denies it but it is true. The NRA and the Citizens Committee for the Right to Keep and Bear Arms say some of the violence is by "anti-Semitic, racists hatemongers, not guns." However, such people will always be with us. Let's keep them from getting guns. The NRA says people kill people, guns don't, but if these people didn't use guns, what would they use? Guns kill, not sticks and stones.

Proposed solutions include: prosecuting parents whose guns were used; suing gun manufacturers; encouraging parents to listen to their children, to help them to stand up for one another, to meet at the school and to talk to one another about their kids' problems. Kids can use the teen help line (401-741-TEEN) to report threats of violence in schools. Other recommendations include high-visibility police patrols to confiscate guns and rewards for turning them in.

Elliot Aronson reduced the competitive nature of the classroom and its potential for making some students feel left behind by introducing the "jigsaw" system, dividing fourth, fifth, sixth and higher grades into small racially and ethnically mixed groups to work on lessons. Each student had to become an expert on a topic important in a larger academic puzzle, hence the name "jigsaw." How well students learned and did on exams depended on how well they worked as a group. After initial resistance students came to like the system, and the groups played together at recess. In *Nobody Left To Hate: Teaching Compassion after Columbine.*, Aronson writes most men and boys convicted of murder suffered the kind of rejection and humiliation the jigsaw system is designed to avert.

On the other hand, Michael Guzy, a retired police detective, writes, "First get the guns, then tackle the root causes." He likens the efforts to prevent a catastrophe by focusing on societal causes instead of gun control to a cardiologist telling a patient in the middle of a heart attack to eat more oat bran and take up jogging.

The NRA continuously rejects reasonable gun controls even though polls show that 75% of the public support gun control. Why doesn't Congress listen to the public? The U.S. is not a frontier. We are reasonably safe in our homes and cars with reasonable precautions and alarms. Why don't they help us with the urban, domestic and school violence caused by guns?

Senators John McCain (R) and Joseph Lieberman (D) are acting together to help control guns. Why don't Dennis Hastert (R) and Delay (R) in the House do the same? They don't because the NRA gives big money to their campaigns. They are bought.

Richard Ford, a hunter, writes the NRA does not speak for him and for many hunters and target shooters who have always accepted government regulation. Hunters must obtain a hunting license, must observe a limit on birds or animals shot, pass a hunter's safety course and wear colored jackets in the field. Hunters do not use assault weapons or handguns. Hunters have no stake in the controversy over restricting felons from gun ownership, outlawing assault weapons and reducing ownership of handguns. Small, inexpensive handguns are preferred by criminals but useless to hunters.

Ford asks: "Why do hunters put up with the NRA and their gibberish which sounds like corrupted logic and bizarre exaggerations?" My father was a hunter and taught me shotgun and rifle safety first. Guns were always carried unloaded and stored unloaded. Shells were locked up.

Present laws to control guns have been better than nothing, but not sufficient. The Brady Handgun Violence Prevention Act of 1993-94 restricted handgun sales. Licensed gun dealers have to observe a waiting period and run a background check on potential purchasers. This law is associated with a reduction in gun suicide rates for those over 55 but with no reduction in homicides or overall suicide rates. The Brady Law has now been extended to shotguns and rifles. Several states passed safe gun storage laws. This seems to prevent unintentional shooting deaths in children under 15. A permit must be obtained to carry concealed guns, and it is unavailable to anyone with a felony conviction or mental illness.

Possession of guns by convicted criminals is a big problem. By law convicted felons can't buy guns but they obtain them anyway from friends and relatives or at gun shows. According to Lacy, this occurs because of the fragmented computer systems and antiquated criminal records in court houses. Information on felony convictions, arrest warrants, restraining orders, dishonorable military discharge and evidence of mental incompetence does not get to the National Instant Background Check System of the FBI. Thus, instant background checks may fail. This is the weak link in the effort to keep guns out of the hands of felons.

As for those convicted of violent misdemeanors, current federal law does not prevent them from buying guns, even though it should. In JAMA the epidemiologist Garen Wintemute, et al. provides evidence that prior misdemeanor convictions are strong predictors of subsequent crimes, some of which are violent. One in five misdemeanants purchasing handguns was charged with a new crime, including violent and firearm-related crimes, within a year of the purchase. Those convicted of violent misdemeanors should not be allowed to buy guns, as is the case in California. Will the U.S. Congress protect the rest of us? Don't hold your breath!

Mayors of New York, Chicago, Los Angeles and Gary, Indiana write in the *New York Times* February 24, 2004 about their efforts to get guns off the streets, noting that Congress is about to undercut them by the Protection of Lawful Commerce in Arms Act. It would shield firearm companies, dealers and trade associations from any form of civil liability. The mayors say we deserve a Congress that makes our lives safer.

How do people get assault weapons—automatic guns? I thought they were outlawed.

They are no longer available for purchase from licensed gun dealers. However, many were stolen years ago and kept. Some were smuggled into the country or stolen from the military.

Two dozen cities, including St. Louis, Detroit, Atlanta and Miami, have filed suits against gun makers. They hold them responsible for gun violence. The Clinton administration planned to sue them also. I am sure the present administration has dropped that plan. The NRA wants states to pass legislation prohibiting cities from suing.

The NRA also is pressing for the elimination of the National Center for Injury Prevention and Control (NCIPC) established at the Center for Disease Control and Prevention (CDCP) in Atlanta, Georgia, over a decade ago. There is now a Science Center for injury control, also under threat of elimination by the government. These agencies have published many useful studies on injuries in fires, drownings, bicycle and car crashes and poisonings but the NRA is opposed to any group whose research may undermine their policies. Their influence is yet another example of the corrupting influence of powerful lobbies.

Table 1

Prevention of Injury

Kind of Injury	Prevention Strategy
Motor vehicle	Stop driving while intoxicated Energy absorbing steering columns Increase padding on contact points Better side impact prevention Both seatbelts and airbags (both are needed) No children in front seats, car seats in the back seat (facing backwards) for small children up to the age of five to six Side air bags No children in cars unattended Safe tires, problems of vehicle design Rest stops—pull off the road if drowsy
Motorcycles (a hazardous means of transportation)	Helmets required Lights on 24 hours a day Crash bars Leg protection Many motorcycle accidents are the result of alcohol and drugs
Pedestrians (youth and elderly)	Divert high-volume traffic from residential areas Luminous attire, for children and the elderly
Bicycle Injuries Automobiles are the problem	Helmets required Separate lane for cyclists
Falls (particularly in the elderly) (Primarily hip fractures)	Prevent osteoporosis by calcium intake throughout life Hormone therapy during menopause Calcium, vitamin D in older adults Weight-bearing exercises Protective hip pads may help Use a walker if unsteady

Poisoning (children and suicides)	Child resistant containers
Poison centers	Warning labels little help
Suicide or accidental death	Decrease engine emissions for carbon monoxide poisoning
problems	Drug safety programs
	Safer drugs to reduce mortality from intentional and unintentional overdoses (particularly for those who are depressed)
	Seratonin uptake inhibitors may be better than tricyclic agents
Fires and scalding	Smoke detectors
	Fire safe cigarettes
	Water heaters—maximum of 50 degrees C
	Frequent checks of propane tanks and connections
	Don't leave children home alone
Drownings	Fence pools
	Swimming skills taught early
	Alcohol in adults
	Flotation devices for all in boats
Firearms	Firearms in the home result in the majority of suicide and homicides
	Gun control is the only answer
Fireworks	Fireworks safety and limited access
Farm accidents	Baler, tractor safety programs.
Garbage and trash compactor deaths	Care and safety.
Bullying	Identify, study, treat and respond.

DOCTORS AND HEALTH PROMOTION

83. Why doesn't my doctor talk to me about maintaining my health, about disease prevention and health promotion? What should I do?

A simplistic answer is that your doctor was taught to focus on diseases rather than health. Have you ever gone to see your doctor because you were healthy and wanted to maintain your health? Probably not. Hospitals now call themselves health centers but few of us go there when we are healthy and feel well and want to stay that way. We think of hospitals as the kind of place denoted in the German word for hospital: *krankenhaus* or sick house.

Our hospitals and health centers, however, do provide services for maintaining health, like screening, advice about nutrition, wellness and fitness programs, child care and other activities. For example, in its *Wellness Connection* newsletter the Putnam Memorial Health Corporation in Bennington, Vermont, provides information about symptoms of a heart attack so you can get care early enough to make a difference. Their offerings include aerobics; diabetes management; information on childbirth, breast feeding, safety and fitness; and support groups for many of life's problems. Most programs do not charge a fee. Some companies will subsidize your participation in wellness and fitness programs. Check your community and hospital for hotlines on transportation and other urgent problems. Take advantage of health services.

In years past, the environment was the primary source for human disease and death, in the form of infectious diseases, toxins, malnutrition, water pollution, mosquitoes and other problems. These threats have been greatly reduced in our society in good part by public health measures.

Now, in developed countries, disease primarily originates in the problems of individuals: arteriosclerosis, obesity, smoking, alcohol, stress, injury, toxins, carcinogens, dietary supplements and other factors. According to Surgeon General David Satcher, human behavior is the most important factor in the public health challenges facing the nation. Speaking at Yale University he said, "There is no way we are going to control costs as long as we focus on treatment of patients after they are sick. There is not enough incentive for health promotion and disease prevention."

Satcher would set these priorities for the near future: 1) addressing mental illness; 2) giving children a healthy start; 3) getting people to take responsibility for their own health; 4) improving our understanding of the health care system and 5) eliminating health disparities related to race, minority status and level of income.

Dr. Lester Breslow describes primary prevention as averting occurrence of disease and secondary prevention as halting progression of a disease from its early unrecognized stage to a more severe one. In 1952, he says, the President's Commission on Health Needs of the Nation noted an individual's responsibility for one's health can be fully effective if society provides access to necessary support and activities. Since then such support has helped bring about the eradication of smallpox and poliomyelitis and the recent decline in lung cancer and mortality (Chapter 16). Health risk factors are decreasing with seat belt use, mammography, adult vaccinations, smoking cessation and reduced alcohol use but the obesity data is disturbing.

In 1979, a U.S. Public Health Service document put forward an approach to health promotion and the Office of Disease Prevention and Health Promotion (ODPHD) was set up in Washington by the U.S. Department of Health and Human Services (DHHS) to provide leadership. The ODPHD provides information for individuals, physicians and public health people in periodic prevention reports. Their major mission is to help with nutrition, tobacco control, occupational safety and health, oral health, control of the spread of HIV, respiratory diseases, asthma, obesity, heart disease, stroke, cancer and other health problems. One of their mottos is "PPIP—Putting Prevention into Practice." Information about their programs can be obtained from the ODPHD, U.S. DHHS, Hubert H. Humphrey Building, Room 738G, 200 Independence Avenue SW, Washington, D.C., 20201, or *http:// odphp.osophs.dhhs.gov.*

Another national program that helps in disease prevention and health promotion is the American Council on Science and Health (ACSH), a consumer education consortium concerned with "issues related to food, nutrition, chemicals, pharmaceuticals, lifestyle, the environment and health." It is an independent nonprofit tax-exempt organization of physicians, scientists and policy advisors, founded in 1978 by scientists concerned that many important public policies related to health and the environment lacked a sound scientific basis. To provide information for debates about public health issues, the ACSH produces a large number of publications and reports on what is real in prevention, health promotion and environmental topics. You may obtain their pamphlets and special reports simply by writing or calling the ACSH, 1995 Broadway, 2nd Floor, New York, NY 10023-5860 or *ACSH@acsh.org.*

Their reports include "Asbestos," "Aspirin and Health," "Biotech Pharmaceuticals," "Chronic Fatigue Syndrome," "Dietary Fiber," "Natural Carcinogens," "Facts about Fats, Hay Fever, Pesticides-Helpful or Harmful," "Priorities in Caring for Your Children," among others. They published the first comprehensive guide on the health consequences of smoking and its irreversible health effects. Take advantage of their publications and activities to keep informed about your health. Look into subscribing as well to the health letters published by many medical schools. (Chapters 56, 66)

F. Douglas Scutchfield and K. T. Hartman state that "Physicians and hospitals should incorporate prevention in their daily practice and be sure patients receive the immunizations, counseling and screening procedures effective in preventing disease." The World Health Organization (WHO) defines health as "physical, mental and social well-being not merely absence of disease and infirmity." Ask your doctor for help with prevention. Good doctors are willing to help but they may get discouraged upon encountering difficulties in trying to get people to stop smoking or lose weight or exercise. A healthy lifestyle is up to you (Chapter 65). All your doctor can do is to advise and encourage you.

STRESS

84. Is stress all bad? What is the best way to deal with it? What is the chronic fatigue syndrome?

Along with its negative connotations, studies of stress also show a positive side. It is what allows us to respond to life, its challenges and its emergencies. In the 1920s the great Harvard physiologist Walter Cannon focused on a short-term effect of stress in describing our built-in response to danger as "fight or flight." Cannon showed that when we experience a shock or perceive a threat, our body responds by releasing hormones that prepare us for physical exertion, for instance by increasing heart rate and blood pressure to deliver more oxygen and blood sugar to the muscles. Do we stay and fight the danger or do we get out of the way?

It was in 1936, however, that modern stress medicine began, with the discoveries of the native Hungarian Hans Selye, then working as an endocrinologist in Montreal and a pioneer in describing the paradox of our physiological systems which, when activated by stress, can on the one hand protect us but on the other hand damage our bodies. Selye described three stages in coping with stresses of many different kinds: First, the body experiences an alarm reaction, ready for "fight or flight;" Next, unable to sustain that heightened state of alarm, it builds a sustained resistance to stress; Then, if beset long enough, it succumbs to exhaustion. For the general reader Selye described stress as both good and bad in *Stress without Distress.*

In 1999 Dr. Bruce McEwen observed that new research has confirmed the protective and damaging effects of stress, noting ". . . the search for biological mechanisms that determine protective versus damaging effects of these mediators is a theme in biobehavioral research." As better suited to the complexity of this search, he replaced the word "stress" with two terms deemed to be more comprehensive. "Allostasis," as defined by Peter Sterling and J. Eyer, means the maintenance of stability through change. "Allostatic load" is the "long-term effect of the physiological response to distress," said McEwen . . . ."Among the many factors that contribute to allostatic load are genes and early development, as well as learned behaviors reflecting life style, choices of diet, exercise, smoking and drinking."

The association of stress with disease has been understood for a long time. The idea that emotions are related to health preceded Hippocrates (the Father of Medicine—500 B.C.) when doctors thought that the "passions" had a role in causing disease, a precursor of our current understanding of signals between the nervous and immune systems. The stress response begins with a signal of alarm to the hippocampus and hypothalamus in the brain, which then secrete a chemical called corticotrophin releasing factor (CRF). CRF tells the pituitary gland to send corticotrophin (adrenocorticotrophin ACTH) to the adrenal glands which release stress hormones—adrenaline and glucocorticoids to the blood to send energy to muscle, increase blood pressure, increase heart rate and activate immune cells.

Stress is particularly associated with heart disease and heart attacks; grumpy old men and anger produce the greatest risk for heart disease. Mental stress, tension, frustration and sadness all increase the risk of decreased blood flow to the heart. Chronic anger, anxiety, loneliness or depression can be lethal to people with coronary artery disease. People with heart disease may be more vulnerable to stress. Thus, it may not be stress that produces heart disease but heart disease that alters response to stress. Cancer may also involve a relationship to stress. Metastatic cancer patients who have a positive outlook and resist the problems of stress seem to live longer and do better, as described by Dr. Bernie Siegel.

You may remember the message of "Adelaide's Lament," in *Guys and Dolls*: the stress of cancelled weddings would lead to a person developing a cold. Indeed, stress changes our immune system and seems to make us more susceptible to infectious diseases, particularly infectious diseases such as colds and upper respiratory infection. The role of stress is being studied not only in infections and cancer but also in the development of many diseases, like asthma, rheumatoid arthritis, multiple sclerosis, uveitis, inflammatory bowel disease and psoriasis. Andrew Weil describes other surprising ways that stress affects health including digestive problems, pain from muscle tension and migraine, sexual and reproductive dysfunction, skin conditions, insomnia and depression.

Stress is recognized as battering the hippocampus. Douglas Bremner, writing in the journal *Biological Psychiatry*, said "Traumatic stress is bad for the brain." Long severe periods of stress may permanently damage the brain.

Michelle Pearson describes the uncertainties of modern life which put people on edge. She believes many people in our society are on the verge of losing it because of an unbearable amount of uncertainty about everything in one's life: job security, marital permanence, parenting styles, social etiquette, medical advice and other problems. She describes not only road rage but voice mail rage, health care rage, and many other cause of anger. Thus, "We are on edge. We are anxious—that converts to rage because rage, as a criminal psychologist once told me, is a more tolerable human emotion than fear." Stress related health problems are very costly in the U.S. The death rate in Eastern Europe has increased because of the stress of economic uncertainty.

The chronic stress of taking care of an elderly spouse or relative increases the risk of mortality. McEwen again: "The wear and tear of daily life, the different kinds of everyday stress-all have an impact on us and our health." Guwer writes, "stress, anxiety and worry help·keep us alive. True fearlessness is a myth. Without fear you die. Thus stress, worry and fear are related and real."

The stress of a diagnosis of cancer can be devastating. Support groups include patients with the same diagnosis. The web also offers support. These sites offer information for cancer patients and their families or referrals to sources of community support: *www.la.wellnesscommunity.org*; *www.drkoop.com*; *www.vitaloptions.org*; *www.acor.org*; *www.oncolink.upenn.edu/psychosocial*; *www.intelihealth.com*; *www.cancercare.org*.

Distressing, threatening events can cause post-traumatic stress disorder (PTSD), a psychological ailment that includes flashbacks, amnesia and psychic distress, persistent disability and comorbidity. While Vietnam and Gulf War veterans are the best-known victims of the disorder, it can occur in anyone affected by such events. It is a worldwide problem particularly in countries torn by conflict. PTSD often begins disguised as something else and may go unrecognized for awhile but after diagnosis can be treated successfully. Treatment includes emotional engagement with the trauma memory, organization of the trauma story and correction of dysfunctional thoughts. All techniques for reducing stress help.

Stress and fatigue are interrelated. Stress can lead to feeling tired all the time. Weil describes causes of fatigue that can be remedied, among them dehydration, low blood pressure, disturbed sleep, low testosterone, thyroid problems, anemia, eye-strain, medications, late night indulgences and simple boredom.

The chronic fatigue syndrome (CFS) is defined by Whiting et al as a range of symptoms of fatigue, headaches, sleep disturbances, difficulties with concentration and mental fatigue. Other symptom complexes grouped under CFS are myalgic encephalomyelitis and postviral fatigue syndrome. The exact cause is not known and the signs and symptoms are variable and make an exact definition difficult.

CFS may begin suddenly and resemble viral infections. It may be related to depression, fibromyalgia or irritable bowel syndrome. Many treatments have been used including drugs, hormone supplements, osteopathy, massage therapy and others. Consistent studies or evidence are lacking but an extensive review by Whiting et al offered two firm conclusions—the most effective present treatments are graded exercise therapy (GET) or cognitive behavioral therapy (CBT). Both are behavioral in nature.

What is the best way to deal with stress?

Interventions to increase social support and enhance coping skills in the workplace and environment will help deal with two important cause of increased stress described by McEwen and colleagues: isolation and lack of control at work. Stay healthy by being social. Reducing stress does not mean you must change your environment. The *Harvard Health Letter* points out, "It may simply mean exercising more, expanding your social circle, reaching out to others, joining a support group or putting traffic jams in perspective." It is clear that a social support network, particularly marriage, family, friendships, membership in churches and other organizations, and satisfying relationships, helps buffer threats of stress. Dr. Leo Galland says, "Strong emotional relationships often increase self-esteem and perceived self efficacy which allow someone to cope better with symptoms and daily stresses and to stick to a healthy lifestyle." As long ago as 1952, Norman Vincent Peale wrote and preached about *The Power of Positive Thinking.*

Herbert Benson described a method of stress control called "The Relaxation Response" in *Timeless Healing, The Relaxation Response, Placebo Effect, Meditation* and other books. The Relaxation Response is an excellent way to help restore order in your life and reduce acute and chronic stress of the environment. Reducing stress can drive blood pressure down. Siegel in *Love, Medicine and Miracles* emphasizes the importance of relaxation and a positive outlook on life. He describes love, kindness, compassion and their relationships to your health. Siegel states you should love yourself and everyone you meet, embrace morality, recognize the value of silence and schedule a regular time each day for silence for 15 minutes, and then help someone who needs support. He writes about emotional expression and disease outcome, indicating "Good social relations seem associated with positive health outcomes."

Self hypnosis is a good way to reduce stress, help control blood pressure and other aspects of one's life. I had personal experience many years ago with the use of self-hypnosis to stop smoking and can verify it can be extremely helpful. One-fifth of the population cannot be hypnotized but for everyone else it is a technique that is easy to learn. Psychologists and/or psychiatrists can teach most individuals. O. Surman describes how you can do it yourself. (Table) Some medical centers have stress-reduction clinics such as that of Dr. Kabat-Zinn at the U. of Mass. He emphasizes "the power of breathing—an exercise in sitting or lying down comfortably, eyes closed, notice the belly moving with breathing, feel breath go in and out, keep your mind on the breathing with no other thoughts for 15 minutes each day." Guy Mittleman warns some methods to lower distress may do more harm than good. The methods may actually increase stress.

Galland describes four pillars of healing as: 1) your relationship with your social support network and your doctor; 2) exercise, rest and nutrition; 3) your environment—safe; 4) detoxification by a healthy liver and intestinal tract. To deal with stress and fatigue Weil suggests that we hit the sack, eat small frequent meals, be active, drink water (6-8 glass a day), breathe for stimulation, try a herbal tonic and multivitamin, think positively, avoid caffeine and alcohol, eat foods rich in magnesium, like whole grains, legumes, nuts, eat foods rich in omega-3 fatty acids, like salmon, walnuts, and flax seeds. Wilson, a psychologist, started a movement of laughter to beat stress. Laughter produces endorphins which counteract stress hormones, helps the immune system, boosts self-confidence, relaxes muscles and relieves pain.

Table

Stress-Dealing with It

Yoga
Transcendental meditation
Voodoo
The Relaxation Response-Herbert Benson
Relaxation-Bernard Siegel
Controlled breathing-Andrew Weil
Self-hypnosis
Psychotherapy

85. What are the health problems of environmental pollution? Is Dioxin really that bad for us? What is asbestosis? What are Black Lung Disease and Silicosis? What are toxins that may be brought home by workers on their clothing and bodies? Is global warming a health problem?

Dioxin is a major environmental pollutant, and exposure to asbestos, lead, mercury and beryllium has been a problem in the workplace. Many other workplace and home hazards are specific for certain jobs and residences, among them mining and black lung disease, silicosis, and asbestosis.

Is dioxin really that bad for us?

Yes, it is very bad. In fact, it may be even worse than you think. Evidence is accumulating that it can cause, or has been associated with, birth defects, learning and developmental problems, immune system abnormalities, impaired development of human reproductive organs, diabetes and endometriosis. It is the most potent agent to cause cancer in animals and very likely in people. A recent report by the EPA concluded getting cancer from dioxin is 10 times greater than previously estimated for the people most exposed, although probably less than that for most of us. Dick Clapp says, "Dioxin is diabolic." He calls it the Darth Vader of toxic chemicals.

Dioxin is a complex compound of 75 chemicals that include dioxins, furans, and PCBs, or polychlorinated biphenyls. Notorious for its use as an herbicide and defoliant in Agent Orange, in Vietnam, dioxin is a by-product in the manufacture of some pesticides, of incineration and of some industrial processes that use chlorine. Insulators and electrical equipment are another source of a constituent of dioxin, PCBs. Fires in old buildings release them into the air.

PCBs were banned in 1997, and regulations to control PCB pollution are helping to reduce it but meanwhile they still get into the environment. They settle from the air to grazing lands and go from there into the bodies of cows and pigs.

Ninety percent of the dioxin that gets into our bodies comes from animal fats: meat, cheese, milk and butter. Lobster "tomalley," the soft green substance in the carapace, contains high levels of dioxin and PCBs. Contaminants accumulate in tomalley, the liver and pancreas of the lobster, and the Maine Bureau of Health recommends against consumption.

Dioxin gets into cells and cell nuclei primarily in body fat. Our bodies get rid of dioxin but very gradually, taking seven years to secrete half the amount present. That is a long time. There is no safe level of dioxin.

How can I decrease my risk from dioxin?

You should avoid eating animal fats, including eggs, dairy products, and fatty fish altogether or at least decrease your intake of them. Fat-free foods and Egg Beaters contain less dioxin. Dwain Winters of the Environmental Protection Agency (EPA) said, "You are what you eat." Your levels of dioxin may be relatively high if you date back to the 1950s and 1960s when environmental levels were higher. Your children's levels will be lower because of EPA regulations. Levels in foods have been reported by the EPA at *www.EPA.gov/neea/pdfs/dioxin/part1and2.htm*—click on Volume 3, Chapter 3.

The presence of dioxin in soil, water and sediments may require cutting back on use of lard and fish as feed for cattle and hogs. PCBs posed a dilemma when found in the bed of the Hudson River—what do you do? The PCB problem has been described as a war between environmentalists and corporate America. The problem is we can't get rid of all of them, no matter what. It is very difficult to track levels, health effects, and body burden.

What are toxins that may be brought home by workers on their clothing and bodies?

Stephanie Armour in USA TODAY lists toxins known to have been unknowingly transported home from construction and general industry sites, among them asbestos, beryllium, cadmium, PCBs, hormone substances such as estrogens, infectious agents such as Giardiasis and Brucellosis, lead, mercury and pesticides. Cases of take-home contamination have occurred in at least 40 industries, including lead smelting, nuclear medicine, chemical manufacturing, construction, and shipbuilding.

Beryllium may cause degenerative lung diseases. Cadmium is linked to lung and prostate cancer; PCBs to acne and perhaps skin cancer, and damage to children's brains, nerves and kidneys; and mercury to tremors and gastrointestinal and neurological problems. Children and spouses of workers have suffered illness, toxicity and even death from toxins brought home from work. A whole community may be affected as was Putney, VT by mercury exposure from a thermometer plant.

Workers exposed to toxins at work should talk with managers about the hazards. If you are exposed to a workplace toxin, leave your work clothes at the workplace and shower before going home. Learn more about workplace toxins from the Occupational Safety and Health Administration (OSHA) at 800-321-6742 and www.osha.gov. Some government environmental policies have worked well. Removing lead from gasoline is one example. Another is the use in automobiles of catalytic converters, which convert exhaust pollutants to normal atmospheric gases like nitrogen, carbon dioxide and water. Sulfur-dioxide emissions from electrical power plants were cut by 50%, saving money in the process.

What is asbestosis?

Exposure to asbestos produces lung scarring and cancer of the lining of the lung, or pleural mesothelioma, and the lung. When inhaled, asbestos fibers become trapped in areas of fibrosis or scars in the lung, a condition called asbestosis that may result in cancers. Exposure to asbestos fibers occurs in chrysotile mines, textile mills, cement factories and oil refineries. The removal of asbestos from mines and other areas should decrease the risk.

What is black lung and silicosis?

Diseases of the lungs called pneumoconioses are caused by inhalation of coal dust and silica or quartz dust from drilling or crushing rock in mines. Black lung disease and coal workers' pneumoconiosis (CWP) is an incurable problem producing scarring in the lungs that decreases lung function and may be disabling and then fatal. Silica exposed workers may develop silicosis, with even more scarring than caused by coal dust, and emphysema, with progressive decrease in lung function. Lung disease can result from the inhalation of dust from any hard mineral, such as aluminum oxide, cadmium oxide, cobalt, graphite, mica, talc and beryllium.

The problems of miners' safety were recognized back in 1881 by Leman. Finally in 1977 Congress passed the Federal Mine Safety and Health Act (MSHA), which protects miners from accidents, explosions and now inhalation of toxic particles. In recent years these problems have been greatly reduced. However, black lung disease still occurs perhaps because unscrupulous companies are not obeying the law. Exposure to diesel fuel particles is also a hazard in mining. Many responsible companies follow the MSHA but much remains to be done to protect workers from these occupational hazards.

Other environmental pollutants found in people include lead, mercury, cadmium, tobacco smoke, pesticides—adlrin, chlordane, hexachlorobenzene, DDT, cotinine from nicotine, and phthalates used to soften plastics. A total of 27 pollutants have been found, many producing effects on us that are not known.

Is tap water a problem?

Tap water should be fluoridated and, of course, safe. You should not need to buy bottled water but many people do as a matter of preference and sometimes taste. In some places dog feces and wild animals can produce contamination as can leaking septic tanks. Arsenic in drinking water could be a problem in the western states but for most of us, this is not a problem.

Is global warming a health problem?

The problem of global warming from carbon dioxide produced by burning fossil fuel, primarily coal, should be high on our environmental agenda. Methane produced by cud-chewing animals is another major contributor to global warming as is methane produced by man in rice paddies and elsewhere. Studies are underway to try to control this by changing cows' diets.

Global warming, cutting down rain forests, and other environmental changes greatly affect the atmosphere, the ozone layer, flooding, ocean level and other phenomena. The year 2003 was the third hottest since 1861. The ice is shifting in the Arctic, and in both the Arctic and Antarctic, glaciers are getting smaller and sea levels are rising. Plant growth and animal migration are affected. The full potential impact on our health is not known.

Scientists disagree about how rapidly global warming is taking place, but they have documented that it is happening, relentlessly. It is of concern to many countries but not to the current U.S. government, which does not seem to want to admit the existence of global warming and its hazards. Could it be that the industrial polluters are strong lobbyists? Senator John McCain (R-AZ) and Senator Joseph Lieberman (D-CT) brought a Climate Stewardship Act to the Senate and it was seven votes shy of passing. The National Resources Defense Council is working hard for this bill and the environment. They are at 40 West 20th Street, New York, NY 10011, phone 212-727-4500 and *www.nrdc.org* or *www.savebiogems.org.*

86. Why do they do research on animals? The poor things suffer and I am opposed to it. Do scientists care about animal comfort?

Research on animals greatly benefits people. The U.S. Public Health Service stated "Virtually every medical achievement over the last century has depended directly or indirectly on research in animals." The elimination of poliomyelitis in our children by vaccination resulted from animal studies, and development of the vaccine required use of tissues from animals. Research on animals has facilitated treatment of heart disease, HIV/AIDS, cancer and bacterial infections. New drugs and even cosmetics must be tested to ensure safety.

Roger Caras, the President of the American Society for the Prevention of Cruelty to Animals, reported to a conference on public responsibility in medical research that most people do not understand what health researchers do. They may not remember the terrible epidemics of childhood diseases now prevented by vaccines developed in animals. Carl Cohen and James V. Parker tell of a grandmother staffing an animal rights booth at a health fair. She was opposed to using anything from animals, not only meat and fur but also medicines. Upon learning that vaccines came from animal research, she said she was also opposed to immunizations. What would happen if epidemics return? "Don't worry," she said, "scientists will find some way by using computers." Ingrid

Newkirk, president and co-founder of People for the Ethical Treatment of Animals, was quoted in *USA Today,* "even if animal research resulted in a cure for AIDS, we'd be against it."

Do scientists care about animal comfort?

Animal comfort is a primary concern in the conducting of experiments. What animals are used in research? The overwhelming majority are rats and mice, although certain experiments require the use of dogs, cats and even primates. In 1990 it was found that animals in scientific research involved only 0.003% of the number of animals consumed for food. Only half as many animals undergo medical procedures in research as do those having operations ordered by pet owners for cosmetic reasons, as reported by Cohen and Parker.

Most scientists use animals bred for research. No investigator would use a sick animal for a research project, and animals must be well cared for and healthy to produce good results. Remember, pets are not used in experimentation. Pet owners need have no concern their pets will be taken and used in medical research. Scientists look for ways to reduce the numbers of animals needed to obtain valid results. They refine experimental techniques and replace animals with other research methods whenever possible.

The key law governing research with animals is the Federal Animal Welfare Act, passed in 1966 and amended several times since then. The NIH and most other federal funding agencies require scientists to use these guides for the care and use of laboratory animals to ensure appropriate standards for care in the laboratory. The 1985 Health Research Extension Act requires all medical research funded through the NIH to conform to the Public Health Service policy on humane care and use of laboratory animals. Very strict controls and rules are observed. Animals must be given an anesthetic before operations, and they must not be allowed to suffer.

Now the American Anti-vivisectionist Society has established an Alternatives Research and Development Foundation. They are opposed to the use of any animals in research. They seek to make research in mice, rats and birds prohibitively expensive and extremely burdensome. Do they believe it is all right to poison and trap rats and mice but not to use them in research? Do they wear leather shoes made from cowhide or eat meat or wear fur coats? Do they refuse to use or depend on modern machines and techniques developed in animals? Do they know that animal shelters, the animal warden and the Humane Society kill animals that are not adopted?

"We eat pigs in some cultures and abhor them in others," says Adrian R. Morrison and "use them in experiments and some have them as pets." He also says, "I believe animal use by humans is natural and no less appropriate in the scheme of things than animal use by other animals." Research in such animals is critical for human health. Should we use people to evaluate new potential therapy? No, animals are better for this.

Morrison gives his first Principles of Research: 1) our first obligation is to our fellow humans; 2) all human beings are persons; 3) animals are not little persons; 4) we have a great obligation to the animals under our control; and 5) good science requires good animal care, but bureaucracy does not necessarily equate with increased welfare. My hope is more scientists will step forward to inform the public of their views on the important societal issue of the use of animals in biomedical research.

More information is available on the Federal Animal Welfare Act at http:\\www.aphis.usda.gov\ac. PHS policies on animals and research can be found on the web at http:\\www.nih.gov\grants\oprr\phspol.htm. Information may also be obtained by writing to Animal Care at the USDA, 4700 River Road, Unit 84, River Dale, MD, 20737-1234, or the NIH office of Protection from Research Risk, 6100 Executive Blvd., MSC 7507, Ste. 3801, Rockville, MD, 20892-7507. The Foundation for Biomedical Research provides publications—Portraits of a Partnership for Life: a remarkable story of research, animals and man. You may obtain answers to frequently asked questions about animal research and the importance of animals and research series from the Foundation for Biomedical Research, 818 Connecticut Ave, NW, Ste. 303, Washington DC, 20006.

DRUGS AND ADDICTION

87. Are we winning the war on drugs? What is an addiction? Is an addiction a sickness or a criminal activity? What are commonly used drugs and recreational drugs? What is the best therapy? Are compulsive behavior and gambling addictions?

We are not winning the war on drugs. In spite of massive expenditures here and overseas, the war on drugs has not limited the flow into this country. Big drug busts and seizures have not done the job. Efforts to eradicate coca (cocaine) and poppy (heroin) plants in Colombia have not worked. Many countries are busier than ever in supplying drugs to the U.S., and illegal drug use in the U.S. is higher and more widespread than ever. Nearly 2 million more Americans used illicit drugs in 2001 than in 2000. More than 16 million Americans are current drug users. Now the focus of the U.S. Government will be to try to decrease the demand for drugs.

What is an addiction?

The Tufts *Health and Nutrition Letter*, in referring to the Diagnostic and Statistical Manual of Mental Disorders, define an addiction as a pattern of substance abuse that leads to at least three of the following symptoms within a 12 month period:

1) Increased tolerance.
2) Withdrawal symptoms.
3) Using the substance more than intended.
4) Inability to control the individual's use of the substance.
5) Expending effort to obtain the substance.
6) Replacing important activities with use of the substance.
7) Continuing to use the substance despite its negative consequences.

In simple terms, addiction is the use of a substance, excluding ordinary foods such as sugar or chocolate, you can't get along without even though it may be harmful. Common addictive drugs are listed in Table 1. Research shows addiction entails two separate processes. One is "passive neuroadaptation:" changes in the brain circuitry as the direct result of drug taking and the other is "the laying down of memory traces," which occurs high in the limbic system of the brain, the Hippocampus. Addiction, according to Johanna Helmuth, relies on the same neurobiological mechanisms that underlie learning and cravings triggered by memory: All drugs bombard the brain's dopamine-mediated reward circuits involved in learning and movement. Long-term abuse can wear out these pathways and lead to memory problems and lack of motor coordination. The entire process involves not just dopamine but also glutamate, which may be more at the root of the matter.

Genetic inheritance contributes to the likelihood of drug addiction. The National Institute of Drug Abuse (NIDA) is now supporting studies to track down this connection, treat earlier those with such a genetic background and use vaccines for prevention. In *Drugs and the Making of the Modern World*, David T. Courtwright writes about problems of addiction surrounding both illegal and legalized drugs.

Is an addiction a sickness or a criminal activity? How should it be treated?

An addiction is an abnormality of brain function brought on by repetitive use of a substance, possibly linked to a genetic background. Thus, it is an acquired illness. Although acquiring or dealing in illegal drugs amounts to criminal activity, the addiction itself is not criminal.

USA TODAY reports on the problems of locking up drug offenders, allegedly at an annual cost of billions of dollars. Most drug offenders in state prisons have no convictions for violence. Half of them have no history of violence or drug dealing. Some still believe prison sentences cut down on drug use. If so, why is it more common now? Would mandatory treatment programs be better? Many people think so.

What are commonly used and recreational drugs?

Marijuana (cannabis) is the most abused drug, and new hallucinogenic herbs are always turning up. Now it is salvia divinorum, a native Mexican sage plant that can be smoked or chewed. Federal agents are concerned about it. Meanwhile, great debate continues about medicinal use of marijuana. Should it be legalized? N. Solowig et al found long-term, heavy use led to impairment in memory and attention that gets worse with increasing years of use.

Use has soared of the so-called club drugs: Ecstasy, CMDMA (3, 4-methylene dioxy methamphetamine), GHD and Rohypnol. At *www.clubdrugs.org* the NIDA gives facts on these club drugs, and the picture isn't pretty. Ecstasy, used by more than 1.4 million people a year, can cause prolonged memory impairment and brain damage ending in death. Its use promotes violent behavior, and under its influence many kids have become drug dealers. Methamphetamine, also known as meth, speed, crack or crystal, is believed to be the fastest-growing illegal drug in this country. Originally grown mostly in California, it is now produced everywhere in the country.

Heroin, cocaine and morphine are well known for causing addiction. Whether smoked as crack or inhaled, cocaine scrambles the brain by attaching to proteins and causing dopamine to flood the nerves. The "date-rape drug," gamma hydroxy butyrate (GMB), can trigger fatal comas. Huffing is sniffing the fumes of glue, air freshener, spray paint and other common household products to get a high. Many contain toluene, which produces a rush for about 45 minutes along with the risk of brain damage. Some kids have died from inhaling fumes from these products.

Prescription drugs are the second most commonly abused types of drugs, according to the 2002 National Survey on Drug Use and Health, with internet advertising as a contributing factor. Prescription drugs, particularly tranquilizers and pain medications, can be abused by illegal use or overuse. New powerful pain drugs have become addictive. These include Oxycontin, a pain reliever sought in so many pharmacy robberies that some pharmacies will no longer stock it. Lortab is another. While FDA approved, these are not safe drugs.

Most commonly abused prescription drugs are: opioids, or narcotic analgesics and morphine, codeine, Oxycontin, Vicodin, Demerol; central nervous system depressants—Nembutal, Valium, Xanax—and central nervous system stimulants—Ritalin, Dexedrine. Creatine and Andro (androstenedione) are supplements that are legal and probably harmless but the question is: Do they help athletes?

The Controlled Substance Act categorizes drugs and substances into the following five schedules based on rankings of their medicinal value and their potential for harmfulness and abuse. Schedule I: heroin and other drugs having the highest potential for abuse with no currently accepted medical use. Schedule II: drugs with a high potential for abuse but with currently accepted medical use like Oxycontin, morphine, Ritalin, and Tylenol with codeine. Schedule III : anabolic steroids. Schedule IV: psychotrophic, anticonvulsant drugs—valium for anxiety, Motofel, an anti-diarrheal drug. Schedule V: the lowest potential for abuse with a currently accepted medical use like Lomotil, Robitussin and similar drugs.

What is the best therapy?

D. Goldman and C. S. Barr write that "addictions are relapsing, remitting, lifelong illnesses notoriously difficult to treat." More than 12,000 Federal treatment centers focus on opioid dependence. To find a treatment center call 1-800-662-HELP-4357 or *http://findtreatments.samhsa.gov/facilitylocatordoc.htm*. These facilities are overwhelmed and cannot take care of everyone. It is estimated that they can take only 180,000 out of more than 800,000 opioid addicts. The Drug Addiction Treatment Act now allows qualified physicians to prescribe drugs for addiction therapy. They use Methadone maintenance therapy, or levomethadyl acetate for heroin and other addictions. Methadone, however, is addictive. Other agents used are buprenomorphine, clonidine and naltrexone.

Office-based physician care can be provided for detoxification. Since addicts often have many other medical problems and complex health needs, physicians should put regular medical care together with drug abuse care. Several agents help with cocaine withdrawal such as propanolol and a cannabinoid (CBI) antagonist, a selective CBI receptor antagonist. Other addictions require physician care, psychiatric care, group therapy and family support and love. Staying in close touch with your kids helps.

Building self-esteem helps counter peer pressure. For more information contact:

NIDA, 6001 Executive Blvd, Room 5213, Bethesda, MD 20892, or call 203-443-1124, or *www.nida.nih.gov* or *www.drugabuse.gov*

Substance Abuse and Mental Health Services Administration, Center for Substance Abuse Treatment, 5600 Fishers Lane, Suite 618, Rockwall II, Rockville, MD 30857 301-443-5052, *www.samhsa.gov/centers/csat/csat.html*

For publications, contact SAMHSA's—National Clearinghouse for Alcohol & Drug Info. 1-800-729-6686, *www.health.org*

White House Office on National Drug Control Policy, Drug Policy Information Clearinghouse PO Box 6000, Rockville, MD 20849, 1-800-666-3332, *www.whitehousedrugpolicy.gov/about/clearingh.html*

Are compulsive behavior and gambling addictions?

They are and have been called behavioral addictions. Other subjects of behavioral addiction include food, sex, shopping, running, and clicking. Mall disorders include excessive eating and shopping and kleptomania.

Gamblers get high and show tolerance and withdrawal symptoms just like drug addicts. Mental health professionals define a pathological gambler as a person who exhibits five or more of the following behaviors:

- Preoccupation with gambling thoughts or plans
- Need to gamble with increasing sums
- Repeated, unsuccessful attempts to cut back or stop
- Irritability when attempting to reduce gambling
- Gambling to escape problems or feelings of helplessness, guilt or anxiety
- "Chasing" losses by trying to get even after losing
- Lying to conceal extent of gambling
- Committing crimes to finance gambling
- Jeopardizing a significant relationship, job or educational or career opportunity because of gambling
- Reliance on others for financial relief.

Gamblers compensate for deficiencies in their brain reward systems by overdoing and getting hooked. Gamblers Anonymous, modeled on Alcoholics

Anonymous, offers treatment. Counseling and drug therapy, such as fluvoxamine (Luvox), an antidepressant, may help. For information call the National Council on Problem Gambling at 1-800-522-4700.

Table 1

Common Addictive Drugs

Cocaine
Heroin
Morphine
Oxycontin
Marijuana
Methamphetamine (speed, crystal meth, ice, crack)
Ecstasy (MDMA)
GHB—Gamma Hydroxy Butyrate—the date rape drug
Ephreda Plant (contains ephedrine)—now banned
Laetrile
Ginseng
Creatine and Andro (androstenedione)

REFERENCES

References for Introduction

1. The Merck Manual—Home Edition. Pocket Books, NY 2000.
2. Harvard Medical School Family Health Guide. Simon and Schuster, NY 1999.
3. Kemper, DW. Healthwide Handbook—A self-care manual for you. Healthwise, Boise, Idaho. 12th edition, 1996.
4. The Physicians Desk Reference (PDR) Family Guide to Encyclopedia of Medical Care. Ballantine Books, NY 1999.
5. The PDR Family Guide to Common Ailments. Ballantine Book, NY 1999.
6. The Doctors Book of Home Remedies for Men. Men's Health Book. Croft Publishing Co. NY 2000.
7. The PDR Family Guide to Natural Medicines and Healing Therapy. Ballantine Books, NY 2000.
8. Fetrow CW, Avila JA. The Complete Guide to Herbal Medicine. Pocket Books, NY 2000.
9. Osler, Sir William Aequanimitas, third edition. Philadelphia, Blakiston 1932.

10. Centers for Disease Control and Prevention Report—Ten great public health achievements—U.S. 1900-1999. JAMA 1999; 281:1481.
11. Lee, TH Paying for the golden age of medicine. Harvard Health Letter. 2000; 25: January.
12. Benson, H. Timeless healing—the power of belief. Simon and Schuster, New York, 1996.
13. Feinstein, AR An additional basic science for clinical medicine: IV. The development of clinimetrics. Ann Int Med 1983; 99:843-848.
14. Cohen J. The traveler's pocket medical guide and international certificate of vaccination. The Travel Clinic, 263 Glen Eira Road, North Caulfield, Melbourne, Victoria, Australia, 2000. *http://www.travelclinic.com.au.*
15. Weil A. Spontaneous Healing. Fawcett Columbine, New York. 1995.
16. Weil A. Eating Well for Optimum Health. Alfred Knopf, New York. 2000.

References Chapter 1

1. Nahrwold, D.L. "Presidential address: Toward physician competency." Surgery 126 (1999): 589-93.
2. Grumbach K, Bodenheimer T. A primary care home for Americans. JAMA 2002; 288:889-893.
3. Roter DL, Hall JA, Aoki Y. Physician gender effects in medical communication. JAMA 2002; 288:756-764.

References Chapter 2

1. Schwartz, A.N., R. Jimenez, T Myers, A Solomon. *Getting the best from your doctor.* New York: Harper Collins, 1998.
2. Frishman, R. "Don't Be a Wimp in the Doctor's Office." *Harvard Health Letter* 21 (1996): 1-2.

References Chapter 3

1. Neergaard L. Same-day doctor visits emerge from the realm of fantasy. The Day, New London, CT. 2001; March 26.
2. Healthcare savvy – when to treat a fever. Consumer Reports on Health. 2002; September. PO Box 56355, Boulder, CO. 80322-6355.

References Chapter 4

1. Gawande, Atul. "Whose Body Is It, Anyway?" The New Yorker (September 1999).

2. Gates, Peter. "How Should Physicians Involve Patients in Medical Decisions?" *JAMA* 283 (May 2000): 2390.
3. Fischer, David, Anita L. Stewart, Daniel A. Bloch, Kate Lorig, Diana Laurent, and Halsted Holman. "Capturing the Patient's View of Change as a Clinical Outcome Measure." *JAMA* 282 (September 1999): 1157-62.
4. Edwards, A., G. Elwyn. "The Potential Benefits of Decision Aids in Clinical Medicine." *JAMA* 282 (1999): 779-80.

References Chapter 5

1. Manian, FA. "Whither continuity of care." *NEJM* 340 (1999): 1362-63.
2. Sox, Harold C. "Independent Primary Care Practice by Nurse Practitioners." *JAMA* 283 (January 2000): 106.
3. Mundinger, Mary O., Robert L. Kane, Elizabeth R. Lenz, Annette M. Totten, Wei-Yann Tsai, Paul D. Cleary, William T. Friedewald, Albert L. Siu, Michael L. Shelanski. *JAMA* 283 (January 2000): 59-68.
4. Bagley, Bruce. "Health Outcomes Among Patients Treated by Nurse Practitioners or Physicians. *JAMA* 283 (January 2000): 2521.
5. Grumbach, Kevin, Coffman, Janet. "Physicians and Nonphysician Clinicians: Complements or Competitors." *JAMA* 280 (September 1998): 825-26.
6. Baggs, Judith Gedney, Madeline H. Schmitt, Alvin I. Mushlin, Pamela H. Mitchell, Deborah H. Eldredge, David Oakes, Alan D. Hutson. "Association between nurse-physician collaboration and patient outcomes in three intensive care units." *Crit Care Med* 27 (1999): 1991-98.
7. Greenfield, Lazar J. "Doctors and Nurses: A Troubled Partnership." *Ann Surg* 230 (1999): 279-88.
8. O'Neal LW. Nurses. St. Louis Met. Med. 2002; Aug:7.

References Chapter 6

1. Epstein et al. "Second Opinion on Biopsies." *J Cancer* (2000).
2. Zuger, A. "Ask Another Doctor? Expect a Chill in the Exam Room." *New York Times*, 4 April 2000, sec. D, p. 7.
3. Tarkan, L. "Value of Second Opinions is Understood in Study of Biopsies." *New York Times*, 4 April 2000, sec. D, pp. 7-8.

References Chapter 7

1. Weingarten, G. *The Hypochondriac's Guide to Life and Death*. New York: Simon and Schuster, 1998.

2. Gordon, L.A. "Munchausen Patients Have Found the Computer." *Med Economics* (October 1997): 33-37.
3. Levinson, W., Ghat R. Gorawara, R. Dueck et al. "Resolving Disagreements in the Patient-Physician Relationship." *JAMA* 282 (1999): 1477-83.
4. Barsky AJ, Ahern DF. Cognitive behavior therapy for hypochondriasis. JAMA 2004; 291:1464-1470.

References Chapter 8 – None

References Chapter 9

1. Tinetti, M.E. "For Older Patients, Attention to the Many Facts of Good Health. Yale Letter on Aging." *Yale University School of Medicine* 1 (1998): 1.
2. Why should you switch from your primary care physician to a geriatrician. Tufts U. Health and Nutrition Letter 2002; Aug:6.
3. Marwick, C. "Cyberinformation for Seniors." *JAMA* 281 (1999): 1474-1477. *Harvard Health Letter* 24 (1999): 6-7.
4. Goodwin, J.S. "Geriatrics and the Limits of Modern Medicine." *New Engl J Med* 340 (1999): 1283-1285.
5. Bury, S.B., Edmunds. "The Death of Humane Medicine and the Rise of Coercive Healthism." *JAMA* 277 (1997): 1244.
6. Cullum C.M., R.N. Rosenberg. "Memory loss-when is it Alzheimer's disease?" *JAMA* 279 (1996):1689-1690.
7. Fratiglione, L. "Influence of social network on occurrence of dementia: a community-based longitudinal study. *Lancet* 355 (2000): 1315-1319.
8. Rosenfeld, I. *Live Now, Age Later.* New York: Warner Books, 1999.
9. Perls T, Silver H. *Living to 100: Lessons in living to your maximum potential at any age.* New York: Basic Books, 1999.
10. Warshofsky, F. "The Methuselah Factor." *Modern Maturity* Nov-Dec (1999): 28-33
11. Harris, J. "Intimations of Immortality." *Science* 288 (2000):59.
12. Richardson C. "The Road Less Traveled." Yale University School of Medicine, New Haven, CT.
13. Rubenstein, L. "Hip protectors—a breakthrough in fracture prevention." *New Eng J Med* 343 (2000): 1562-1563.
14. Asch, S.M., E.M. Sloss, C. Hogan et al. "Measuring underuse of necessary care among the elderly/Medicare beneficiaries." *JAMA* 284 (2000): 2325-2333.
15. El-Sohemy, Ahmed. "Statin Drugs and the Risk of Fracture." *JAMA* 274 (2000): 1921-1922.
16. Chandler, Julie M. et al. "Low Bone Mineral Density and Risk of Fracture in White Female Nursing Home Residents." *JAMA* 284 (2000): 972-977.

17. Wallace, Robert B. "Bone Health in Nursing Home Residents." *JAMA* 284 (2000): 1018-1019.
18. Olson, Lars. "Combating Parkinson's Disease–Step Three." *Science* 290 (2000): 721-724.
19. Parkinson Study Group. "Pramipexole vs Levodopa as Initial Treatment for Parkinson Disease: A Randomized Controlled Trial." *JAMA* 284 (2000): 1931-1938.
20. Hargrave TD. Who says when its time to turn in the car keys? AARD – MM 2001; March-April: 32-34.
21. Wright AP. Steady on your feet. AARP Bulletin 2001; Nov:19-20.
22. Engelhart MJ, Geerlings ML, Ruitenberg A, et al. Dietary intake of anti-oxidants and risk of Alzheimer's Disease. JAMA 2002; 287:3223-3229.
23. Helmuth L. New Alzheimer's treatment that may ease the mind. Science 2002; 297:1260-1263.
24. Gill TM, Baker DI, Gottschalk M, et al. A program to prevent functional decline in physically frail, elderly persons who live at home. New Engl J Med 2001; 347:1068-1074.
25. Feskanich D, Singh V, Willett WC, et al. Vitamin A intake and hip fractures among postmenopausal women. JAMA 2002; 287:47-54.
26. Reid IR, Brown JP, Burckhardt P, et al. Intravenous Zoledronic Acid in postmenopausal women with low bone mineral density. N Engl J Med 2002; 346:653-661.
27. Osteoporosis prevention, diagnosis and therapy. JAMA 2001; 285:785-795.
28. Chestnut CH. Osteoporosis, an underdiagnosed disease. JAMA 2001; 286:2865-2866.
29. Barzilai N, Atzmon G, Schechter C, et al. Unique lipoprotein phenotype and genotype associated with exceptional longevity. JAMA 2003; 290:2030-2040.

References Chapter 10

1. Fox E "Predominance of the Curative Model of Medical Care." *JAMA* 278 (1997): 761-763.
2. Billings JA, S. Block. "Palliative care in undergraduate medical education." *JAMA* 278 (1997) 733-738.
3. Kassirer JP. "Our Stubborn Quest for Diagnostic Certainty: A Cause of Excessive Testing." *New Engl J Med* 22 (1989): 1489-1491.
4. Tierney WM., Miller ME, McDonald CJ. "The Effect on Test Ordering of Informing Physicians of the Charges for Outpatient Diagnostic Tests." *New Engl J Med* 322 (1990): 1499-1504.
5. Goldman L "Changing Physicians' Behavior: The Pot and the Kettle." *New Engl J Med* 322 (1990): 1524-1525.

6.   Sheps SB, Schechter MT. "The Assessment of Diagnostic Tests: A Survey of Current Medical Research." *JAMA* 252 (1984): 2418-2422.

References Chapter 11

1.   Antman K, Sheas C. "Screen mammography under age 50." *JAMA* 281 (1999): 1470-1472.
2.   Center for Disease Prevention and Health Promotion. Screening for colorectal cancer—U.S. 1997. *JAMA* 281 (1999): 1581.
3.   Petty TL "Screening Strategies for Early Detection of Lung Cancer. The Time is Now." *JAMA* 284 (2000): 1977-1979.
4.   Frazier AL, Colditz GA, Fuchs CS, Kuntz KM. "Cost-effectiveness of Screening for Colorectal Cancer in the General Population." *JAMA* 284 (2000): 1954-1961.
5.   Liu, S et al. "Whole Grain Consumption and Risk of Ischemic Stroke in Women. A Prospective Study." *JAMA* 284 (2000): 1532-1534.
6.   Is that a mole or a melanoma? Consumer Reports on Health. 2002; July:1,4
7.   Brody L. Fast, safe, painless. Readers Digest. 2002; April:110-115.
8.   Traverso G, Shuber A, Levin B, et al. Detection of APC mutations in fecal DNA from patients with colorectal tumors. NEJM 2002; 346:311-320.
9.   Edwards A, Elwyn G. The potential benefits of decision aids in clinical medicine. JAMA 2999; 282:779-780.
10.   Imperiale TF, Wagner DR, Lin CY. Results of screening colonoscopy among persons 40 to 49 years of age. NEJM 2002; 346:1781-5
11.   Detsky AS. Screening for colon cancer – can we afford colonoscopy? NEJM 2001; 345:607-608.
12.   The pros and cons of the screening tests. Harvard Health Letter. 2001; March:4-5.

References Chapter 12

1.   Stedman's abbreviations, acronyms and symbols. Williams and Wilkins, NY 1992.
2.   Garb S. Abbreviations and acronyms in medicine and nursing. Springer, NY 1976.
3.   Massman J. Dictionary of medical and health acronyms. Gleneida, NY. 1991.
4.   Baue AE. Its acronymania all over again. Arch of Surgery 2002; 137:486-489.

References Chapter 13:

1.   Trotter G. Medicine's response to ethnic differences. Healthcare Ethics. 1997; 7:6-7.

2. Salmon DA, Haber M, Gangarosa EJ. Health consequences of religious and philosophical exemptions from immunization laws. JAMA 1999; 282:47-53.
3. Spence RK. Blood management policies for Jehovah's Witnesses. The Am J of Surg. 1995; 170:6A 14-15S.
4. Watanabe MD. NIH sets up Minority Health Center. The Scientist 2001; February 5:6.
5. Kagawa-Singer M, Blackhall LJ. Negotiating cross-cultural issues at the end of life. JAMA 2001; 286:2993-3001

References Chapter 14

1. Diseases we can prevent. Nutrition Action Healthletter. 1999; 26:3-9.
2. Clements M, Hales D. How healthy are we? Parade Magazine 1997; Sept 7:4-9.
3. Schardt D. Rating your risk of heart disease and stroke. Nutrition Action Healthletter. 1998; November:9-12.
4. Kumar A, Short J, Parillo JE. Genetic factors in septic shock. JAMA 1999 282;6:579-581.
5. Bion JF, Brun-Buisson C. Introduction – infection and critical illness: genetic and environmental aspects of susceptibility and resistance. Int Care Med 2000 26:S1-S2.

References Chapter 15

1. Malacrida R, Bettelini CM, Degrata, et al. Reasons for dissatisfaction: A survey of relatives of intensive care unit patients who died. Crit Care Med 1998; 26:1187-1193.
2. Chung KC, Hammill JB, Kim HM, et al. Predictors of patient satisfaction in an outpatient plastic surgery clinic. Surgical Forum 1999:545-546.
3. Kenagy JW, Berwick DM, Shore MF. Service quality in health care. JAMA 1999; 281:661-665.
4. Smith MA, Atherly AJ, King RL, Pacala JT. Peer review of the quality of care. JAMA 1997; 278:1573-1578.
5. Prager LO. Doctors advised to listen when patients speak on health care. American Medical News. 1998; February 23;10.

References Chapter 16

1. Detsky AS, Redelmeier DA. Measuring health outcomes-putting gains into perspective. New Engl J Med 1998; 339:402-404.
2. Satcher D. Immunization a must: Protects all. USA Today, 1999; August 19.
3. Manning A. Kids in USA get 21 shots before starting first grade. USA Today, 1999; August 3.

4. 10 Great Public Health Achievements From the Centers of Disease Control and Prevention, United States 1900-1999. JAMA 1999; 281:1481-1483.

5. Centers for Disease Control impact of vaccines universally recommended for children – United States 1900-1998.

6. Marwick C. Calling the shots. IOM report calls for immunization revisions. JAMA 2000; 284:683-4.

7. Koplan JP, Fleming DW. Current and future public health challenges. JAMA 2000; 284:1696-1698.

8. Salmon DA, Haber M, Gangarosa, et al. Health consequences of religious and philosophical exemptions from immunization laws. JAMA 1999; 282:47-53.

9. Delayed supply of influenza vaccine and adjunct ACIP influenza vaccine recommendations for the 2000-01 influenza season. Medical news from the CDC. JAMA 2000; 284:687-690.

10. Gellin BG, Schaffner W. The risk of vaccination. New Engl J of Med 2001; 344:372-373.

11. Dales L, Hammer SJ, Smith NJ. Time trends in autism and in MMR immunization coverage in California. JAMA 2001; 284:1183-1185.

12. Edwards KM. State mandates and childhood immunization. JAMA 2000; 284:3171-3173.

13. Feikin DR, Lezotte DC, Hamman RF, et al. Individual and community risks of measles and pertussis associated with personal exemptions to immunization. JAMA 2000; 284:3145-3150.

14. Michaud CM, Murray CSL, Bloom BR. Burden of disease – implications for future research. JAMA 2001; 284:535-539.

15. Nathanson N, Fine P. Poliomyelitis eradication – a dangerous end game. Science 2002; 296:269-270.

16. Fauci AS. Smallpox vaccination policy – the need for dialogue. N Engl J Med 2002; 346:1319-1320.

17. Flu Shots. Harvard Health Letter. 2000; 25:1.

18. DeFrancesco L. Augism on the rise. The Scientist 2001; May 14:16 and 18.

19. Wolfe RM, Sharp LK, Lipsky MS. Content and design attributes of anti-vaccination websites. JAMA 2002; 287:3245-3248.

20. The flu vaccine remains the best way to prevent and control flu. FDA Consumer 2001; Nov/Dec:17.

21. Meadows M. Vaccine shortages: An update. FDA Consumer. 2002; Sept-Oct:12-14.

22. Meadows M. Understanding vaccine safety. FDA Consumer 2001; July-Aug:18-23.

23. Marwick C. Merits, flaws of live virus flu vaccine debated. JAMA 2000; 283:1814-1815.

24. Rappuoli R, Miller HI, Falkow S. The intangible value of vaccination. Science 2002; 297:937-939.

25. Ada G. Vaccines and vaccination. N Eng J Med 2001; 345:1042-1053.
26. Oram RJ, Daum RS, Seal JB, et al. Impact of recommendations to suspend the birth dose of Hepatitis B virus vaccine. JAMA 2001; 285:1875-1879.
27. Bicknell WJ. The case for voluntary smallpox vaccination. N Eng J Med 2002; 346:1323-1325.

References: Chapter 17

1. Stunkard AP. A method of evaluating a therapeutic agent. Am J Psychiatry 1950; 107:46307.
2. Enserink N. Can the placebo be the cure? Science 1999; 284:238-240.
3. Trussell J. Pills or placebo? Science 1999; 284-913.
4. Siegel B. Love, medicine and miracles. Harper Rowe, NY 1896.
5. Weil A. Spontaneous healing. Fawcett Columbine, NY, 1995.
6. Weil A. Health and healing. Houghton Mifflin, Boston, 1988.
7. Weil A. Natural health, natural medicine: A comprehensive manual for wellness and self care. Houghton, Mifflin, Boston 1995.
8. Benson H, Stark M. Timeless healing – the power and biology of belief. Scribner, NY, 1996.
9. Benson H, Beary J, Carol MP. The relaxation response. Psychiatry 1975; 37:37-46.
10. Benson H, Epstein MD. The placebo effect – a neglected asset in the care of patients. JAMA 1975; 232:1225-27.
11. Benson H, Stuart I eds. The wellness book. The comprehensive guide to maintain health and treating stress-related illness. Fireside Simon and Schuster, NY 1992.
12. Weiner NO. The harmony of the soul mental health and moral virtue reconsidered. State University of NY, Albany, NY. 1993.
13. Ludwig G. The restoration of order. Concordia Publishing House, St. Louis 1999.
14. Benson H. Wired for God. Harvard Medical Alumni Bulletin Summer 1996.
15. Hellmich N. Anorexia, bulimia signal a troubled body and soul. USA Today 2000; July 15.
16. Rayl AJS. Humor: A mind-body connection. The Scientist 2000; 14:1-18.
17. Koenig HG. Religion, spirituality and medicine: Application to clinical practice. JAMA 2000; 284:1708.
18. Koenig HG, Cohen HJ, George LB, et al. Attendance at religious services, interleukin 6, and other biologic indicators of immune function in older adults. Int. Psychiatry Med 1997; 27:233-360.
19. Nordenberg T. The healing power of placebos. FDA Consumer 2000; Jan-Feb: 14-17.

20. Spiro H. The.Power of Hope. Yale U Press, New Haven, CT 1998.
21. Siegel B. Peace, Love and Healing. Harper and Row, NY 1989.
22. Faith and Healing – Making a place for spirituality. Harvard Health Letter. 1998; 23:February.
23. Bunk S. Mind-body research matures. The Scientist. 2001; June 11:8,18.

References Chapter 18

1. Callahan M. Eight symptoms you must not ignore. Readers Digest 1997; July:54-60.
2. Newman J. Six critical symptoms. Readers Digest 2001; June:112-117.
3. Eastman P. Now, do-it-yourself care symptoms not to treat yourself. Your Health 2002; Jan:12.

References Chapter 19

1. Dunteman E. When should an alogolist be consulted? St. Louis Met. Med. 1999, January.
2. Kim JS. The use of acupuncture in managing pain. St. Louis Met. Med. 1999, January.
3. Society of Critical Care Medicine opposes bill that could curtail pain management, palliative care. SCCM Forum 1998; 10:1&11.
4. Gureje O, von Rorff M, Simon GE, et al. Persistent pain and well-being. JAMA 1998; 280:147-151.
5. Gawande A. The pain perplex. The New Yorker 1998; Sept. 21: 86-94.
6. Crews JC. Multimodal pain management strategies for office-based and ambulatory procedures. JAMA 2002; 288:629-632.

References: Chapter 20

1. Papas CA. Unlike women, many men avoid doctors even when feeling pain. USA Today 1999; June 15.
2. Dunteman E. When should an alogolist be consulted? St. Louis Met. Med. 1999, January.
3. Creighton C. Pain and pain management. St. Louis Met. Med. 1999, January.
4. Kim JS. The use of acupuncture in managing pain. St. Louis Met. Med. 1999, January.
5. Page SL. Advances in pain medicine. St. Louis Met. Med. 1998, November.
6. Gureje O, von Rorff M, Simon GE, et al. Persistent pain and well being. JAMA 1998; 280:147-151.

References Chapter 21 – None

References Chapter 22

1. Portman RM. Patient privacy recommendations: What do they mean? Bulletin of American College of Surgeons 1997; 82:15-55.
2. Hodge JG, Gostin LO, Jacobson PD. Legal issues concerning electronic health information. JAMA 1999; 282:1466-1471.
3. Today's Debate – Congress fails to repair breaches in access to health records. USA Today 1999; Aug. 20:14a.
4. Appelbaum PS. Threats to the confidentiality of medical records – No place to hide. JAMA 2000; 283:795-797.
5. Friedrich MJ. Preserving privacy, preventing discriminiation becomes the province of genetics experts. JAMA 2002; 288; 815-819.

References Chapter 23

1. Nathanson N, Auerbach JD. Confronting the HIV pandemic. Science 1999; 284:1619.
2. Cohen J. The scientific challenge of Hepatitis C. Science 1999; 285:26-30.
3. Mascola JR. Herpes simplex virus vaccines – why don't antibiotics protect? JAMA 1999; 284(4):379-380.
4. Corey L, Langenberg AGM, Ashley R, et al. Recombinant Glycoprotein vaccine for the prevention of genital HSV-2 infection. JAMA 1999; 282(4):331-340.
5. Chua KB, Bellini WJ, Rota PA, et al. Nipah virus: A recently emergent deadly paramyxovirus. Science. 2000; 288:1432-1435.
6. Enserink M. New York's lethal virus came from Middle East, DNA suggests. Science. 1999; 286:1450-1451.
7. Infectious diseases – here to stay. Harvard Health Letter 2000; 25:January #3.
8. Daszak P, Cunningham AA, Hyatt AD. Emerging infectious diseases of wildlife. Science 2000; 287:443-449.
9. Raoult D, Birg M, LaScola B, et al. Cultivation of the bacillus of Whipple's disease. New Eng J Med. 2000; 342:620-5.
10. Chase M. Hepatitis A outbreaks in the U.S. are target of vaccine campaigns. Wall Street Journal. 2999; November 12:B1.
11. Manning A. One antibiotic shot may thwart Lyme. USA TODAY 2001; May 20.
12. Zimmer C. Do chronic diseases have an infection root? Science 2001; 293:1975-1977.
13. Choiniere P. Study shows new treatment highly successful against hepatitis C virus. The Day – New London, CT 2001; Oct 2.

14. Cohen J. Report of new hepatitis virus has researchers intrigued and upset. Science 1999; 285:644-645.
15. Norman R. Fifth Disease: An uncommon name for a not uncommon virus. The Day, New London, CT 2001; April 9.
16. Higgins A. Gabon outbreak confirmed as deadly Ebola. The Day, New London, CT 2001; Dec 10.
17. Osterhelm M. Emerging infections – another warning. New Eng J Med. 2000; 342:1280-1281.
18. Enserink M. Malaysian researches trace Nipah virus outbreak to bats. Science 2000; 289:518-9.
19. Binder S, Levitt AM, Sacks JJ. Emerging infectious diseases: Public health issues for the 21st century. Science 1999; 284:1311-1313.
20. Hander FH. Helicobacter pylori and critical illness: A passive bystander or cause of disease. Crit Care Med. 1999 27:1385-86.
21. Wilmore DW. Polymerase chain reaction surveillance of microbial DNA in critically ill patients: Exploring another new frontier. Annals of Surg 1998; 277:10-11.
22. Update: Outbreak of Rift Valley Fever. JAMA 2000; 284:2989-2990.
23. Protracted outbreaks of cryptosporidiosis associated with swimming pool use. JAMA 2001; 285:2967-2968.
24. Fatal illnesses associated with a new world arenavirus. JAMA 2000; 284:1234-1238.
25. Lewis R. The infection – chronic disease link strengthens. The Scientist 2000; September 4:1,16,17.
26. Hawker FH. Helicobacter pylori and critical illness. Crit Care Med 1999; 27:1385-1386.
27. Manning A. USA's "disease detectives" track epidemics worldwide. USA TODAY 2001; July 25.
28. Enserink M, Pennisi E. Researchers crack malaria genome. Science 2002; 295:1207.
29. Bren L. Trying to keep "Mad Cow Disease" out of U.S. Herds. FDA Consumer. 2001; March-April:13-14.
30. Enserink M. Intensified battle against Foot and Mouth appears to pay off. Science 2001; 292:410.
31. Tan L, Williams MA, Khun MK, et al. Risk of transmission of bovine spongiform encephalopathy to humans in shells. JAMA 1999; 281:2330-2339.
32. Balter M. Tracking the human fallout from 'Mad Cow Disease'. Science 2000; 289:1452-1454.
33. Manocha S, Walley KR, Russell JA. Severe acute respiratory distress syndrome (SARS): A critical care perspective. Crit Care Med 2003; 31:2684-2692.

References Chapter 24 – None

References Chapter 25

1. JAMA Patient page, Generalized anxiety disorder. JAMA 2000; 283:3156.
2. Wartik N. Depression comes out of hiding. NY Times 2000; June 25:1-4.
3. Pace B, Glass RM. Generalized anxiety disorder. JAMA 2000; 283:3156.

References Chapter 26

1. Adams HC. A primer on food-borne illness investigations. St. Louis Metropolitan Medicine 2000; August 12-13.
2. Sheffer AL, Braus P. Food Allergies: When edibles become the energy. Harvard Health Letter 1997; July:4-5.
3. Williams JD, Drucker BJ. Our food is safe (honest). St. Louis Metropolitan Medicine 2000; August:11.
4. Winter G. Contaminated food makes millions ill despite advances. NY Times 2001; March 18:1 and 20.
5. Sheffer AL, Braus P. Food Allergies : When Edibles Become the Enemy. Harvard Health Letter 1997;July:4-5.
6. Ebbeling WJ. Food allergy diagnosis. Nutrition research. 1992; 12:137-144.
7. Schardt D. Food allergies. Nutrition Action Healthletter. 2001; April:10-13.
8. Long A. The nuts and bolts of peanut allergy. N Engl J Med 2002; 346:1320-1322.

References Chapter 27

1. Appleby, J. "Who Do You Call: 911 or Your HMO?" USA Today, 24 August 1999.
2. Gambill, GL. "When to Call an Ambulance-No Easy Answers." St. Louis Metropolitan Medicine Metro Medicine (1997).
3. Culley, L. "Increasing the Efficiency of Emergency Medical Services by Using Criteria-Based Dispatch." 24 Ann Emer Med (1994): 867-72.
4. Shapiro MJ. Are emergency rooms being traumatized? St. Louis Metro Medicine 1997; Sept 20-21.
5. Nagurney JT, Gregg DW. Making good use of the emergency room. Harvard Health Letter 1997 Special supplement. October 9-12.
6. Appleby S. E.R. Conditions: Critical. USA Today 2000: Feb 4.

References Chapter 28A

1. Wallis, L.A., editor. Textbook of Women's Health. Philadelphia, PA: Lippincott, Williams & Wilkins, 1998.
2. "Ensuring good mammograms." Cancer 39 (1999): 68-69.

3. Antman, K., S. Shea. "Screening mammography under age 50." *JAMA* 281 (1999): 1470-1472.
4. Grabrick, D.M., L.C. Hartmann, J.R. Cerhan et al. "Risk of breast cancer with oral contraceptive use in women with a family history of breast cancer." *JAMA* 284 (2000): 1791-1798.
5. Schrag, D., K.M. Kuntz, J.E. Garber, J.C. Weeks. "Life expectancy gains from cancer prevention strategies for women with breast cancer and BRCA1 or BRCA2 mutations." *JAMA* 283 (2000): 617-624.
6. Franks, A.L., K.K. Steinberg. "Encouraging News from the SERM Frontier." *JAMA* 281 (1999): 2243-2244.
7. Ettinger, B., D.M. Black, B.H. Mitlak. "Reduction of vertebral fracture risk in postmenopausal women with osteoporosis treated with Raloxifen." *JAMA* 282 (1999): 637-645.
8. Vastiag, B. Consensus panel recommendations for treatment of early breast cancer. JAMA 2000; 284:2707-2708.
9. Mendelsohn, M.E., R.H. Raras. "The Protective Effects of Estrogen on the Cardiovascular System." *NEJM* 340 (1999): 1801-1808.
10. Cain, J.M., M.K. Howett. "Preventing Cervical Cancer." Science 288 (2000): 1752-1754.
11. Berchuck, Andrew, Joellen M. Schildkraut, Jeffrey R. Marks, P. Andrew Futreal. "Managing Hereditary Ovarian Cancer Risk." Supplement to *Cancer* 86 (1999): 2517-2524.
12. Twickler, D.M., T.B. Forte, R. Santos-Ramos, D. McIntire, P. Harris, D. Scott. "The Ovarian Tumor Index Predicts Risk for Malignancy." *Cancer* 86 (1999): 2280-90.
13. Woloshin, Steven, Lisa M. Schwartz. "Invited commentary: Early-stage breast cancer treatment for elderly women—does one size fit all?" *Surgery* 128 (2000): 865-867.
14. Smith, MA, Shimp, LA. 20 Common problems in women's health. McGraw-Hill, St. Louis 2000.
15. DeAngelis, CD, Winker, MA. Women's health – filling the gaps. JAMA 2001; 285: 1508-1509.
16. Buring, JE Women in clinical trials – A portfolio for success. New Eng J Med 2000; 343:505-506.
17. Altkorn, D, Vokes, T. Treatment of postmenopausal osteoporosis. JAMA 2001; 285: 1415-1417.
18. Anttila, J, Saikku, P, Koskela, P, et al. Serotypes of chlamydia treatments and risks for development of cervical squamous cell carcinoma. JAMA 2001; 285: 47-51.
19. Rodriguez, C, Patel, AV, Calle, E, et al. Estrogen replacement therapy and ovarian cancer mortality in a large prospective study of U.S. women. JAMA 2001; 285:1460-1465.

20. Speizer F, Manson J, et al. Healthy women, healthy lives. Simon & Schuster, NY 2001.
21. Marchbanks PA, McDonald JA, Wilson HG, et al. Oral contraceptives and the risk of breast cancer. N Engl J Med 2002; 346:2025-2032.
22. Kauff ND, Satagopan JM, Robson ME, et al. Risk reducing salpingo-oophorectomy in women with BRCA1 or BRCA2 mutation. N Engl J Med 2002; 346:1609-1615.
23. Boyd NF, Dite GS, Stone J, et al. Heritability of mammographic density, a risk factor for breast cancer. N Engl J Med 2002; 347:886-894.
24. Veronesi U, Cascinelli N, Mariani L, et al. Twenty year follow-up of a randomized study comparing breast-conserving surgery with radical mastectomy for early breast cancer. N Engl J Med 2002; 347:1227-1232.
25. Active lifestyle cuts breast cancer risk. Health News 2001; Oct.
26. Morris KT, Johnson N, Krasikov N, et al. Genetic counseling impacts decision for prophylactic surgery for patients perceived to beat high risk for breast cancer. Am J Surg 2001; 181:431-433.
27. Nelson HD, Humphrey LL, Nygren P, et al. Postmenopausal hormone replacement therapy. JAMA 2002; 288:872-881.
28. Tarkon L. Treatment in the wings: New drugs could replace even Tamoxifen. NY Times 2002; April 9.
29. Chen CL, Weiss NS, Newcomb P, et al. Hormone replacement therapy in relation to breast cancer. JAMA 2002; 287:734-741.
30. Hlatky MA, Boothroyd D, Vittinghoff E. Quality of life and depressive symptoms in postmenopausal women after receiving hormone therapy. JAMA 2002; 287:591-597.
31. Wassertheil-Smoller S, Hendrix SL, Limacher M, et al. Effect of estrogen plus progestin on stroke in postmenopausal women. JAMA 2003; 289:3673-2684.
32. Lacey JV, Mink PJ, Lubin JH, et al. Menopausal hormone replacement therapy and risk of ovarian cancer. JAMA 2002; 288:334-341.
33. Kim JH, SKates SJ, Uede T, et al. Osteopontin as a potential diagnostic biomarker for ovarian cancer. JAMA 2002; 287:1671-1679.
34. Koutsky LA, Ault RA, Wheeler CM, et al. A controlled trial of a human papillomavirus type 1b vaccine. N Engl J Med 2002; 347:1645-1651.
35. Mandelbatt JS, Lawrence WF, Womack SM, et al. Benefits and costs of using HPV testing to screen for cervical cancer. JAMA 2002; 287:2371-2381.
36. Wald A, Langenberg AGM, Link K, et al. Effect of condoms on reducing the transmission of herpes simplex virus type 2 from men to women. JAMA 2001; 285:3100-3106.
37. Stanberry LR, Spotswood LS, Cunningham AL, et al. Glucoprotein-D-adjuvant vaccine to prevent genital herpes. N Engl J Med 2002; 347:1652-1661.

38. Davidson NE, Helzlsquer KJ. Good news about oral contraceptives. N Engl J Med 2002; 346:2078-2079.

39. Bren L. Alternatives to hysterectomy. FDA Consumer 2001; Nov-Dec.

References Chapter 28B

1. McConnell JD, Bruskewitz R, Walsh P, et al. The effect of finasteride on the risk of acute urinary retention and the need for surgical treatment among men with benign prostatic hyperplasia. N Engl J Med 1998; 333:557-563.

2. Catalone WJ, Partin AW, Slawin KM, et al. Use of the percentage of free prostate-specific antigen to enhance differentiation of prostate cancer from benign prostatic disease. JAMA 1998; 279:1542-1547.

3. Gunby P. Prostate cancer's complexities of causation, detection, and treatment challenge researchers. JAMA 1997; 227:1580-1581.

4. D'Amico AV, Whittington R, Malkowicz, SB, et al. Biochemical outcome after radical prostatectomy, external beam radiation therapy or interstitial radiation therapy for clinically localized prostate cancer. JAMA 1998; 280:969-974.

5. Chodak GW. Comparing treatments for localized prostate cancer – persisting uncertainty. JAMA 1998; 280:1008-1010.

6. Stanford JL, Feng Z, Hamilton AS, et al. Urinary and sexual function after radical prostatectomy for clinically localized prostate cancer. JAMA 2000; 283:354-360.

7. Goldstein I, Lue TF, Padma-Nathan H, et al. Oral Sildenafil in the treatment of erectile dysfunction. N Engl J Med 1998; 338:1397-1404.

8. Prostate cancer: Sometimes the best treatment is no treatment. Focus on Healthy Aging. Mt. Sinai School of Med 2002; Aug.

9. Fowler FJ, Collins MM, Albertsen PC, et al. Comparison of recommendations by urologists and radiation oncologists for treatment of clinically localized prostate cancer. JAMA 2000; 283:3217-3222.

10. Exercise and the prostate: Can you run away from trouble? Harvard Men's Health Watch 2001; May.

11. Diets and prostate cancer: More on selenium and other nutrients. Harvard Men's Health Watch 1998; Dec.

12. Is there a male menopause – and will hormones help? Harvard Men's Health Watch 2001; June.

13. Rolata G. Testosterone replacement therapy in men is widespread but untested. The Day (New London, CT) 2002; Aug 19.

14. Castellsaque X, Bosch FX, Munoz N, et al. Male circumcision, penile human papilloma virus infection and cervical cancer in female partners. N Engl J Med 2002; 346:1105-1112.

15. Vaughan ED, Jr. Medical management of benign prostatic hyperplasia – are two drugs better than one? N Engl J Med 2003; 349:2449-2451.

References Chapter 29

1. Mack MJ. Minimally invasive and robotic surgery. JAMA 2001; 285:568-572.
2. Baue AE. Minimal surgical procedures. In Baue AE, Faist E, Fry D, editors. Multiple organ failure. Springer, NY 2001; Chapter 55:545-561.
3. Vergano D. The operation you get often depends on where you live. USA TODAY 2000; Sept 19:1 and 9A
4. Vergano D. Good times toll up high surgery rates in Louisiana and Texas. USA TODAY 2000; Sept 19:9D.
5. Welch CE. What is surgery? Am J of Surg 1987; 154-463.
6. Ernst CB. Surgery, the abused word. Surg Gyn Obstet 1975; 140:608.
7. Allen CJ. Surgeries. Arch Surg 1996; 131:128.
8. Baue AE. "How many surgeries have you done?" J Am Coll of Surg 2002.

References Chapter 30

1. Surgery – Tips about having surgery. Harvard Health Letter 2000; Nov:6-7.
2. Godfrey TM. Who's afraid of the big bad knife? The Day, New London, CT 2000; Aug 7:C1-2.

References Chapter 31

1. Stern C. Before you go into the hospital. Parade Magazine 1997; May 4:6-8.
2. Looser rules for fasting before surgery. Tufts University Health and Nutrition Letter. 2002; July:2.
3. Davis D. Patients want X to mark surgery spot. USA TODAY 2001.
4. Before you go under the knife, go on the offensive. Focus on Healthy Aging. Mt. Sinai School of Medicine 2002; April:7.

References Chapter 32

1. Hsiao WC, Braun P, Becker ER, Thomas SR. The resource-based relative value scale. JAMA 1987; 258:799-802.
2. Roe BB. Sounding board – rational remuneration. New Engl J Med 1985; 313:1286-1289.
3. Radovsky SS. Sounding board – U.S. medical practice before Medicare and now – differences and consequences. 1990; 332:263-267.
4. Ingelhart JK. Health care policy report – The American health care system – expenditures. 1999; 340:70-76.
5. Humphries C. Health policy – many patients unaware how their doctors get paid or not. Harvard Medical Alumni Bulletin Spring 2001.

6.   Hemanway D, et al. Physicians responses to financial incentives – evidence from a for-profit ambulatory care center. N Eng J Med 1990-322:1059-1063.
7.   Zuger A. Dissatisfaction with medical practice. N Engl J Med 2004; 350:69-75.

References Chapter 33 – None

References Chapter 34 – None

References Chapter 35

1.   Ferber D. Superbugs on the hoof? Science 2000; 288:792-794.
2.   Black H. Agricultural antibiotics scrutinized. The Scientist. 2000; June 12:1 and 14.
3.   Khurshid MA, et al. Staphylococcus aureus with reduced susceptibility to Vancomycin. JAMA 2000; 283:597-600.
4.   Hawkey PM. Mechanisms of resistance to antibiotics. Int Care Med 2000; AS9-13.
5.   Gonzales R, Steiner JF, Sander B. Antibiotic prescribing for adults with colds, upper respiratory infections and bronchitis by ambulatory care physicians. JAMA 278; 1997:901-904.

References Chapter 36

1.   Bogardus ST Jr, Holmboe EE, Jekel JF. Perils, pitfalls and possibilities in talking about medical risks. JAMA 1999; 281:1037-1041.
2.   Hatcher CR. Hands on approach to patient grievances. Bulletin of the American College of Surgeons. 1997; 39-41.
3.   Glaberson W. Looking for attention with a billion-dollar message. NY Times 1999; July 18:3.
4.   Mohr JC. American medical malpractice in historical perspective. JAMA 2000; 283:1731-1737.
5.   Appleby J. Insurer, hospitals try apologies for errors. USA TODAY March 5, 2003.
6.   Rubin R. Fed-up obstetricians look for a way out. USA TODAY 2003.
7.   Hickson GB, et al. Patient complaints and malpractice risk. JAMA 2002; 287:2951-2957.

References Chapter 37

1.   Barger-Lux MJ, Heaney RP. For better or worse: the technological imperative in health care. Soc Med. 1896; 22:1313-1320.
2.   Fuchs VR. The growing demand for medical care. New Eng J Med. 1968; 279:192.

References Chapter 38

1. Kalb PE. Health care fraud and abuse. JAMA 1999; 282:1163-1168.
2. Sage WM. Fraud and abuse law. JAMA 1999; 282:1179-1182.
3. Ariyan S. Of mice and men – honest and integrity in medicine. Annals of Surg. 1994; 220:745-750.
4. Kaiser J. A misconduct definition that finally sticks. Science 1999; 286:391.

References Chapter 40

1. Keating NL, Zaslavsky AM, Ayanian JZ. Physicians' experiences and beliefs regarding informal consultation. JAMA 1998; 280:900-901.

References Chapter 41

1. Spiro H, Curnen MGM, Peschel E. St. James D (eds). Empathy and the practice of medicine. New Haven: Yale University Press, 1993.
2. Sarr MG. Warshaw AL. How well do we communicate with patients as surgeons? Surgery 1999; 126:126.
3. Hafferty FW. Letters from my mother and her friends. Acad Med 1997; 72:839-840.
4. Schmidt SA. When you come into my room. JAMA 1969; 276:512.
5. Battista C. Medical school chaplain promotes a curriculum of caring. Yale Med Winter-Spring 1998;44.
6. Ashmore JD. Emily Post has surgery. The Pharos. Winter 1997; 35-36.
7. Bellet P, Maloney MJ. The importance of empathy as an interviewing skill in medicine. JAMA 1991; 266:1831-1832.
8. Williams TF, Cabot, Peabody and the care of the patient, Bulletin of the history of medicine. 1950;24:462-481.
9. Roter DL, Steward M, Putnam SM, et al. Communication patterns of primary care physicians. JAMA 1997; 277:350-356.
10. Hundert EM. On entering the profession. Harvard Medical Alumni Bulletin 1997 Autumn: 21-16.
11. Scotti MJ Jr. Medical school admissions criteria – the needs of patients matter. JAMA 1997; 278:1196-1197.
12. Ludmerer KM. Instilling professionalism in medical education. JAMA 1999; 282:881-882.
13. Ludmerer KM. Time to heal. Oxford University Press, Oxford, England. 1999.
14. Bellet PS, Maloney MJ. The importance of empathy as an interviewing skill in medicine. JAMA 1991; 266:1831-1832.
15. Ellis FJ. Medical schools need to re-examine their core values. Academic Physician and Scientist 1997; Nov-Dec:1-7.

References Chapter 42

1. Weil A. Spontaneous healing 1995, Ballantine Books, New York.
2. Weil A. Eating well for optimum health. Alfred A. Knopf, New York, 2000.
3. Wetzel MS, Eisenberg DM, Kaptchuk TJ. Courses involving complementary and alternative medicine at US medical schools. JAMA 1998; 280(9):784-787.
4. Eisenberg DM, David RB, Ettner SL, et al. Trends in alternative medicine use in the United States, 1990-1997. JAMA 1998;280(18):1569-1575.
5. Astin JA. Why patients use alternative medicines: Results of a national study. JAMA 1998;279(19):1548-1553.
6. Gordon JS. Call for a new medicine. Harvard Medical Alumni Bulletin 1996;16-33.
7. The practitioner's guide to integrative therapies. St. Louis Metropolitan Medicine 1998;24-28.
8. Angell M, Kassirer JP. Alternative medicine – the risks of untested and unregulated remedies. N Engl J Med 1998;339(12):839-841.
9. Bove G, Nilsson N. Spinal manipulation in the treatment of episodic tension-type headache: A randomized controlled trial. JAMA 1998;280(18):1576-1577.
10. Cherkin DC, Deyo RA, Battie M, Street J, Barlow W. A comparison of physical therapy, chiropractic manipulation, and provision of an education booklet for the treatment of patients with low back pain. N Engl J Med 1998;339(15):1021-1029.
11. Collacott EA, Zimmerman JT, White DW, Rondone JP. Bipolar permanent magnets for the treatment of chronic low back pain. JAMA 2000;283:1322-1325.
12. Smaglik P. Office of alternative medicine gets unexpected boost. The Scientist. 1997;Nov 10:7.
13. Fetrow CW, Avila JR. The complete guide to herbal medicine pocket books. Simon-Schuster, NY 2000.
14. Ulett GA, Evidence based acupuncture for pain control. St. Louis Metropolitan Med 1999; Jan:24-25.
15. Harvard Health Letter Alternative Medicine 2000;25:1.
16. Fontanarosa PB, Lundberg GD. Alternative medicine meets science. JAMA 1998; 280:1618-1619.
17. NIH consensus development panel on acupuncture: acupuncture. JAMA 1998;280(17):1518-1524.
18. Solomon PR, Adams F, Silver A, et al. Ginko for memory enhancement. A randomized controlled trial. JAMA 2002; 288:835-840.
19. De Smet, PAGM. Herbal Remedies. N Engl J Med 2002; 347:2046-2056.
20. Ernst E, Pittler MH, Stevinson C, White C. ed. Alternative and complementary medicine. The desktop guide to complementary and alternative medicine: An evidenced-based approach. Harcourt Publishers, Ltd, St. Louis, MO. 2001.
21. Chopra D. Perfect Health. Three Rivers Press, NY. 1991, 2000.

22. Brody JE, Grady D. The NY Times Guide to Alternative Health. Times Books-Henry Hott, NY.. 2001.

23. Morris CA, Avom J. Internet marketing of herbal products. JAMA 2003; 290:1505-1509.

24. DeAngelis CD, Fontanarosa PB. Drugs alias dietary supplements. JAMA 2003; 290:1519-152.

References Chapter 43

1. Leape LL, Cullen DJ, Clapp MD, et al. Pharmacist participation on physician rounds and adverse drug events in the intensive care unit. JAMA 1999;282:267-270.

2. Sternberg S: $23 million fen-phen verdict raises pressure for settlements. USA Today, 1999; Monday, August 9:5D.

3. Monane M, Mathias DM, Nagle BA, Kelly MA. Improved prescribing patterns for the elderly through an online drug utilization review intervention. JAMA 1998; 280:1249-1252.

4. Schweiger AB. The five most common drug mistakes. Woman's Day 1997; 10/7:66-70.

5. Tanner L. JAMA: Doctors heavily influenced by drug firms. The Day, New London, CT 2000:A1 and A5.

6. Dieperink ME, Drogemullo L. Industry sponsored grand rounds and prescribing behavior. JAMA 2001; 285:1443-1444.

7. DeAngelis CD. Conflict of interest and the public trust. JAMA 2000; 284:2237-2238.

8. Cho MK, Shobara R, Schissel A, Rennie D. Policies on faculty conflicts of interest at U.S. Universities. JAMA 2000; 284:2203-2208.

9. McNeil DJ, Jr. Selling cheap 'generic' drugs, India's copycats irk industry. NY Times 2000; Dec 1:1and 14.

10. Cauchon D. Americans pay more, here's why. USA Today 1999; Nov 10:1-2A.

11. Angell M. The pharmaceutical industry – To whom is it accountable? New Eng J Med 2000; 342:1902-1904.

12. Saving money on prescription medicines. Consumer Reports on Health. 2001; 13:1 and 4.

13. Tanouge E. U.S. has developed an expensive drug habit; now, how to pay for it. Wall Street Journal. 1998; Nov 16:A1 and 10.

14. Drugmakers gifts to doctors finally get needed scrutiny. USA TODAY 2002; Oct 14:14A.

15. Schwartz LM, et al. Marketing medicine to the public: A readers guide. JAMA 2002; 287:774-775.

16. Rosenthal MB. Promotion of prescription drugs to consumers. N Eng J Med 2002; 346:498-505.

17. Drazen J. The consumer and the learned intermediary in health care. N Eng J Med 2002; 346:523-524.
18. Appleby J. Glaxo wants to keep cheap drugs out of USA. USA TODAY 2003; March 7.
19. Mello MM, Studdert DM, Brennan TA. The pharmaceutical industry versus Medicaid – Limits on state initiatives to control prescription-drug costs. N Engl J Med 2004; 350:608-613.
20. Inglehart JK. The new Medicare prescription-drug benefit – A pure power play. N Engl J Med 2004; 350:826-832.

References Chapter 44

1. Taheri P, Butz DA, Greenfield LJ. Length of stay has minimal impact on the cost of hospital admission. J Am Coll Surgeons 2000; 191:123-130.
2. Schwartz WB, Mendelson DN. Hospital cost containment in the 1980s: Hard lessons learned and prospects for the 1990s. N Eng J Med 1991; 324:1037-1042.
3. Begg CB, Cramer LD, Hoskins WB, Brennan MF. Impact of Hospital Volume on Operative Mortality for Major Cancer Surgery. JAMA 1998;280:1747-1751.
4. Allison JJ, Kiefe CI, Weissman NW, et al. Relationship of hospital teaching status with quality of care and mortality for Medicare patients with acute MI. JAMA 2000; 284:1256-1263.
5. Magid DJ, Calonge, Rumsfeld JS, et al. Relation between hospital primary angioplasty volume and mortality for patients with acute MI treated with primary angioplasty versus thrombolytic therapy. JAMA 2000; 284:3131-3138.
6. Jollis JG, Romano PS. Volume-outcome relationship in acute myocardial infarction. JAMA 2000; 284:3169-3171.
7. Schrag D, Cramer LD, Bach PB. Influence of hospital procedure volume on outcomes following surgery for colon cancer. JAMA 2000; 284:3028-3035.
8. Taylor DH Jr, Whellan DJ, Sloan FA. Effects of admission to a teaching hospital on the cost and quality of care for Medicare beneficiaries. New Eng J Med 1999; 340:293-299.

References Chapter 45

1. Souba, WW. The commercialization of American medicine: Are we headed for curing without caring. J of Surg Res 1997; 67:1-3.
2. Kassirer. Academic medical centers under siege. N Eng J Med 1994; 331:1370-72.
3. Woolhandler S, Himmelstein DV. Where money is the mission: investor owned care. N Engl J Med 1999; 341:444-446.

4. Reinhardt UE. Hippocrates and the "securitization" of patients. JAMA 1997; 277:1850-1851.
5. Emanuel L. Bringing market medicine to professional account. JAMA 1997; 277:1004-1005.

References Chapter 46

1. Jastremski CA, Harvey M. Making changes to improve the intensive care unit experience for patients and their families. New Horizons 1998; 6(1):99-118.
2. Paris JJ, Muir JC, Reardon FE. Ethical and legal issues in intensive care. J Intensive Care Med 1997; 12:298-309.
3. Franklin CM. Deconstruction of the black box known as the intensive care unit. Crit Care Med 1998; 26(8):1300-1301.
4. Baue RD, Baue AE. Clinics, technology and ethics in critical care. APICE 13, A. Gullo, Editor. Springer-Verlag Italiano, Milano 1999:13-19.
5. Habet KJ, Calvin JE. Intensive care units in the era of managed care. Current Opinion in Crit Care 1996; 2:313-318.
6. Carlet J. Quality assessment of intensive care units. Current Opinion in Crit Care 1996; 2:319-325.
7. Azoulay E, Chevret S, Leleu G, et al. Half the families of ICU patients experience inadequate communication with physicians. Crit Care Med 2000; 28:3044-3049.
8. Fontes Pinto Novacs MA, Knobel E, Book AM, et al. Stressors in ICU: Perceptions of the patient, relatives and health care team. Int Care Med 1999; 25:1421-1426.
9. Jurkovich GJ, Pierce B, Pananen L, Rivara FP. Giving bad news: the family perspective. J of Trauma 2000; 48:865-872.
10. Rotondi AJ et al. Patients recollections of stressful experiences while receiving prolonged mechanical ventilation in an intensive care unit. Crit Care Med 2002; 30:746-752.
11. Lange MP. Family stress in the intensive care unit. Crit Care Med 2001; 29:2025-2026.

References Chapter 47

1. Leape LL. Error in medicine. JAMA 1994; 272(23):1851-1857.
2. Leape LL, Woods DD, Hatie MJ, et al. Promoting patient safety by preventing medical error. JAMA 1998; 280(16):1444-1447.
3. Cullen DJ, Sweitzer BJ, Bates DW, et al. Preventable adverse drug events in hospitalized patients: A comparative study of intensive care and general care units. Crit Care Med 1997; 25(8):1289-1297.

4. Leape LL, Brennan TA, Laird N, et al. The nature of adverse events in hospitalized patients: results of the Harvard Medical Practice Study II. N Engl J Med 1997; 324(6):377-384.
5. Lazarou J, Pomeranz BH, Corey PN. Incidence of adverse drug reactions in hospitalized patients: a meta-analysis of prospective studies. JAMA 1998; 279(15):1200-1205.
6. Steinhauer J. So the brain tumors on the left, right? New Y Times 2000; April 11:25.
7. Patient, protect thyself. Harvard Health Letter 2000; Feb 3.
8. Hughes CM. How many deaths are due to medical errors? JAMA 2000; 287:2187.
9. Cole T. Medical errors versus medical injuries. JAMA 2000; 284:2175-2177.
10. Krizek TJ. Surgical error-ethical issues of adverse events. Arch Surg 2000; 135:1359-1366.
11. Brenna TTA. The Institute of Medicine Report on Medical Errors – Could it do harm? New Eng J Med 2000; 342:1123-1125.
12. Gostin L. A public health approach to reducing error – medical malpractice as a barrier. JAMA 2000; 283: 1742-1743.
13. Voelk R. Hospital collaborative creates tools to help reduce medication errors. JAMA 2001; 286:3067-3069.
14. Amon E. Communication strategies for reducing hospital error and professional liability. St. Louis Met Med 2002; Feb.
15. Maisel WH et al. Recalls and safety alerts involving pacemakers and implantable cardioverters-defibrillator generators. JAMA 2001; 286:793-799.
16. Vastag B. Hospitals get safety improvement task list. JAMA 2000; 286:661-662.
17. Zhan C, Miller MR. Excess length of stay, charges and mortality attributable to medical injuries during hospitalization. JAMA 2003; 290:1868-1874.

References Chapter 48

1. Portman RM. Patient privacy recommendations: What do they mean? Bulletin of American College of Surgeons 1997; 82:15-55.

References Chapter 49

1. Cook D, Rocker G, Marshall J, et al. Withdrawal of mechanical ventilation in anticipation of death in the intensive care unit. New Engl J Med 2003; 349:1123-1132.
2. McKhann C. A time to die. The place for physician assistance. In support of physician-assisted suicide. Yale U Press, 1995.

3. Groenewoud JH, et al. Clinical problems with the performance of euthanasia and physician-assisted suicide in the Netherlands. NEJM 342: 2000:551-556.
4. Granzini L, et al. Physicians experiences with the Oregon death with dignity act. NEJM 342; 2000:557-563.
5. Angell M. The Supreme Court and physician-assisted suicide – the ultimate right. NEJM 336; 1997:50-53.
6. Foley KM. Competent care of the dying instead of physician-assisted suicide. NEJM 336; 1997:54-57. van der Maas PJ, et al. Euthanasia, physician-assisted suicide, and other medical practices involving the end of life in the Netherlands 1990-1995. NEJM 335; 1996:1699-16705.
7. Pellegrino ED. Doctors must not kill. J Clin Ethics 3, 1992:95-102.
8. Hoyt JW. Medical futility. Crit Care Med 1995; 23(4):621-622.
9. Council on Ethical and Judicial Affairs, American Medical Association: Medical futility in end-of-life care: Reports of the council on ethical and judicial affairs. JAMA 1999; 281(10):937-941.
10. Angell M. The supreme court and physician-assisted suicide – the ultimate right. N Engl J Med 1997; 336:50-53.
11. Lynn J. No: suicide issue diverts us from the real problems. Bulletin AARP, May 1999:29-31.
12. Alpers A, Lo B. Does it make clinical sense to equate terminally ill patients who require life-sustaining interventions with those do not? JAMA 1997; 277(21):1705-1708.
13. Hendin H, Rutenfrans C, Zylicz Z. Physician-assisted suicide and euthanasia in the Netherlands: Lessons from the Dutch. JAMA 1997; 277(21):1720-1722.
14. Emanuel LL. Facing requests for physician-assisted suicide: Toward a practical and principled clinical skill set. JAMA 1998; 280(7):643-647.
15. Quill TE, Lo, Bernard, Brock DW. Palliative opinions of last resort, stopping eating and drinking, terminal sedation, physician-assisted suicide and voluntary active euthanasia. JAMA 1997; 278:2099-2104.
16. Emanuel EJ, Fairclough DL, Emanuel LL. Attitudes and desires related to euthanasia and physician-assisted suicide among terminally ill patients and their caregivers. JAMA 2000; 284:2460-2468.
17. Silver P. Teaching physicians about end of life decisions: We need to do a better job. Crit Care Med 2000; 28:3769-3700.
18. Steinhauser KE, Christakis NA, Clipp EC, et al. Factors considered important at the end of life by patients, family, physicians and other care providers. JAMA 2000; 284:2476-2482.
19. Bernabel R, Bambassi G, Lapane K, et al. Management of pain in elderly patients with cancer. JAMA 1998; 279:1877-1882.
20. Daaleman TP, van de Creek L. Placing religion and spirituality in end of life care. JAMA 2000; 284:2514-2517.

21. Lynn J. Learning to care for people with chronic illness facing the end of life. JAMA 2000; 284:2508-2511.
22. Quill J. Initiating end of life discussions with seriously ill patients. JAMA 2000; 284:2502-2507.
23. Brietbart W, Rosenfeld B, Pessin H, et al. Depression, hopelessness and desire or hastened death in terminally ill patients with cancer. JAMA 2000; 284:2907-2911.
24. Baue RD (1990) The patient as a person: Ethical considerations of patients with multiple organ failure. In: Baue AE, Multiple organ failure: Patient care and prevention. Mosby-Year Book, St. Louis pp 512-514.
25. Baue AE, Baue RD (1996) Ethics in critical care medicine. Medical decision making in critical care – a patient as a person. In: Gullo A. editor. Anesthesia, Pain, Intensive Care and Emergency Medicine. Springer-Verlag, Italiano-Milano, Italy, pp 969-974.
26. Finucane TE, Christmas C, Travis K. Tube feeding in patients with advanced dementia. JAMA 1999; 282:1365-1370.
27. Luce JM, Levy MM, Carlet JM. Editors. Compassionate end-of-life care in the intensive care unit. Crit Care Med. 2001; 295 suppl. 2:N1-N61.
28. Donahoo JD. Spirituality and the role of the chaplain in palliative care. The Guthrie Journal. Sayre, PA 2000; 69:124-132.
29. Prendergast TJ, Puntillo KA. Withdrawal of life support – Intensive caring at the end of life. JAMA 2002; 288:2732-2740.
30. Helft PR, Siegler M, Lantos J. The rise and fall of the futility movement. N Engl J Med 2000; 343:293-296.
31. Nielsen EZ. Up the slope: Physician-assisted suicide and the infamous slippery slope. The Pharos. 2001:4-11.
32. Schulz R, Beach SR, Lind B, et al. Involvement in caregiving and adjustment to death of a spouse. JAMA 2001; 285:3123-3129.

References Chapter 50

1. Lears L. Advance directives revisited: ethical instruments or useless documents. Health Care Ethics USA, Center for Health Care Ethics, St. Louis University Medical Center, 1998;6:2-3.
2. Silverman HJ, Lanken PN. Advanced directives: are they filing their purpose? Current Opinion in Critical Care 1996;2:337-343.
3. Tonelli MR. Pulling the plug on living wills—a critical analysis of advanced directives. Chest 1996;110:816-822.
4. Teno JM, Lynn J, Phillips RS, et al. Do formal advanced directives affect resuscitation decisions and the use of resources for seriously ill patients? J Clin Ethics 1994;5:23-35.
5. Emmanuel LL, Emanuel CJ. The Medical Directive. JAMA 1989; 261:2388-2393.

6. Perkins HS. Time to move advanced care planning beyond advance directives. Chest 2000; 117:1228-1231.
7. Gearon CJ. Families fight doctors over living wills. The States. AARP Modern Maturity 2000; Sept:9-11.
8. Perkins HS. Time to move advance care planning beyond advance directives. Chest 2000; 117:1228-1231.

References Chapter 51

1. Pastores SM, Halpern NA. Autopsies in the ICU: We still need them! Crit Care Med 1999; 27, 2:235-236.
2. Blosser SA, Zimmerman HE, Stauffer JL. Do autopsies of critically ill patients reveal important findings that were clinically undetected? Crit Care Med 1999. 26;8:1332-1336.
3. Belzberg H, Rivkind AI. It always pays to make a diagnosis: To autopsy or not to autopsy? Crit Care Med 1998. 26;8:1299-1300.

References Chapter 52

1. Kubler-Ross, E. 1969. On Death and dying. New York: Macmillan.
2. Friedrich MJ. Hospice care in the United States: A conversation with Florence S. Wald. JAMA 1999; 281:1683-1685.
3. Goldenberg I. Hospice: To humanize dying. Bulletin of the American College of Surgeons, 1979; 64:6-9.
4. Leigner LM. St. Christopher's Hospice, 1974 – Care of the dying patient. reprinted in JAMA 2000; 284:2426.
5. National Hospice Organization: Standards of a Hospice program of care. Hospice J 1994; 9:39-74.
6. Lynn J. Serving patients who may die soon and their families. JAMA 2001; 284:925-932.
7. AARP "Solving nursing home problems: A guide for families" (D17065) Send for at AARP Fulfillment, EE01522, 601 E. St. NW, Washington, DC 20249.
8. Gomby DS. Promise and limitations of home visitation. JAMA 2000; 284:1430-1431.
9. Mitka M. Home modifications to make older lives easier. JAMA 2001; 286:1699-1700.

References Chapter 53

1. O'Rourke K. Is managed care unethical? Health Care Ethics, USA St. Louis U Health Sciences Center 1995; 3:1 and 8.
2. Taheri PA, Butz D, Griffes LC, et al. Physician impact on the total cost of care. Annals of Surgery 2000; 231:432-435.

3. Inglehart JK. Medicare and prescription drugs. N Engl J Med 2001; 344:1010-1015.

4. Baker DW, Sudano JJ, Albert JM, Borawski EA, Dor A. Lack of health insurance and decline in overall health in late middle age. N Engl J Med 2001; 345:1106-1112.

5. Wells S. "Medical necessity": A question of definition. Bulletin American College of Surgeons 1999; 84:4-5.

6. Himmelstein DU, Wolhandlerr S, Hellander I, Wolfe SM. Quality of care in investor-owned vs. not-for-profit HMOs. JAMA 1999; 282:159-63.

7. Bodenheimer T, Lo B, Casalino L. Primary care physicians should be coordinators, not gatekeepers. JAMA 1999; 281:2045-49.

8. Starfield B. Is U.S. health really the best in the world? JAMA 2000; 284:483-486.

9. Ayanian JZ, Weissman JS, Schneider EC, et al. Unmet health needs of uninsured adults in the United States. JAMA 2000; 284:2061-2069.

10. Holl-Allen RTJ. Health care delivery in the United Kingdom and the United States. Archives of Surgery 1998; 133:1124-1125.

11. Rosenbaum S, Frankford DM, Moore B, Bozi P. Who should determine when health care is medically necessary? New England J of Med 1999; 340:229-232.

12. Appleby J. Insurers report healthy earnings. USA Today 2000; Aug 4:B1.

13. Willing R. HMO cut costs at the expense of care, plaintiff says. USA Today 2000; Feb 23: 12A.

14. Kassirer JP. Doctor discontent. New England J of Med 1998; 339:1545-1544.

15. Grumbach K, Selby JV, Damberg C, et al. Resolving the gatekeeper conundrum. JAMA 1999; 282:261-266.

16. Weaver P. Green light for suits against HMOs but not in federal courts. AARP Bulletin 2000; Sept:9 and 12.

17. Pear R. U.S. demands to review Medicare mailings by HMOs. New York Times 2000; March 19:20.

18. Angell M. Patients rights bills and other futile gestures. New England J of Med. 2000; 342:1663-1664.

19. McGinley L. Humana faces suit on matters of coverage. Wall St. Journal 1999; Oct 5:A3.

20. Koop CE. Dr. Koop's Guide to Managed Care. Readers Digest 1999; Sept:78-83.

21. Kassirer JP, Angell M. Risk adjustment or risk avoidance? New England J of Med. 1998; 339:1925-1926.

22. Young JA. Managed care provides foundation for quality health system. St. Louis Post Dispatch 1998; Oct 11:B3.

23. Lipina DD. Despite heavy criticism HMOs offer many benefits. St. Louis Post-Dispatch 1998; Oct 31:30.

24. Moore G. Managed care can rescue academic health centers. Harvard Medical Alumni Bulletin 1998-99 Winter:8.

References Chapter 54

1. O'Rourke K, Rev. Guilds, not unions, may be best choice for doctors. St. Louis Post-Dispatch 1999; March 18: B7.
2. Reardon TR. AMA to continue push for "patients bill of rights" American Medical News 1997; Dec 22/27:17,19.
3. One clear and determined voice for quality patient care. Your Guide to the AMA 1999; Chicago, IL.
4. Seutchfield FD, Benjamin R. The role of the medical profession in physician discipline. JAMA 1998; 279:1915-1916.
5. Brennan TA. Hospital peer review and clinical privileges action. JAMA 1999; 282:381-382.

References Chapter 55

1. Cohn J. The international flow of food. FDA Consumer 2001; Jan-Feb:25-31.
2. Formanek R, Jr. Highlights of FDA food safety efforts. FDA Consumer 2001; March-April:15-17.
3. Black H. Agricultural antibiotics scrutinized. The Scientist 2000; 14:1-5.
4. Bunk S. FDA and industry improve cooperation. The Scientist 2000; March:17.
5. Rubin R. Pills on the pedestal – Vioxx and Celebrex. USA Today 2001; Feb 6.
6. Industry distortion of the FDA. NY Times 2004; Dec 8, A30.
7. Rubin R. Arthritis drug adds warning label. USA TODAY Dec 10-12, 2004.
8. Meadows M. The power of acutance. FDA Consumer 2001; March-April:18-23.
9. Meadows M. FDA issues public health advisory on Phenylpropanolamine in drug products. FDA Consumer 2001; Jan-Feb:9.
10. Rubin R. Strokes linked to cough syrup, weight loss aid. USA Today 2001: Feb.
11. Marshall E. Planned Ritalin trial for tots heads into uncharted waters. Science 2000; 290:1280-1282.
12. McGinnis JM, Lee PR. Healthy people at mid decade. JAMA 1995; 273:1123-1129.
13. Satcher, D. Eliminating global health disparities. JAMA 2000, 284(22):2864-2865.
14. Greider K. Why the FDA didn't see it coming. AARP Bulletin Dec 2004; 45:3-4.
15. Marwick C. Healthy People 2010 Initiative launched. JAMA 2000; 283:989-990.
16. Feigal DW, et al. Ensuring safe and effective medical devices. N Engl J Med 2003; 348:191-192.
17. Prescriptions for drug safety. Consumer Reports on Health 2003; March 1;4-6.
18. Rudolf PM, Bernstein IBC. Counterfeit drugs. New Engl J Med 2004; 350:1384-1386.
19. Should I enroll in a clinical trial? Harvard Health Letter. Jan 2004.

References Chapter 56

1. Marwick C. Cyberinformation for seniors. JAMA 1999;286:1474-1477.
2. Jadad A, Gagliardi A. Rating health information on the internet. JAMA 1998;279:611-614.
3. Henkel J. Buying drugs online. FDA Consumer 2000; Jan-Feb:25-29.
4. Phan A. On-line health help is unreliable. USA Today, Tuesday, August 10, 1999
5. Koop CE. Dr. Koop's Guide to Managed Care. Reader's Digest 1999;Sept:78-83.
6. Moyninhan R, Bero L, Ross-Degnan D, et al. Coverage by the news of the benefits and risks of medication. New Engl J of Med 2000;342:1645-1650.
7. Lacey J. Media coverage of drugs often misleading. Harvard Medical School Alumni Bulletin 2000;Fall:3.
8. Gawande A. Mouse hunt: forget cancer. Is there a cure for hype? The New Yorker, Dec 1998; 5-6.
9. Marshall E. The power of the front page of the New York Times. Science 1998;280:996-997.
10. Steinbrook R. Medical journals and medical reporting. New Engl J of Med 2000;342:1668-1691.
11. Carrns A. Cyberchondriacs get what goes around on the internet now. The Wall Street Journal. 1999;Oct 5A1 and A6.

References Chapter 57

1. Grumbach K. Primary care in the United States – The best of times, the worst of times. New Engl J of Med 1999;241:2008-2010.
2. Forrest CB, Whelan EM. Primary care safety net delivery sites in the United States. JAMA 2000; 284:2077-2083.
3. Barnett PG, Midtling JE. Public policy and the supply of primary care physicians. JAMA 1989; 262:2864-2868.

References Chapter 58

1. Voelker R. Activist Young says "gathering storm" will propel a single-payer movement. JAMA 1998;280:1467-68.
2. Lamm RD. Marginal medicine. JAMA 1996;280:931-33.
3. Carlton JG. Finding ways to provide access to health care for all citizens. St. Louis Post-Dispatch, Imagine St. Louis, Sunday, May 30, 1999, p. B1.
4. Appleby J. Health costs going out of control report says. USA TODAY. 2001; March 8:3B.
5. Davis R. Appleby J. Report: Health system broken. USA TODAY 2001; March 24:1.

6. Freudenheim M. Alarmed at rising number of uninsured Americans, coalition forms. NY Times 2002; Feb 9.
7. Sternberg S. Study blames 18,000 deaths in USA on lack of insurance. USA TODAY 2002; Oct 7.
8. Winslow R. One patient, 34 days in the hospital, a bill for $5.2 million. Wall St J 2001; Aug 2.
9. Finkel. Complications—$145,000 for a kidney. NY Times 2001; May 27.
10. Fuchs VR. What's ahead for health insurance in the US. N Engl J Med 2002; 346:1822-1824.

References Chapter 59

1. O'Rourke K. Ethical issues in health care. St. Louis University Center for Health Care Ethics. Health Care Ethics USA XVIII/8 April 1997.
2. Russo E. A look back at NBAC. The Scientist 1999; Oct 11:4-5.
3. Kassirer J. Is managed care here to stay? New Eng J Med. 1997; 276:1014.
4. President's Commission for the Study of Ethical Problems in Medicine. Securing Access to Health care. Gov. Printing Office, Washington, DC. 1983:22-23.
5. Angelos P. Ethical guidelines in surgical patient care. J of Am College of Surgeons 1999; 188:55-58.
6. O'Rourke K. Surrogate decision making – Ethical issues. Health care Ethics— USA. St. Louis U Center for Health Care Ethics, 221 N. Grand Blvd, St. Louis, MO 63103. 1998; 6:#3.

References Chapter 60

1. Korenman SG, Berk R, Wenger N, Lew V. Evaluation of the Research Norms of Scientists and Administrator's Responsible for Academic Research Integrity. JAMA 1998;279:41-47.
2. Angelos P. Ethical Guidelines in Surgical Patient Care. J Am Coll Surg 1999; 188:55-58.
3. Hanlon CR. Ethics in Surgery. J Am Coll Surg 1999; 186:41-49.
4. Pellegrino ED. Interests, obligations and justice: Some notes toward an ethic of managed care. J Clin Ethics 1995; 6:312-317.
5. Ethical Issues in Managed Care. Council on Ethical and Judicial Affairs of the AMA. JAMA 1995; 213:330-335.
6. Hundert EM. On entering the profession. Harvard Medical Alumni Bulletin, Autumn 1997; 23-26.
7. Baker R, Caplan A, Emanuel L, Latham SR. Crisis, ethics in the American Medical Association, 1847 and 1997. JAMA 1997; 278:163-164.
8. Peabody F. The care of the patient. JAMA 1927; 88:877-882.

9. Baue RD. The patient as a person: ethical considerations of patients with multiple organ failure. In: Baue AE: Multiple organ failure: patient care and prevention. Mosby Yearbook: 1990:512-514.

10. Kassirer JP. Managing Care – Should we adopt a new ethic? New Engl J Med 1998; 339:397-398.

References Chapter 61

1. Nyman DJ, Sprung CL. Informed consent in intensive care. Curr Opin Crit Care 1996; 2:331-336.

2. Katz J. Reflections on informed consent: 40 years after its birth. J Am Coll Surg 1988; 186:466-474.

3. Shuster E. 50 years later: the significance of the Nuremberg Code. New Engl J Med 1997; 337:1436-1440.

4. Marwick C. Protecting subjects of clinical research. JAMA 1999; 28:516-175.

5. Baue R. The patient as a person: Ethical considerations of patients with multiple organ failure. In: Baue AE. Multiple Organ Failure, Mosby-Yearbook, St. Louis, MO 1990, pp. 512-514.

6. Baue RD. Ethical considerations of MODS, SIRS, and MOF. In: Baue AE, Faist E, Fry D. (eds.), Springer, NY 2000; pp 663-671.

7. Annas GJ. A national bill of patients' rights. New Engl J Med 1998; 338:695-699.

8. Gamble JN. Under the shadow of Tuskegee: African Americans and health care. Am J Public Health 1997; 87:1773-1778.

9. Webb SA. Are randomized controlled trials ethical in critically ill patients? Crit Care Med 2000; 28:1246-1248.

10. Morse MA, Califf RM, Sugarman J. Monitoring and ensuring safety during clinical research. JAMA 2001; 285:201-205.

11. Paasche-Orlow MK, Taylor HA, Brancati FL. Readability standards for informed-consent forms as compared with actual readability. N Engl J Med 2003; 348:721-726.

References Chapter 62

1. Annas GJ. A national bill of patients' rights. New Engl J Med 1998; 338:695-699.

2. Nader R. Yes: HMOs currently face no liability. AARP Bulletin, 1999; September.

3. Jacobson D, Pomfred SD. ERISA litigation and physician autonomy. JAMA 2000; 283:921-926.

4. Angell M. Patients' Rights Bill and other futile gestures. New Engl J Med 2000; 342:1663-1664.

5. Today's debate: Suing HMOs. USA TODAY 2000; February 25.

6. Pear R. Insurance groups to merge in battle over patients' rights. New York Times 2000; December 1:A21.
7. Gostin LO. National health information privacy: Regulations under the Health Insurance Portability and Accountability Act. JAMA 2001; 285:3015-3021.

References Chapter 63

1. Fairfield H. With the Human Genome Project, Biology Joins the Ranks of Big Science. New York Times 2000; June 27.
2. Pennisi E. Finally the Book of Life and Instructions for Navigating It. Science 2000; 288:2304-2307.
3. Collins FS, McKusick VA. Implications of the Human Genome Project for Medical Science. JAMA 2001; 285:540-544.
4. Sternberg J. Cell Transplant Saves Dying Heart. USA Today 2000; Nov. 13:8D.
5. Bunwol TF, Watanabe AM. Genetic information, Genomic Technology and the Future of Drug Discovery. JAMA 2001; 285:551-555.
6. Yan H, Kinzler KW, Vogelstein B. Genetic Testing – Present and Future. Science 2000; 289:1890-1892.
7. Lewin T. Boom in Genetic Testing Raises Questions on Sharing Results. New York Times 2000; July 21:A1 and 14.
8. Sullivan A. Promotion of the Fittest. New York Times Magazine. 2000; Aug. 23:16-17.
9. Friedrich MJ. Genetic Screening to Offset Adult Disease. JAMA 2000; 284:2308.
10. Holtzman NA, Marteau TM. Will Genetics Revolutionize Medicine. New Eng. J. Med. 2000; 343:141-144.
11. Marshall E. Families Sue Hospital, Scientist for Control of Canavan Disease. Science 2000; 290: 1062.
12. Koopman WJ. Prospects for Autoimmune Disease. JAMA 2001; 285:648-650.
13. Stephenson J. Genetic Test Information Fears Unfounded. JAMA 1999; 282:2197-98.
14. Lerman C, Hughes C, Trock BJ, et al: Genetic Testing in Families with Hereditary Nonpolyposis Colon Cancer. JAMA 1999; 281(17): 1618-1622.
15. O'Rourke K. Genetic Testing: Ethical Issues. St. Louis Metropolitan Medicine 1998 August; 14-15.
16. Haddad FF, Yeatman TJ, Shivers SC, Reintgen DS. The Human Genome Project: A Dream Becoming a Reality. Surgery 1999; 125:575-580.
17. Holtzman NA. Are Genetic Tests Adequately Regulated? Science 1999; 286:409.
18. Fuller BP, Kahn JE, Barr PA, et al. Privacy in Genetics Research. Science 1999; 285:1359-1361.

19. Sternberg S. Complete Proteins Separate Humans from Creatures of the Field. USA Today 2001; Feb 12:6D.
20. Thompson L. Human Gene Therapy – Harsh Lessons, High Hopes. FDA Consumer 2000; Sept/Oct:19-24.
21. Woo SLC. Gene Therapy Researchers Bright Fields, Pitfalls and Promises. FDA Consumer 2000; Sept/Oct:40.
22. Stephenson J. Gene Therapy Trials Show Clinical Efficacy. JAMA 2000; 283:589-590.
23. Kling J. Genetic counseling. The human side of science. The Scientist. 1999; July:19-20.
24. Burke W. Genetic Testing. N Engl J Med 2002; 347:1867-1875.
25. Noguchi P. Risks and benefits of gene therapy. N Engl J Med 2003; 348:193-194.

References Chapter 64

1. Bouma H III. Ethical considerations in human cloning. Surgery 1999; 125:468-470.
2. Vogel G. Company gets rights to cloned human embryos. Science 2000; 287:559.
3. Healey BP. Editorial: The asexual revolution of Dolly the lamb. J. Women's Health 1998; 7(1):1-2.
4. Butler D. Dolly researcher plans further experiments after challenges. Nature 1998; 391:825-826.
5. Prather RS. Pigs is pigs. Science 2000; 289:1886-1887.
6. Kestenbaum D. Cloning plan spawns ethics debate. Science 1998; 279:315.
7. McLaren A. Cloning: Pathways to a pluripotent future. Science 2000; 288:1775-1780.
8. Pickrell J. Experts assess plan to help childless couple. Science 2001; 291:2061-2063.

Stem-cell Research

1. Juengst E, Fossell M. The ethics of embryonic stem cells – now and forever, cells without end. JAMA 2000; 284:3180-3184.
2. Vogel G. Can adult stem cells suffice? Science 2001; 292:1820-1822.
3. Marshall E. Ethicists back stem cell research, White House treads cautiously. Science 1999; 285:502.
4. Stone R. UK backs use of embryos, sets vote. Science 2000; 289:1269-1270.
5. Daji EH, Leiden JM. Gene and stem cell therapies. JAMA 2001; 285:545-600.
6. Korn D. The NIH guidelines on stem cell research. Science 2000; 289:1877.
7. Friedrich MJ. Debating pros and cons of stem cell research. JAMA 2000; 284:681.

8. Shapiro HT. Ethical dilemmas and stem cell research. Science 2000; 285:2065.
9. Vogel G. Bush squeezes between the lines on stem cells. Science 2001; 293:1242-1245.
10. Juengst E, Fossel M. The ethics of embryonic stem cells. JAMA 2000; 284:3180-3184.
11. Milpied N, Deconinck E, Gaillard F, et al. Initial treatment of aggressive lymphoma with high dose chemotherapy and autologous stem cell support. N Engl J Med 2004;350:1287-1295.
12. Genetically modified foods
13. Goldman KA. Bioengineered food – safety and labeling. Science 2000; 290:457-458.
14. Fischer KS, Barton J, Khush GS, et al. Collaborations in rice. Science 2000; 290:279-280.
15. Kaiser J. Panel urges further study of biotech corn. Science 2000; 290:1867.
16. Patient plant breeders harvest food prize. Science 2000; 289:1871.
17. Normile D. Hopes grow for hybrid rice to feed developing world. Science 2000; 288:429.
18. Thompson L. An interview with Dr. Jane E. Henney. FDA Consumer 2000; Jan-Feb:19-23.
19. Kaiser J. Transgenic crop report fuels debate. Science 2000; 288:245-247.
20. Paleritz BA, Lewis R. Fears or facts? A viewpoint on GM crops. The Scientist 1999; October 11:10.
21. Lewis C. Kind of fish story – the coming of biotech animals. FDA Consumer 2001; Jan-Feb:15-20.
22. Devine K. GM food debate gets spicy. The Scientist 2000; October 30:10 and 33.
23. Wolfenbarger LL, Phifer PR. The ecological risks and benefits of genetically engineered plants. Science 2000: 290:2088-2098.
24. Moffat AS. Can genetically modified crops go greener? Science 2000; 290:253-254.
25. Brown WA. Facts, beliefs and genetically modified food. The Scientist 2000; April 17:39.
26. Cowan CA, Klimmanskkaya I, McMahon J, et al. Derivation of embryonic stem-cell lines from human blastocysts. N Engl J Med 2004; 350:1353-1356.

References Chapter 65

1. Myers J, Prakash M, Froelich V, et al. Exercise capacity and mortality among men referred for exercise testing. N Engl J Med 2002; 346:793-801.
2. Should you have a stress test before you exercise. Harvard Men's Health Watch 2002; 6:April.

3. No Sweat: New guidelines for moderate exercise. Harvard Men's Health Watch 2001; 6:Dec.
4. Hakim AA, Petrovitch H, Burchfield CM, et al. Effects of walking on mortality among non-smoking retired men. N Engl J Med 1998; 338:94-99.
5. Blair SN, Kohl HW, Barlow CE, et al. Changes in physical fitness and all cause mortality. JAMA 1995; 273:1093-1098.
6. Paffenbarger RS, Jr, Hyde RT, Wing AL, et al. The association of changes in physical activity level and other lifestyle characteristics with mortality among men. N Engl J Med 1993; 328:538-545.
7. Exercise for everyone. Harvard Men's Health Watch. 1999; January:7-8.
8. Strength training. Harvard Men's Health Watch. 200; 5:1-4.
9. Gill TM, Dipietro L, Krumholz, HM. Role of exercise testing and safety monitoring for older persons starting an exercise program. JAMA 2000; 284:342-349.
10. Hu FB, Stampfer MT, Colditz GA, et al. Physical activity and risk of stroke in women. JAMA 2000; 283:2961-2967.
11. Lee I-M, Hsich C-C, Paffenbarger RS, Jr. Exercise intensity and longevity in men: The Harvard Alumni Health Study. JAMA 1995; 273:1179-1184.
12. Manson JE, Hu FB, Rich-Edwards JW. A prospective study of walking as compared with vigorous exercise in the prevention of coronary heart disease in women. N Engl J Med 1999; 341:650-658.
13. Breslow L. Private health and public medicine. Pharos of AOA. 1969; April:44-48.
14. Mitka M. Aging patients are advised "stay active to stay alert". JAMA 2001. 285; 19:2437-2438.

References Chapter 66

1. Jacobson MF. Follow the money. Nutrition Action Health. 2000; 27:Oct. p2.
2. Diet and health – Ten mega trends. Nutrition Action Newsletter 2001; Jan-Feb:3-12.
3. Jacobson MF. Diet and disease: Time to act. Nutrition Action Healthletter. 1999; Dec:2.
3. Diseases we can prevent. Nutrition Action Healthletter. 1999; Dec 3-9.
4. Jacobson MF. Meat labeling: Help. Nutrition Action Newsletter. 2001: April 2.
5. Horowitz B. Can fast-food titans thrive on healthful fare? USA TODAY 2002; Sept 30.
6. Tarnower H, Baker SS. The complete Scarsdale diet. Bantam Books, NY 1980.
7. Mediterranean diet: A fish connection. Harvard Health Letter 1997; April:1-2.
8. Leibman B, Hurley J. Healthy Foods. Nutrition Action Healthletter. 1875 Conn. Avenue NW, Suite 300, Washington, DC 20009-85728.

9. Jacobson MF. Popular diets: Untested. Nutrition Action Healthletter. 2000; May. Vol 27:2.
10. Brody J. The New York Times Book of Health. Random House, NY 1997.
11. Hellmich W. Diet authors square off. USA TODAY 2000; Feb 24:1-2.
12. Little accord on a round table of diet experts. New York Times 2000; Feb 25:A13.
13. Barnard ND, Nicholson A, Howard JL. The medical costs attributable to meat consumption. Prev Med 1995; 24:646-655.
14. Bren L. New dietary guidelines. FDA Consumer 2000; Sept-Oct:10.
15. Kumanyika S. Improving our diet – Still a long way to go. NEJM 1996; 335:738-739.
16. Connor WE, Connor SJ. Should a low fat-high carbohydrate diet be recommended for everyone? NEJM 1997; 337:562-563.
17. Ornish, D. Dr. Dean Ornish's program for reversing heart disease. PCRM Market Place, PO Box 99, Summertown, TN 38483.
18. Benson H, Stuart EM. The wellness book – Fireside. Simon and Schuster, NY.
19. Atkins RC. Dr. Atkins New Diet Revolution. Avon Press, NY.
20. Whaler A. Dropping the diet myths. Green Mountain at Fox Run, Brattleboro Weekend Reformer. 1999; July 17-18:25.
21. Liebman B. Fat – fine tuning the message – the DASH diet. Nutrition Action Healthletter. 1998; March:1-7.
22. Hellmich N. Restaurants dish out days worth portions. USA TODAY 2001; Feb 1:1D.
23. The new four food groups – for optimal nutrition. Physicians Committee for Responsible Medicine. 5100 Wisconsin Avenue, NW, Suite 404, Washington, DC 20016
24. Cram P, Nallamothu BK, Frederick AM, et al. Fast food franchises in hospitals. JAMA 2002; 287:2945-2946.
25. Schlosser E. Fast Food Nation. Harpers Collins, NY 2002.
26. Jacobson MF, Hurley J. Restaurant confidential. Workman Publishing, NY. 2002.
27. Schneeman BO. Book Review: Food politics: How the food industry influences nutrition and health. N Engl J Med 2002; 346:2017-2018.
28. Weil A. The lowdown on low-carb diets. Self Healing. 2002; Nov.
29. Ware JH. Interpreting incomplete data in studies of diet and weight loss. N Engl J Med 2003; 348:2136-2137.
30. Agatston A. The South Beach Diet. Random House NY 2003 Rodale 2003.

References Chapter 67

1. Greider L. Most trendy diets fail in the long run. AARP Bulletin 2001; June 3.
2. Hellmich N. Pudgy kids need family allies to fight battle of the bulge. USA TODAY 1999; Aug 31:8D.

3. Serdula MK, Mokdad AH, Williamson DF. Prevalence of attempting weight loss and strategies for controlling weight. JAMA 1999. 282:1353-1358.
4. Hellmich N. He fights a heavyweight bout. George Blackburn. USA TODAY 2000, June 15:1D.
5. Friedman JM. Mapping the brain's food-intake circuitry. Howard Hughes Med Inst. Research News 2004: Dec 20.
6. Campfield LA, Smith FJ, Burn P. Strategies and potential molecular targets for obesity treatment. Science. 1998. 280:1383-1390.
7. Gura T. Tracing leptins, partners in regulating body weight. Science 2000, 287:1738-1741.
8. Stephenson J. Knockout science: Chubby mice provide new insights into obesity. JAMA 1999. 282:1507-1508.
9. McCarthy P. Scientists finding evidence of caloric restriction's benefits. The Scientist 1997, May 26. 11-14.
10. Weindruch R, Sohal RS. Caloric intake and aging. New Engl J Med 1997; 337:986-994.
11. Calle EE, Thun MJ, Petrelli JM, et al. Body-mass index and mortality in a prospective cohort of US adults. New Engl J Med. 1999; 341:1097-1105.
12. Williamson DF. The prevention of obesity. New Engl J Med. 1999; 341:1140-1141.
13. Allison DB, Fontaine KR, Manson JE, et al. Annual deaths attributable to obesity in the United States. JAMA 1999; 282:1530-1538.
14. Fat Trapper maker to refund $10 million. USA TODAY. 2000, April 27:7D.
15. Adams C. FDA urges consumers to avoid using product sold as fat-loss supplement. Wall Street Journal. 1999, November 12:B6.
16. Fen-phen controversy hints at a larger drug problem. USA TODAY. 1999, August 9:12A.
17. Hellmich N. Pitching pills that lighten wallets. USA TODAY. 1999, August 16:6D.
18. $23 million fen-phen verdict raises pressure for settlements. USA TODAY. 1999, August 9:5D.
19. Ingeslby TV, Henderson DA, O'Toole T, Dennis DT The continuing epidemic of obesity in the United States. JAMA 2000. 184:1650-1651.
20. Mokdad AH, Serdula MK, Dietz WH, et al. The spread of the obesity epidemic in the United States, 1991-1998. JAMA 1999. 282:1519-1522..
21. Galuska DA, Will JC, Serdula MK, Ford ES. Are health care professionals advising obese patients to lose weight? JAMA 1999. 282; 16:1576-1578.
22. Walsh T, Devlin MJ. Eating disorders: progress and problems. Science 1998; 280:1387-1390.
23. Anderson RE, Crespo CJ, Bartlett SJ, et al. Relationship of physical activity and television watching with body weight and level of fatness among children: results from the Third National Health and Nutrition Examination Survey. JAMA 1998 279:938-942.

24. Robinson TN. Reducing children's television viewing to prevent obesity. JAMA 1999; 282:1561-1567.

25. Heymsfield SB, Greenberg AS, Fujioka K. Recombinant Leptin for weight loss in obese and lean adults. JAMA 1999. 282; 16:1568-1575.

26. Atwood C. Eating disorders expert proposes fat tax on foods. Harvard Medical School Alumni Magazine 1997. p. 36.

27. Kassirer JP, Angell M. Losing weight – an ill-fated new year's resolution. New Engl J Med. 1998. 338:52-54.

28. Fletcher AM. Secrets of the diet masters. Bottom Line. 1998, October 1.

29. Schardt D. Fat burners. Nutrition Action Healthletter. 1999, July/August:9-11.

30. Branson R, Potoczna N, Kral JG, et al. Binge eating as a major phenotype of melanocortin 4 receptor gene mutations. N Engl J Med 2003; 348:1096-1103.

31. Wirth A, Krause J. Long-term weight loss with sibutramine. JAMA 2001; 286:1331-1339.

32. Gadde KM, Franciscy DM, Wagner II HR, et al. Zonisamide for weight loss in obese adults. JAMA 2003; 289:1820-1825.

33. Cummings DE, Weigle DS, Frayo RS, et al. Plasma ghrelin levels after diet-induced weight loss or gastric bypass surgery. N Engl J Med 2002; 346:1623-1630.

34. Livingston EH. Obesity and its surgical management. Am J Surg 2002; 184:103-113.

35. Helmich N. 10 ways to make it a habit to eat less, eat better and exercise more. USA TODAY 2004; Jan 6.

36. Brownell K. Food fight: The inside story of the food industry. America's obesity crisis and what we can do about it. McGraw-Hill 2004.

37. Ramos EJ, et al. Is obesity an inflammatory disease? Surgery 2003; 134:329-335.

38. Korner J, Liebel RL. To eat or not to eat – how the gut talks to the brain. N Engl J Med 2003; 349:926-928.

References Chapter 68

1. HDL: The "good" (but complex) cholesterol. Harvard Health Letter 1997; 8:September.

2. Rigotti A, Krieger M. Getting a handle on "good" cholesterol with the high-density lipoprotein receptor. New Engl J Med 1999; 342:2011-2013.

3. Ridker PM, Stampfer MJ, Rifai N. Novel risk factors for systemic atherosclerosis. A comparison of C-reactive protein, fibrinogen, homocysteine, lipoprotein (a), and standard cholesterol screening as predictors of peripheral arterial disease. JAMA 2001; 285:2481-2485.

4. Stamler J, Daviglus ML, Garside DB, et al. Relationship of baseline serum cholesterol levels in 3 large cohorts of younger men to long-term coronary, cardiovascular, and all-cause mortality and to longevity. JAMA 2000; 284:311-318.

5. Liebman B. The chocolate myth factory. Nutrition Action Healthletter. 2001; March:7-9.
6. Jacobson MF. How much sugar? Labels should say. Nutrition Action Healthletter. 2000; September:2.
7. Is sugar bad for you? Harvard Health Letter. 2001; 26.
8. Liebman B. Sugar. The sweetening of the American diet. Nutrition Action Healthletter 1998; November:3-8.
9. DeBarros A. Fast-food highway hazards. USA TODAY 2001; June 1:7D.
10. Donahue D. Read this and you won't want fries – or anything. USA TODAY. 2001; February 1:6D.
11. Hurley J, Liebman B. Behind bard. Dr. Atkins and friends take the wrap. Nutrition Action Healthletter. 2000; October:13-15.
12. Jacobson MF. Tax junk foods. Nutrition Action Healthletter. 2000; December:2.
13. Hu FB, Stampfer MJ, Rimm EB, et al. A prospective study of egg consumption and risk of cardiovascular disease in men and women. JAMA. 1999; 281:1387-1394.
14. Raising "good" cholesterol. Harvard Health Letter. 1998; January:3.
15. Smaglik P. Oat bran could lower cholesterol , replace fat. The Scientist. 2001; 77:February.
16. Lauer MS, Fontanarosa PB. Updated guidelines for cholesterol management. JAMA. 2001; 285:2508-2509.
17. Knopp RH, Walden CE, Retzlaff BM, et al. Long-term cholesterol-lowering effects of 4 fat-restricted diets in hypercholesterolemic and combined hyperlipidemic men. JAMA. 1997; 278:1509-1515.
18. Pearson TA. Lipid-lowering therapy in low-risk patients. JAMA. 1998; 279:1659-1661.
19. Ornish D. Low fat diets. New Engl J Med. 1998; 338:127.
20. Taubes G. New study says low-fat diet can lower blood pressure. Science. 1997; 276:350.
21. Ridker PM, Stampfer MJ, Hennekens CH. Plasma concentration of lipoprotein(a) and the risk of future stroke. JAMA. 1995; 273:1269-1273.
22. Berthold HK, Sudhop T, von Bergmann K. Effect of a garlic oil preparation of serum lipoproteins and cholesterol metabolism. A randomized controlled trial. JAMA. 1998; 279:1900-1906.
23. Sacks FM, Pfeffer MA, Moye LA, et al. The effect of Pravastatin on coronary events after myocardial infarction in patients with average cholesterol levels. New Engl J Med. 1996; 335:1001-1009.
24. Downs JR, CLearfield M, Weis S, et al. Primary prevention of acute coronary events with Lovastatin in men and women with average cholesterol levels. JAMA. 1998; 279:1615-1622.

25. LaRosa JC, He J, Vupputuri S. Effects of statins on risk of coronary disease. A meta-analysis of randomized controlled trials. JAMA. 1999; 282:2340-2346.
26. Lewis C. Health Claim – For foods that could lower heart disease risk. FDA Consumer. 2000; November/December:11.
27. Jacobson MF. Trans fat: Hidden killer. Nutrition Action Healthletter. 2000; January/February:2.
28. Libman B, Hurley J. The best-dressed list. Picking a salad dressing. Nutrition Action Healthletter. 2000; September:12-15.
29. Blackburn H. Sounding Board – Olestra and the FDA. New Engl J Med. 1996; 334:984-986.
30. Bad fats, good fats: New insights into diet and health. Harvard Men's Health Watch. 2000; 4:2-3.
31. Grundy SM. Early detection of high cholesterol levels in young adults. JAMA. 2000; 284:365-367.
32. The new margarines: Can they help your heart? Harvard Men's Health Watch 2002; Feb:1.
33. Albert MA, Danielson E, Rafai N, et al. Effect on statin therapy on C-reactive protein levels. JAMA 2001; 286:64-70.

References Chapter 69

1. Mizock BA. Homocysteine and critical illness. Crit Care Med 2000; 28:1229-1230.
2. Schindler K, Zauner G, Buchmayer H, et al. High prevalence of hyperhomocysteinemia in critically ill patients. Crit Care Med 2000; 28:991-995.
3. Nygard O, Nordehaug JE, Refsum H, et al. Plasma homocysteine levels and mortality in patients with coronary artery disease. NEJM 1997; 337:230-236.
4. Stacey M. The fall and rise of Kilmer McCully. NY Times Magazine 1997; August 10:25-29.
5. McCully RS. Homocysteine, folate, vitamin B6 and cardiovascular disease. JAMA 1998; 279:392-393.
6. Tice JA, Ross E, Coxson PG, et al. Cost-effectiveness of vitamin therapy to lower plasma homocysteine levels for the prevention of coronary heart disease. JAMA 2001; 286:936-943.

References Chapter 70

1. Taking stock of antioxidants. Harvard Health Letter 2002; 27:Feb.
2. Weil A. Why take supplements if you eat a healthy diet? Self Healing Premier Issue 1999; Nov.

3. Vitamin D needed for muscles as well as bone. Tufts U Health and Nutrition Letter 2002; June.

4. Ten super foods you should eat. Nutrition Action Health Letter. 2000: December.

5. Lamberg L. Melatonin potentially useful but safety, efficacy remain uncertain. JAMA 1996; 276:1011-1014.

6. Losonczy KH, Harris TB, Havlik RS. Vitamin E and vitamin C supplement use and risk of all – cause and coronary heart disease mortality in older persons. Am J Clin Nutr 1996; 64:190-196.

7. Vitamin prescriptions for healing. Prevention Magazine Health Books, Rodale Press, Inc., Emmaus, PA 18098

8. Schardt D. Magnesium. Nutrition Action Health Letter 1998; December:9-11.

9. Liebman B. Multiple choice – How to pick a multi-vitamin. Nutrition Action Health Letter 1999; 26:18.

10. Oakley GP. Eat right and take a multivitamin. New Engl J Med 1998; 338:1060-1061.

11. Liebman B. Do you know your vitamin ABCs? Nutrition Action Health Letter 1999; 26:16.

12. Honein MA, Paulozi LJ, Matthews TJ, et al. Impact of folid acid. JAMA 2001; 285:2981-2986.

13. Rimm EB, Willett WC, Hu FB, et al. Folate and vitamin B6 from diet and supplements and risk of coronary artery disease among women. JAMA 1998; 279:359-365.

14. Napier K. Facts and fiction about vitamin E. Harvard Health Letter. 1996; 22:1-3.

15. Flavenoids, the next new thing? Harvard Health Letter 2000; December:6.

16. Greenberg ER, Sporn MB. Antioxidant vitamins, cancer, and cardiovascular disease. New Engl J Med 1996; 334:1189-1190.

17. How much protein is enough? Consumer Reports on Health 2001; Feb.

18. Barnard ND, Nicholson A, Howard JL. The medical costs attributable to meat consumption. Prev. Med 1995; 24:646-655.

19. Are you getting too much vitamin A? Harvard Health Letter 2002; March.

20. Grant JM, Shouten EG, Kok FO. Effect of daily vitamin E and multivitamins on acute respiratory tract infections in elderly persons. JAMA 2002; 288:715-721.

21. Freedman JE. Antioxidant versus lipid altering therapy – some answers, more questions. N Engl J Med 2001; 345:1636-1637.

References Chapter 71

1. Wolk A, Manson JE, Stanpher MJ, et al. Long-term intake of dietary fiber and decreased risk of coronary heart disease among women. JAMA 1999; 281:1998-2004.

2. Fuchs CS, Giovannucci EL, Colditz GA, et al. Dietary fiber and the risk of colorectal cancer and adenoma in women. New Engl J of Med 1999; 340:169-176.
3. Ludwig DS, Pereira MA, Korenke CH, et al. Dietary fiber, weight gain, and cardiovascular disease risk factors in young adults. JAMA 1999; 282:1539-1546.
4. Rimm EB, Ascherio A, Giovannucci E, et al. Vegetable, fruit and cereal fiber intake and risk of coronary artery disease among men. JAMA 1995; 274:447-451.
5. Wynder EL, Stellman SD, Zang EA. High fiber intake – Indicator of a healthy lifestyle. JAMA 1996; 274:486-487.
6. Choosing whole grains: Trickier than you think. Tufts U Health and Nutrition Letter 2002; July 4-5.
7. Ripsin CM, Keenan JM, Jacobs DR, et al. Oat products and lipid lowering – a meta-analysis. JAMA 1992; 267;3317-3325.
8. Jacobs DR Jr, Marquart L, Salvin J, et al. Whole-grain intake and cancer: an expanded review and meta-analysis. Nutr Cancer 1998; 30:85-96.
9. Glore SR, Van Treeck D, Knehaus AW, et al. Soluble fiber and serum lipids – a literature review. J Am Dietet Assoc 1994; 94:425-436.

References Chapter 72

1. Ornish D, Scherwitz LW, Billings J, et al. Intensive lifestyle changes for reversal of coronary artery disease. JAMA 1998; 260:2001.
2. Medicare will pay for low-fat diet as an alternative to heart surgery. The Associated Press, St. Louis Post-Dispatch 1999; October 2.
3. Superko HR. Surprising new clinical lessons from the regression trials. Educational Highlights. American College of Cardiology 1996; 11:1-5.
4. Vegetarianism – should you or shouldn't you? Harvard Health Letter 1999; 24:7.
5. Liebman B. DASH, A diet for all seasons. Nutrition Action Health Letter 1997; Oct:10-12.
6. Good for the heart but not for the prostate. Harvard Men's Health Watch. 2002; Jan:1-3.

References Chapter 73

1. Should you be eating garlic for your health? Harvard Health Letter 2000; December 7.
2. Gillman MW, Cupples A, Gagnon D, et al. Protective effect of fruits and vegetables on development of stroke in men. JAMA 1995; 273:1113-1117.
3. Joshipura KJ, Ascherio A, Manson JZ. Fruit and vegetable intake in relation to risk of ischemic stroke. JAMA 1999; 282:1233-1239.

4. Smith-Warner SA, Spiegelman D, Youn SS, et al. Intake of fruits and vegetables and risk of breast cancer. JAMA 2001; 285:769-776.
5. High blood pressure – the end of an epidemic. Nutrition Action Health Letter. 2000; December 3:3.
6. Brody J. Book of health. New York Times 1998:202-206.
7. Is your diet colorful enough? Consumer Reports on Health. 2002; Sept.
8. Heber D. Eat by color. Readers Digest 2002; May:138-147.
9. Weil A. Sea weeds: The wonder vegetables. Self Healing 2002; July:1-3.
10. Weil A. The power of produce. Self Healing 1999; July 1-6, 7.

References Chapter 74

1. Schardt D, Corcoran L. Beat the heat. Nutrition Action Health Letter. 1998; June:10-11.

References Chapter 75

1. Preventing cancer. Harvard Men's Health Watch, 1998; November.
2. Sauerwein K. New book that suggests diet can help prevent breast cancer causes stir. St. Louis Post-Dispatch, 1998; December 26:11.
3. Liebman B. Diet and cancer: The big picture. Nutrition Action Health Letter 1998; 10:3-7.
4. Mehta JL. Antioxidants and vitamins in your patient with coronary artery disease. ACC Educational Highlights. Winter 1998; 6-10.
5. Losonczy KG, Harris TB, Havilk RJ. Vitamin E and vitamin C supplement use and risk of all cause and coronary heart disease mortality in older persons: the established populations for epidemiologic studies of the elderly. A J Clin Nutr 1996; 64:190-196.
6. Hennekens CH, Buring JE, Manson JE, et al. Lack of effect of long-term supplementation with beta-carotene on the incidence of malignant neoplasms and cardiovascular disease. New Engl J Med 1996; 334:1145-1149.
7. Diet and prostate cancer: New grains of hope. Harvard Men's Health Watch 2001; March.
8. Brody JD. Book of health. New York Times Company, NY 1998; 202-206.
9. Omenn GS, Goodman GE, Thornquist MD, et al. Effects of beta-carotene and vitamin A on lung cancer and cardiovascular disease. New Engl J Med 1996; 334:1150-1155.
10. Prostate cancer – what can you do to lower your risk? Harvard Health Letter 2001; March.
11. Perlman JM. Hocus-Focus-Can diet protect your eyes? Nutrition Action Health Letter 2000; July-august.

12. Guidelines on diet, nutrition and cancer prevention: Reducing the risk of cancer with healthy food choices and physical activity. American Cancer Society. Ca-A Journal for clinicians 1996; 46:325-341.
13. Prevention – fighting cancer with food. Harvard Health Letter 1997; 23:December.
14. Cancer, diet and funding – food or pharmaceuticals. The Scientist 1999; 13:September 27.
15. Thompson L. Trying to look sunsational? FDA Consumer 2000; July-August.
16. Skin cancer – Is sun screen an enabler? Harvard Health Letter 2000; 25:July.
17. Malignant melanoma: The dark side of sunshine. Harvard Men's Health Watch 1999; 3:July.
18. The infection connection. Consumer Reports on Health. 2002; 14:Aug.
19. Weight and cancer: More links uncovered. Tufts U Health and Nutrition Letter. 2002; Sept 1 and 8.

References Chapter 76

1. Liebman B. Salt; coincidence or conspiracy. Nutrition Action Health Letter. 1998, June, 9.
2. Whelton P, Appel LJ, Espeland MA, et al. Sodium reduction and weight loss in the treatment of hypertension in older patients (TONE). JAMA 1998; 279:839-878.
3. Alderman MH, Cohen H, Madhavan S. Dietary sodium intake and mortality. Lancet 1998; 351:781-785.
4. New guidelines – recommendations updated for hypertension. Harvard Health Letter 1998; January.
5. Appel LJ, Moore TJ, Obarzanek, et al. A clinical trial of the effects of dietary patterns on blood pressure. New Engl J Med 1997; 336:1117-1124.
6. Sacks FM, Svetley LP, Vollmer WM, et al. Effects on blood pressure of reduced dietary sodium and the DASH diet. New Engl J Med 2001; 344:3-10.
7. He J, Ogden LG, Vupputuri S, et al. Dietary sodium intake and subsequent risk of cardiovascular disease in overweight adults. JAMA 1999; 282:2027-2034.
8. Graudal NA, Gallee AM, Garred P. Effects of sodium restriction on blood pressure, renin, aldosterone, etc. JAMA 1998; 279:1383-1391.
9. Brody J. Lick the salt habit and your body will thank you. The Day – New London, CT 2001; May 14.
10. Taubes G. The political science of salt. Science 1998; 281:898-907.
11. Wickelgren I. Mutation points to salt recycling pathway. Science 2000; 289:23-26.
12. Do it yourself: Monitoring blood pressure at home. Harvard Men's Health Watch 1999; 4:December.

13. Stassen JA, Thijs L, Fagard R, et al. Predicting cardiovascular risk using ambulatory blood pressure. JAMA 1999; 282:539-546.
14. Sheps SG, Dart RA. New guidelines for prevention, detection, evaluation and treatment of hypertension. Chest 1998; 113:263-265.
15. Siegel D, Lopez J. Trends in antihypertensive drug use in the U.S. JAMA 1997; 278:1745-1748.
16. Moser M. Why are physicians not prescribing diuretics more frequently in the management of hypertension. JAMA 1998; 279:1813-1816.
17. Whelton PK, He J, Cutler, JA. Effects of oral potassium on blood pressure. JAMA 1997; 277:1624-1632.
18. Perry HM, Davis BR, Price TR, et al. Effect of treating isolated systolic hypertension on the risk of developing stroke. JAMA 2000; 284:465-471.
19. Weil A. Take control of high blood pressure. Self Healing. 2000; March.
20. High blood pressure – the end of an epidemic. Nutrition Action Newsletter 2000; Dec:3-8.
21. Blood pressure drug helps prevent stroke. Health News 2002; May:6.
22. Blood pressure perils. Consumer Reports on Health. 2002; Sept:1,4-6.

References Chapter 77

1. Albert CM, Hennekens CH, O'Donnell CJ, et al. Fish consumption and risk of sudden cardiac death. JAMA 1998; 279:23-28.
2. Ascherio A, Rim EB, Stampfer, MJ, et al. Dietary intake of marine N-3 fatty acids, fish intake and the risks of coronary disease amongst men. New Engl J Med 1995; 332:977-982.
3. Katan MB. Fish and heart disease. New Engl J Med 1995; 332:1024-1025.
4. Daviglus ML, Stamler J, Orencia AJ, et al. Fish consumption and the 30 year risk of fatal myocardial infarction. New Engl J Med 1997; 336:1045-1053.
5. Iso H, Rexrods KM, Stampfer MJ, et al. Intake of fish and omega-3 fatty acids and risk of stroke in women. JAMA 2001; 285:304-312.
6. Fish: Weighing the risks and benefits. Consumer Reports on Health. 2001; April 13:1,4.
7. Evidence for fish/heart health connection strengthens even more. Tufts U Health and Nutrition Letter 2002; June:3.
8. Weil A. Eating well, the Mediterranean way. Self Healing 2001; Feb 1:6-7.
9. So just how much fish is safe? Tufts U Health and Nutrition Letter. 2002; Jan:8.

References Chapter 78

1. Henkel J. Soy-health claims for soy protein, questions about other components. FDA Consumer 2000; May-June:12-20.

2. Dairy versus soy milk. Harvard Health Letter 2001; Feb:7.
3. A chink in the armor of soy's healthy reputation. The Scientist 2002; June 10.
4. Heartening news about soy foods. Consumer Reports on Health 2002; Nov:9.
5. Crouse JR, Morgan T, Terry JG, et al. A randomized trial comparing the effect of casein with that of soy protein containing varying amounts of isoflavones. Arch Int Med 1999; 159:2070-2076.
6. Anderson JW, Johnstone BM. A meta-analysis of the effects of soy protein intake on serum lipids. N Eng J Med 1995:Aug 3.
7. Weil A. Isoflavones: The secret of soy. Self Healing 1999; Nov.

References Chapter 79

1. Chemical cuisine. Nutrition Action Health Letter. March 1999; pages 4-9.
2. Brophy B, Schardt D. Functional foods. Nutrition Action Health Letter April 1999; 3-7.
3. Silverglald B. Nutrition Action Health Letter. April 1999; 4.
4. Jacobson MI. Fooling with food. Nutrition Action Health Letter 1999; April:2.
5. Functional foods. Nutrition Action Newsletter 2000; Nov:2.
6. Weil A. Functional foods: A mixed bag of groceries – second opinion. Self Healing. 2000; Nov.
7. Jacobson MF, Silvergladle B. Functional foods; health boon or quackery? Brit Med J 1999; 319:205-206.

References Chapter 80

1. Camargo CA Jr, Stampfer MJ, Glynn RJ, et al. Moderate alcohol consumption and risk of angina pectoris or myocardial infarction in U.S. male physicians. Annals of Int Med 1997; 126:372-375.
2. Gaziano JM, Buring JE, Breslow JL, et al. Moderate alcohol intake, increased levels of high-density lipoprotein and its subfractions, and decreased risk of myocardial infarction. NEJM 1993; 329:1829-1834.
3. Berger K, Ajani UA, Kase CS, et al. Light to moderate alcohol consumption and the risk of stroke among U.S. male physicians. NEJM 1999; 341:1557-1564.
4. Mukamal KC, Maclure M, Muller JE, et al. Prior alcohol consumption and mortality following acute myocardial infarction. JAMA 2001; 285:1965-1970.
5. Friedman GD, Klatsky AL. Is alcohol good for your health? NEJM 1993; 329:1882-1883.
6. Weil A. Is wine a health tonic? Self Healing 1998; Dec.
7. Schermer CR, Qualls CR, Brown CL, et al. Intoxicated Motor Vehicle Passengers. Arch Surg 2001; 136:1244-1248.

8. Smith GS, Kayl PM, Hadley JA, et al. Drinking and recreational boating fatalities. JAMA 2001; 280:3974-3980.
9. Johnson BA, Roache JD, Javors MA, et al. Ondansetron for reduction of drinking among biologically predisposed alcoholic patients. JAMA 2000; 284:963-971.

References Chapter 81

1. Rigotti NA, Lee JE, Wechsler H. U.S. college students use of tobacco products. JAMA 2000; 284:699-705.
2. Thun MJ, Apicella LF, Henley SJ. Smoking and other risk factors as the cause of smoking attributable deaths. JAMA 2000; 284:705-712.
3. Vergan D. Teens may be hooked within first days of smoking. USA TODAY 2000; September 12.
4. Ferry LH, Grissino LM, Runfold PS. Tobacco dependence curricula in U.S. undergraduate medical education. JAMA 1999; 282:825-829.
5. Clark PI, Natanblut SL, Schmitt CL, et al. Factors associated with tobacco sales to minors. JAMA 2000; 284:729-734.
6. Stephenson J. A "safer" cigarette? Prove it, say critics. JAMA 2000; 283:2507-2508.
7. Kusnet D. U.S. v. Joe Camel. NY Times 2001; March 25.
8. Kessler D. A question of intent. Public Affairs, New York 2001.
9. Glantz LH, Annas GJ. Tobacco, the Food and Drug Administration and Congress. New Engl J of Med. 2000; 343:1802-1806.
10. Mitka M. Anti-tobacco forces seek first international treaty. JAMA 2000; 284:1502-1503.
11. Rubin R. Female smoking deaths double. USA TODAY 2001; March 28.
12. Christen WG, Glynn RJ, Ajani UA, et al. Smoking cessation and risk of age-related cataract in men. JAMA 2000; 284:713-716.
13. Bondurant S. Putting proof behind the promise of new tobacco products. The Scientist 2001; March 19.
14. Chartrand S. Patients – a company promotes a nicotine vaccine it says can prevent an addiction to smoking. New York Times 2001; May 28.
15. Mitka M. Surgeon General's newest report on tobacco. JAMA 2000; 284:1366-1369.
16. Avery S. There's no magic formula for kicking smoking habit. Naples, Florida Daily News, 2001; June 10.
17. Cutting back on cigarettes may not help. USA TODAY 2000; January 3.
18. Halim NS. Tobacco settlement: Where's the money? The Scientist, 1999; 13:November 8.
19. Doll, R. Pioneer in tobacco research receives first Winslow medal. Yale Medicine 2001; Spring.

20. Tobacco interests poised for big gains from Bush. USA TODAY 2001; February 5.
21. Murdock NH. What is good health? St. Louis Met Med 2001; March.
22. Farkas AJ, Gilpin EA, White MM, Pierce, EP. Association between household and workplace smoking restrictions and adolescent smoking. JAMA 2000; 284:717-722.
23. Morrison AB. Counteracting cigarette advertising. JAMA 2002; 287:3001-3003.
24. Rubin R. Fewer teens smoke cigarettes but Ecstasy use rises. USA TODAY 2001; Dec 5.
25. Bauer UE, Johnson TM, Hopkins RS, Brooks RH. Changes in youth cigarette use and intentions following implementation of a tobacco control program. JAMA 2000; 284:723-728.
26. King C, Siegel M. The master settlement agreement with the tobacco industry and cigarette advertising in magazines. New Engl J Med 2001; 345:504-511.
27. Meckler L. Government says the number of new teen-age smokers is dropping dramatically. The Day, New London, CT 2001; October 5.
28. Weil A. Calling it quits: 10 strategies to stop smoking. Self-Healing 2000; December.
29. Otsuka R, Watanabe H, Hiraba K, et al. Acute effects of passive smoking on the coronary circulation in healthy young adults. JAMA 2001; 286:436-441.
30. Treating tobacco use and dependence. Public Health Service, U.S. Dept HHS 2000, June.
31. Fiore MC, Hatsukami DK, Baker TB. Effective tobacco dependence treatment. JAMA 2002; 388:1768-1771.
32. Annual smoking attributable mortality, years of potential life lost and economic costs. U.S. 1995-1999. JAMA 2002; 287:2355-2356.
33. Gross CP, Soffer B, Bach PB, et al. State expenditures for tobacco control programs and the tobacco settlement. N Engl J Med 2002; 347:1080-1086.

References Chapter 82

1. Winston FK, Durbin DR. Buckle Up! is not enough. JAMA 1999; 281:2070-2072.
2. Lyznicki JM, Doege TC, Davis RM, Williams MA. Sleepiness, driving and motor vehicle crashes. JAMA 1998; 279:1908-1913.
3. Myer AA. Death and disability from injury: A global challenge. J Trauma 1998; 44:1-12.
4. Rivara FP, Grossman DC, Cummins P. Injury prevention. New Engl J Med 1997; 337:543-548, 613-618
5. Tyroch AH, Kaups KL, Suc LP, et al. Pediatric restraint use in motor vehicle collisions. Arch Surg 2000; 135:1173-1176.

6. Holder HD, Gruenewald PJ, Ponicki WR, et al. Effect of community-based interventions on high-risk drinking and alcohol-related injuries. JAMA 2000; 284:2341-2347.

7. Li G. Child injuries and fatalities from alcohol-related motor vehicle crashes. JAMA 2000; 283:2291-2292.

8. Satcher D. Injury: An overlooked global health concern. JAMA 2000; 284:950.

9. McCartt AT. Graduated driver licensing systems. Reducing crashes among teenage drivers. JAMA 2001; 286:1631-1632.

10. Chen LH, Baker SP, Braver ER, Li G. Carrying passengers as a risk factor for crashes fatal to 16 and 17 year old drivers. JAMA 2000; 283:1578-1582.

11. Baler and compactor-related deaths in the workplace-United States, 1992-2000. JAMA 2001; 285:2441-2443.

12. Spivak H, Prothrow-Stith D. The need to address bullying – an important component of violence prevention. JAMA 2001; 285:2131-2132.

13. Cole TB, Flanagin A. What can we do about violence? JAMA 1999; 282:481-483.

14. Wintemute GJ, Drake C, Beaumont JJ, et al. Prior misdemeanor convictions as a risk factor for later violent and firearm-related criminal activity among authorized purchasers of handguns. JAMA 1998; 280:2083-2087.

15. Kellermann AL, Somes G, Rivara SP, et al. Injuries and deaths due to firearms in the home. J Trauma 1998; 45:263-267.

16. Cook PJ, Ludwig J. Gun violence: The real costs. JAMA 2001; 286:605-606.

17. Cook PJ, Lawrence BA, Ludwig J, Miller TR. The medical costs of gunshot injuries in the United States. JAMA 1999; 282:447-454.

18. Ford R. Armed but not alarmed. NY Times 2000; March 21.

19. Cole TB. Medical societies unite against firearm injuries. JAMA 2001; 285:2068-2069.

20. Guzy MW. First get the guns, then tackle root causes. St. Louis Post-Dispatch 1999; April 22.

21. Jackman GA, et al. Seeing is believing: What do boys do when they find a real gun? Pediatrics 2001; 177:1247-1250.

22. Lacy T. Thousands of felons manage to buy guns. USA TODAY 2001; March 29.

23. Brady S, Brady J, Cole TB. Handgun purchasers with misdemeanor convictions. JAMA 1998; 280:2120-2121.

24. Wintemute GJ. Relationship between illegal use of handguns and handgun sales volume. JAMA 2000; 284:566-567.

25. Cole, TB. Complementary strategies to prevent firearm injury. JAMA 2001; 285:1071-1072.

26. Ludwig J, Cook PJ. Homicide and suicide rates associated with implementation of the Brady handgun violence prevention act. JAMA 2000; 284:585-591.

27. Sherman LW. Gun carrying and homicide prevention. JAMA 2000; 283:1193-1195.

28. Teret, SP, Webster DW, Vernick JS, et al. Support for new policies to regulate firearms. New Engl J Med 1998; 339:813-818.
29. Wintemute GJ. The future of firearm violence prevention. JAMA 1999; 282:475-478.
30. Sorenson SB. Regulating firearms as a consumer product. Science 1999; 286:1481-1482.
31. Kassirer JP. Private arsenals and public peril. New Engl J Med 1998; 338:1375-1376.

References Chapter 83

1. Scutchfield FD, Hartman, KT. Physicians and preventive medicine. JAMA 1995; 273:1150-1151.
2. Breslow L. From disease prevention to health promotion. JAMA 1999; 281:1032-1033.
3. Satcher D, Hull FL. The weight of an ounce. JAMA 1995; 273:1149-1150.
4. Prevention Reports. U.S. Dept. Health and Human Services. *http:// odphp.oso.phs.dhhs.gov/pubs/prevrpt.*
5. Nelson DE, Bland S, Powell-Griner E, et al. State trends in health risk factors. JAMA 2002; 287:2659-2667.
6. Dexter PR, Perkins S, Overhage JM, et al. A computerized reminder system to increase the use of preventive care. N Engl J Med 2001; 345:965-970.

References Chapter 84

1. Spiegel D. Healing words. Emotional expression and disease outcome. JAMA 1999; 281:1328-1329.
2. Siegel BF. Love, kindness, compassion and your health. Bottom Line Personal, 1998; July:1.
3. Mental stress and respiratory infections. Harvard Men's Health Watch. 1999; January:5-6.
4. Emotions and health – Can stress make you sick? Harvard Health Letter 1998; 23:1-3.
5. Glaser R, Rabin B, Chesney M, et al. Stress-induced immunomodulation. JAMA 1999; 281:2268-2270.
6. McEwen BS. Protective and damaging effects of stress mediators. New Engl J Med 1998; 338:171-179.
7. Selye H. Stress. A syndrome produced by diverse innocuous agents. Nature 1936; 138:32-40.
8. Sterling P, Eyre J. Allostasis: A new paradigm to explain arousal pathology. In: Fisher S, Reason J, eds. Handbook of life stress, cognition and health. New York: John Wiley, 1998:629-649.

9. Selye H. Stress without distress. JB Lippincott Co, Philadelphia and New York, 1936.
10. Benson H, Stuart EM. The wellness book. Simon & Schuster, New York 1992.
11. Weil A. Spontaneous healing. Fawcett Columbine New York, 1995.
12. Siegel BF. Love, medicine and miracles. Perennial Library. Harper and Row, NY 1985.
13. Kiecolt-Glaser JK, Glaser R. Chronic stress and mortality among older adults. JAMA 1999; 282:2259-2260.
14. Stone R. Stress: The invisible hand in eastern Europe's death rates. Science 2000; 288:1732-1733.
15. Benson H. Timeless Healing. The relaxation response. Fireside, NY 1996.
16. Gullette ECD, Blumenthal JA, Babyak M, et al. Effects of mental stress on myocardial ischemia during daily life. JAMA 1997; 277:1521-1526.
17. Mittleman MA, Maclure M. Mental stress during daily life triggers myocardial ischemia. JAMA 1997; 277:1558-1559.
18. Kabat-Zinn J. Full catastrophe living. Delacorte Press, New York, 1998.
19. Davidson JRT. Recognition and treatment of posttraumatic stress disorder. JAMA 2001; 286:584-588.
20. Whiting P, Bagnall AM, Sowden AJ, et al. Interventions for the treatment and management of chronic fatigue syndrome. JAMA 2001; 286:1360-1368.

References Chapter 85

1. More information about dioxins from the EPA. *www.EPA.gov/ncea/dioxin-htm.*
2. Armour S. Workers unwittingly take home toxins. USA Today 2000; Oct 5:1 and 4.
3. Armour S. Vermont town feels effects of mercury. USA Today 2000; Oct 5:6
4. The National Institute for Occupational Safety and Health website *www.cdc.gov/niosh* for information on chemical and other workplace hazards or call 800-356-4674.
5. Banks DE, Wang M, Parker J. Asbestous exposure, asbestosis and lung cancer. Chest 1999; 115:320-321.
6. Wang X, Yano E. Pulmonary dysfunction in silica exposed workers: A relationship to radiographic signs of silicosis and emphysema. American J of Industrial Med 1999; 36:299-306.
7. Lewis R. The PCB Dilemma. The Scientist 2001; March 19:1 and 14.
8. Joyce S. Major issues in miners health. Environmental Health Perspectives 1998; 106:A 538-543.
9. Kaiser J. Just how bad is Dioxin? Science 2000; 288:1941-1944.
10. Bullers AC. Bottle water better than the tap? FDA Consumer 2002; July-Aug.
11. Watson T. Water pollution linked to dog do. USA TODAY 2002; July 27.

12. Penuelas J, Filella I. Responses to a warming world. Science 2001; 294:793-795.
13. Cabanes C, Cazenae A, Le Provost C. Sea level rise during the past 40 years. Science 2001; 294:840-842.
14. Kaiser J. Second look at arsenic finds higher risk. Science 2001; 293:2189.
15. Vastag B. CDC unveils first report on toxins in people. JAMA 2001; 284:1827-1828.

References Chapter 86

1. Conn PM, Parker J. Animal rights: Reaching the public. Science 1998; 282:1417.
2. Questions people ask about animals in research – Bulletin of the American Physiological Society. 9650 Rockville Pike, Bethesda, MD 20814-3991.
3. Fishbein EA. What price mice. JAMA 2001; 285:939-941.
4. Glickman D. Regulations for the use of laboratory animals. JAMA 2001; 285:941.
5. Morrison AR. Developing an ethical view on the use of animals in biomedical research. The Physiologist 2002; June:135-144.

References Chapter 87

1. War on drugs strategy changed. The Day, New London, CT 2001; May 16.
2. Lewis C. Online Laetrile vendor ordered to shut down. FDA Consumer 2000; March/April.
3. Holden C. Zapping memory center triggers drug craving. Science 2001; 292:1039.
4. Helmuth J. Beyond the pleasure principle. Science 2001; 294:983-984.
5. Linking genes to addiction. Yale Medicine 2001; Summer.
6. Courtwright DT. Forces of Habit. Drugs and the making of the modern world. Harvard U Press, Cambridge, MA 2001.
7. Time to revisit costly drug policy of locking up drug offenders. USA TODAY 2002; Sept 30.
8. Easton S. Incarceration aids drug fight. USA TODAY 2002; Sept 30.
9. Club Drugs – GHB. FDA Consumer 2000; March/April.
10. Solowig N, Stephens RS, Roffman RA. Cognitive functioning of long-term heavy cannabis users seeking treatment. JAMA 2002; 287:1123-1131.
11. Beware of 'Club Drugs'. FDA Consumer 2000; March/April.
12. Vastag B. Ecstasy experts want realistic messages. JAMA 2001; 286:777.
13. Nieves E. Drug labs in valley hideouts feed nation's habit. NY Times 2001; May 13.
14. Steinberg D. Why can't the brain shake cocaine? The Scientist 2001; May 28.

15. Goldman D, Barr CS. Restoring the addicted brain. N Engl J Med 2002; 347:843-844.

16. Meadows M. Prescription drug use and abuse. FDA Consumer 2001; Sept/Oct.

17. Fiellin DA, O'Connor PG. Office-based treatment of opioid-dependent patients. N Engl J Med 2002; 347:817-822.

18. Laine L, Hauck WH, Gourevitch MN, et al. Regular outpatient medical and drug abuse care and subsequent hospitalization of persons who use illicit drugs. JAMA 2001; 285:2355-2365.

19. Weisner C, Merbens J, Parthasarathy S. Integrating primary medical care with addiction treatment. JAMA 2001; 286:1715-1723.

20. Holden C. 'Behavioral' addictions: Do they exist? Science 2001; 294:980-982.

BVG